ELECTRODIAGNOSIS IN NEW FRONTIERS OF CLINICAL RESEARCH

Edited by **Hande Turker**

Electrodiagnosis in New Frontiers of Clinical Research
http://dx.doi.org/10.5772/56664
Edited by Hande Turker

Contributors

Koichi Kaneda, Yuji Ohgi, Mark McKean, Brendan Burkett, Adalgiso Coscrato Cardozo, Mauro Gonçalves, Camilla Hallal, Nise Marques, Gonzalo A. Garcia, Ryuhei Okuno, Kenzo Akazawa, Juhani Partanen, Dr.Hande Turker, Hasan Sozen, Charles S Layne, Amir Pourmoghaddam, William H. Paloski, Daniel O'Connor, Yunfen Wu, María Ángeles Martínez Martínez, Pedro Orizaola Balaguer, Toshiaki Suzuki, Satoru Kai, Koji Nakabayashi, Maria-Fernanda Lorenzo Gómez, Andre Kohn, Ruwan Chandra Gopura, Sanjaya Vipula Bandara, Malin Gunasekara, Sanath Jayawardane, Gladys Onambele-Pearson, Gerard McMahon, Christopher Morse, Adrian Burden, Keith Winwood, Daniel Stashuk, Tameem Adel

Published by InTech

Janeza Trdine 9, 51000 Rijeka, Croatia

Copyright © 2013 InTech

Notice

Publishing Process Manager Marija Radja
Technical Editor InTech DTP team
Cover InTech Design team

Additional hard copies can be obtained from orders@intechopen.com

Electrodiagnosis in New Frontiers of Clinical Research, Edited by Hande Turker
p. cm.
ISBN 978-953-51-1118-4

For EU product safety concerns:
IN TECH d.o.o., Prolaz Marije Krucifikse Kozulić 3, 51000 Rijeka, Croatia,
info@intechopen.com or visit our website at intechopen.com.

Meet the editor

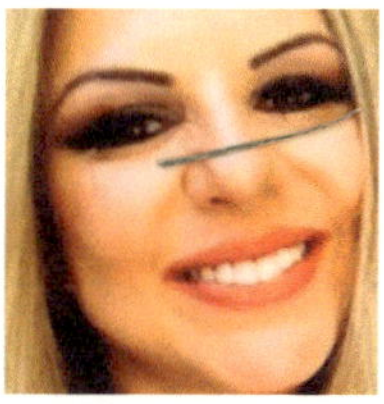

Hande Turker is a neurologist and a clinical neurophysiologist. She has been dealing with electromyography and evoked potentials for nearly twenty years. She is the author of many publications including several book chapters on evoked potentials and electromyography. Her main interests other than clinical neurophysiology are neuropathic pain and botulinum toxin injections in movement disorders. She has been working at Ondokuz Mayis University, Samsun, Turkey since 2003. She is an associate professor and lecturer and teaches electromyography and evoked potentials at the university where she founded the ''Evoked Potentials Lab'' and directed the EMG and EP Unit between 2003 and 2010.
She is also the author of Intech book chapters ''Middle and long latency auditory evoked potentials and their usage in fibromyalgia and schizophrenia'' and ''Neurological complications of hypothyroidism''.

Contents

Preface

During a long perios of time, clinical neurophysiology has expanded and developted new fields.However, the number of specialists of clinical neurophysiology is still limited. Well-qualified and detailed books or monographs on this field are in demand. Contribution of the authors from different countries who are sharing their experience and their own data will increase the attention and focus on clinical neurophysiology.

I am pleased to contribute to the book, "Electrodiagnosis in New Frontiers of Clinical Research" edited by Dr Hande Turker who I know personally and I have followed her academic progress for long time. I had the opportunity to work with her in our Department of Clinical Neurophysiology. She is always full of original ideas and the curiosity that science demands.

In this book chapters relate to different aspects of clinical neurophysiology. I am sure that the book will cover an important necessity of clinical neurophysiologists.

Gulseren Akyuz, M.D., Professor
Department of Physical Medicine and Rehabilitation and Clinical Neurophysiology
Marmara University School of Medicine
Istanbul, TURKEY

From the Editor

Utilization of electrodiagnosis; namely electromyography (EMG), nerve conduction studies, late responses, repetitive nerve stimulation techniques, quantitative EMG and evoked potentials, has long been discussed in many text books as basic principles. However the usage of electroneuromyography is rather new in some aspects when compared with tasks of daily practise. This book, we believe, will cover and enlighten those aspects where electrodiagnosis has begun to play important roles nowadays.

The book begins with an overview of the application of EMG in neurological disorders, a chapter by Faranak et al, where the role of EMG in neurological practise is explained thoroughly.The chapters by Suzuki et al, and Partanen J. describe late responses in cerebrovascular diseases and spontaneous activation in EMG respectively.

After these three basic chapters, there comes an interesting chapter on spinal cord neurophysiology by Kohn et al. The chapter, as stressed in its introduction part, provides conceptual and methodological background for researchers and clinicians who use EMG to study human spinal cord neurophysiology.

The chapter "Clinical Quantitative Electromyography" by Stashuk and Adel aims to provide an overview of different electromyographic techniques stressing quantitative EMG. A review and comparison of applications of EMG techniques for clinical decision concludes the chapter.

The next chapter by Cardozo et al summarizes a very important, yet mostly underestimated subject: Age related neuromuscular adjustments assessed by EMG. The chapter serves its aim and provides a global understanding of EMG parameters used to identify the age related neuromuscular fatigability alterations.

The seventh chapter by Layne C. et al, introduces a novel analysis technique "Synergos" to provide a quantitative index of multiple muscle activation, using surface electromyography from multiple muscles as the input variables. This new technique is important because it may have the potential to be used as a clinical tool to assess abnormalities in the neuromuscular system and monitor the effectiveness of treatments for these disorders.

How deep should you squat to maximise a holistic training response? This striking question's answer is investigated in a research by Gladys et al. Their chapter provides electromyographic, energetic, cardiovascular, hypertrophic and mechanical evidence for its well written findings.

The ninth chapter by Sozen H. and me, focuses on the use of surface electromyography in sports and exercise and gives information about studies concerning the comparison of muscle activation during elliptical trainer, treadmill and bike exercise by using surface EMG as a comparative test.

"Evoked EMG makes measurement of muscle tone possible by analysis of the H/M ratio", say Satoru K and Nakabyaski K. They describe a quite new perspective by using known electrodiagnostic procedures.

I believe that the chapter which follows is interesting, not only for electromyographers, but also for people who deal with underwater sports. This chapter by Kaneda et al, concludes that an investigation of muscle activity during exercise in water provides beneficial information for a broad range of participants, coaches and researchers.

Assistive Robots are one of the rising trends of our age and Gopura et al inform us about the recent trends in EMG-based control methods for assistive robots. I believe that our readers will find this chapter extremely interesting especially for the future directions that the authors propose.

A very distinguished chapter about biorobotics follows the above chapter. Garcia G. et al, present us a 3D graphical simulator they devised which mimics the behaviour of the Osaka Hand. The results are very exciting: Three sound-limbed subjects and a subject with double upper-limb amputation at wrist level were able to control the finger angle naturally and accurately by using this rehabilation system.

The last chapter which is written by Lorenzo-Gomez MF et al, describe an interesting task performed with EMG. Their chapter is about electromyographic treatment in women with chronic inflammatory disorders of the urinary tract. I believe that this chapter will provide a new perspective for both urologists and electromyographers.

This book may of course have errors despite our obsessive reviews and efforts. But all in all, I think that it provides the reader with interesting up-to-date data while summarizing some basic electrodiagnostic knowledge.

As a last remark, I want to thank all the authors of this book for their amazing works, to our publishing process manager Ms Marija Radja, without whom I would not be able to edit this book and finally to my dear mentor and teacher Prof. Dr. Gulseren Akyuz who has written a preface for the book during her very busy schedule.

I dedicate this book to all the people from whom I have learned a lot of things in this life. To my teachers, my patients, my students, my residents, my parents and mostly to my beloved husband Dr. Cuneyt Turker. I know I could not manage life and my career without him.

I wish and hope that this book will be useful for anyone who wants to read about new perspectives in electrodiagnosis. I also hope that it will arouse a new and great inspiration for researchers working on this field.

Assoc. Prof. Dr. Hande Turker MD, MS
Lecturer, Neurologist and Clinical Neurophysiologist
Ondokuz Mayıs University School of Medicine
Department of Neurology
Samsun, Turkey

Chapter 1

Overview of the Application of EMG Recording in the Diagnosis and Approach of Neurological Disorders

Yunfen Wu, María Ángeles Martínez Martínez and
Pedro Orizaola Balaguer

Additional information is available at the end of the chapter

http://dx.doi.org/10.5772/56030

1. Introduction

The Electromyography (EMG) is a neurophysiological technique for examining the electrical activity of skeletal muscles. The source of electrical signal in EMG is the muscle membrane potential. The muscle fibers innervated by the axonal branches of a motor neuron form a motor unit (MU). The muscle fibers of each motor unit are intermingled with fibers of other MUs [1]. The summation of action potentials of MUs is called motor unit action potential (MUAP) [2]. The biosignal recorded from a muscle or its fibers reflects the anatomical and physiological properties of the motor system. As such, EMG recording and analysis are powerful neurophysiological techniques that can be employed to: a) identify the health status of the motor system; b) localize and typify peripheral and central abnormalities and lesions; c) determine the temporal course and the severity of motor system abnormalities, and d) determine and evaluate the effectiveness of treatment strategies.

Muscle activity can be detected during resting state or during voluntary movement. In addition, induction of compound action potential (CMAP) and motor evoked potential (MEP) can be obtained by means of peripheral nerve stimulation (PNS) and cortical stimulation, respectively. While PNS provides measurement of integrity of the peripheral motor system, cortical stimulation through techniques such as Transcranial Magnetic Stimulation (TMS), permit examining the integrity of the corticospinal tract.

Furthermore, the value of EMG recording as an Intraoperative neuromonitoring method has been described since the late 1970´s [3]. To date, EMG recording is a useful technique to prevent neurological damage during diverse surgical procedures.

2. EMG recording techniques

EMG devices record the electrophysiological activity of MUs. EMG recordings can be performed by means of intramuscular (needle) or non-invasive (surface) electrodes.

2.1. Needle EMG (nEMG)

nEMG permits local recording from deep muscles by means of insertion of a needle electrode into the muscle tissue. The needle insertion point is located by identifying anatomic landmarks which may be confirmed through the proper contraction of the selected muscle. nEMG can be used to assess individual MUs and has greater sensitivity and accuracy in the recording of high-frequency signals such as different types of spontaneous activity [4].

However, nEMG has several limitations. First, it reflects the activity of only a small number of active MUs whose fibers are close to the position of the detection site (not representative of all the fibers in the MU, due to its small detection volume). An adequate sample is needed to ensure adequate power (sensitivity and specificity) of the analysis of MUAPs. Moreover, standard sample size is difficult in exploring small muscles [5]. Second, nEMG is painful especially during muscle activation, and prolonged nEMG recording is not possible. In rare cases, local trauma (e.g., pneumothorax) could occur during the examination of some delicate regions [6]. Furthermore, nEMG is time and temperature sensitive. In this regard, the detected signal in nEMG may vary as a function elapsed time from the onset of the nerve injury [7]. Since the temperature exerts a profound influence on neuromuscular transmission and propagation of the action potential along the muscle fibers, a low temperature at the examination area modifies the parameters and characteristics of the recorded signals [8].

2.2. Surface EMG (sEMG)

sEMG is a technique to measure muscle activity noninvasively using surface electrodes placed on the skin overlying the muscle, and has several advantages. First, sEMG recording is painless, especially when used in the absence of peripheral nerve stimulation. Furthermore, sEMG electrodes record from a wide area of muscle territory providing a more global view of MUs. Finally, it allows prolonged simultaneous recordings of muscle activity from multiple sites.

However, sEMG has a relatively low-signal resolution, is highly susceptible to movement artifacts [9] and body temperature. In addition, sEMG signals are dominated by the contributions of superficial MUs, while deeper MUs are not assessed; conditions that increase skin resistance subsequently disturb the sEMG signal (e.g. obesity and edema).

3. EMG study

3.1. Muscle voluntary contraction recording

In depolarization, the summation of action potentials of the MUs (MUAPs) can be assessed by analysis of their parameters (fig. 1).

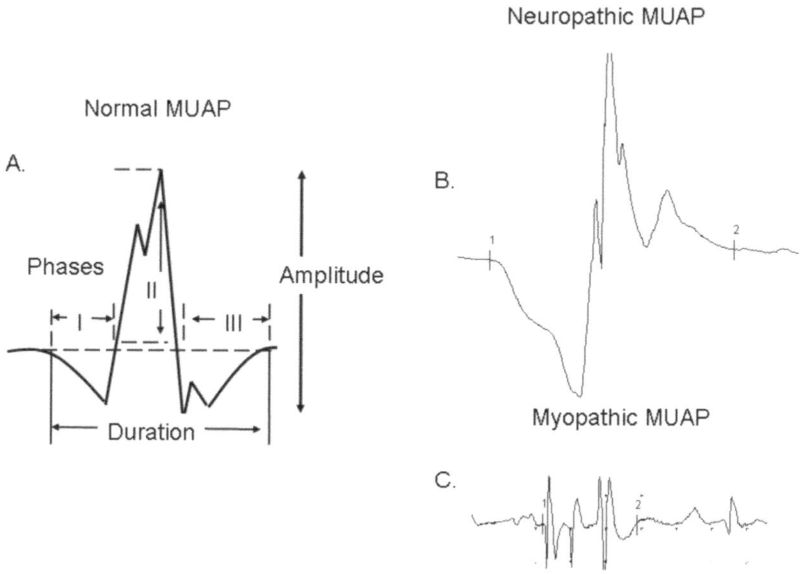

Figure 1. Morphology and parameters of a motor unit action potential (MUAP) measured during nEMG recording. A. A normal MUAP with three phases. B. A polyphasic, high amplitude and enlarged MUAP recorded in chronic neuropathy with reinnervation. C. In some myopathic and neuromuscular junctions (NMJ) disorders, the resulted MUAPs are of short duration, small amplitude and also polyphasic.

Duration is measured from the initial deflection from baseline to the terminal deflection back to baseline; it reflexes the synchrony and also the muscle fiber density in an MU. The average duration of MUAPs increases from infancy to adult (related to the increased width of the endplate zone), and even more during old age; the percentage depends on the specific muscle [2,10]. Abnormalities of MUAP duration can be shown in pathological conditions:

- Short-duration MUAPs are often detected in disorders with loss of muscle fibers [11].
- Long-duration MUAPs are typically found in chronic neuropathic disorders and polymyositis [12,13].
- A mixed pattern (coexisting MUAPs of long and short duration) can be observed in rapidly progressing motor neuron disease and chronic myositis [14].

Morphology (number of phases) is defined as the number of baseline crossings of an MUAP and reflects the firing synchrony of the muscle fibers within an MU. Normally, an MUAP has two to four phases. A MUAP of more than four phases is named polyphasic potential. MUAPs with abnormal morphology can be recorded in neuromuscular disorders:

- An abnormally increased polyphasia is a non-specific signal of both myopathic and neuropathic disorders [2,12].
- Satellite potentials are observed in subacute processes and result from denervated muscle fibers that are reinervated by collateral sprouts from adjacent unmyelinated or thinly myelinated fibers in early reinnervation stage [15].

Stability of the firing of all muscle fibers of the MU reflects the effective transmission across the neuromuscular junctions (NMJs) corresponding to each generated action potential. Abnormalities on MUAP stability indicate increased variability of an MUAP, either in its amplitude, morphology or both; this finding can be shown in primary disorders of the NMJ (e.g., myasthenia gravis, Lambert-Eaton syndrome); as well as often being observed as secondary phenomena in neuropathic (e.g., early reinnervation) or myopathic disorders.

A special technique called "single fiber EMG (SFEMG)" allows assessment of the abnormalities in the physiological variation of transmission time in the motor end-plate, and in the propagation velocity along the muscle and nerve fibers. This method is based on obtaining a single muscle fiber action potential by means of a special electrode with a small recording area. SFEMG is the most sensitive test to demonstrate an impaired neuromuscular transmission in myasthenia gravis. However, this technique is not specific in differentiating between myopathies and neuropathies, or between pre- and postsynaptic NMJ disorders [16-18].

Amplitude is commonly measured from peak to peak. It is proportional to the distance from the recording electrode to the muscle fiber, reflecting only those few depolarized fibers nearest to the recording electrode [19]. The progressive loss of MUs, unless in some muscle groups as of the seventh decade of life, results in MUAPs of smaller amplitude [20].This phenomenon is especially noticeable in extensor digitorum brevis muscle. An MUAP can show abnormal amplitude in the following conditions:

- Reduced amplitude of MUAP is a usual finding in some myopathies.
- In chronic neuropathies, the MUAP amplitude can be increased due to reinnervation process [12].

Recruitment refers to the increase of the firing rate from incorporation of additional MUs [21,22]. MUAP recruitment is reduced primarily in neuropathic diseases and rarely in severe end-stage myopathies [12] (fig 2).

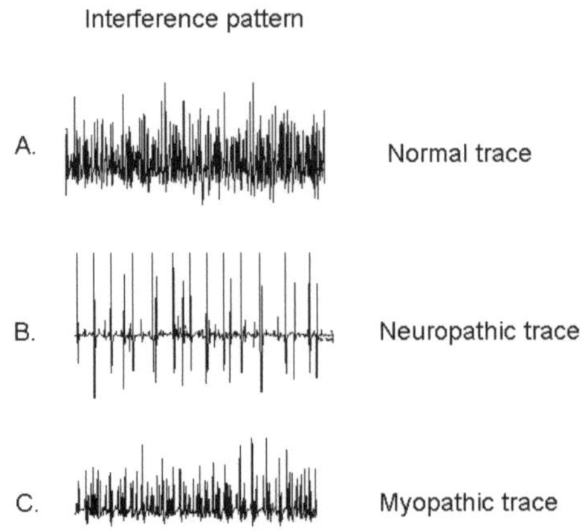

Figure 2. EMG signals recorded from maximum muscle contraction.

Activation is a measurement of the ability to increase firing rate. It depends on the effort exerted by the patient and the examined muscle (e.g. gastrocnemius muscle has some difficulty in its activation). This is a central process [21]. Poor activation may be seen in diseases of the central nervous system (CNS) or as a manifestation of provoked pain (poor collaboration during nEMG).

3.2. Resting state recording

At resting state, muscle activity can be recorded using either intramuscular (needle) or non-invasive (surface) detection systems. The difference between these two detection modalities is based on the volume conductor that separates the muscle fibers from the recording electrodes.

In a healthy muscle at rest, spontaneous physiological activity can be recorded by means of nEMG:

- End-plate potentials: result from the synchronization of miniature end-plate potentials, and can be recorded near the end-plate zone.
- Insertional activity: induced by mechanical depolarization of muscle fiber due to needle electrode insertion (fig 3).

Abnormal spontaneous activity provides information about the topography, diagnosis, time course (spontaneous activity is detected in acute and sub-acute stages of the nerve lesion) and also about the severity in neurogenic, myopathic and NMJ disorders [14,23,24] (fig. 3).

The most described abnormal spontaneous activities include:

- Fibrillation potentials, positive sharp waves, complex repetitive and myotonic discharges resulting from single denervated muscle fibers with an unstable membrane potential that fire individually without axonal stimulation.
- Fasciculation, neuromyotonic and myokymic discharges generating from disturbance of a group of muscle fibers.

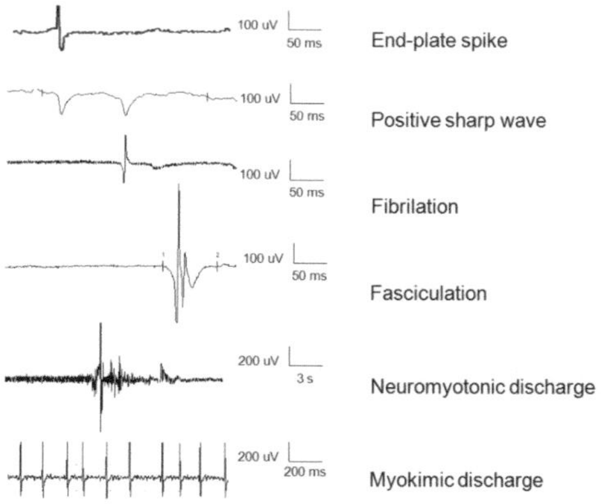

Figure 3. Some examples of spontaneous activity (nEMG recording).

On the other hand, resting sEMG recording is helpful in differentiating several types of tremors, myoclonus, and dystonia. The mean rectified sEMG signal varies linearly with the force generated at constant length and velocity. This linear relationship is maintained even in pathological conditions. sEMG may be used to classify movement disorders through measurement of frequency and amplitude of MUAPs. This technique can provide information about MU recruitment and synchronization, and also determine the relationship of the involved muscles, whether antagonists discharge simultaneously or alternately to produce some movement disorders [9,25-27] (fig 4).

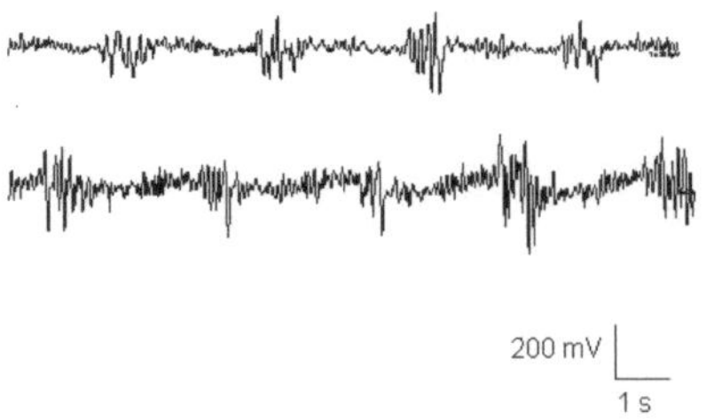

Figure 4. In resting sEMG recording, an alternative movement at 4-5 Hz over extensor (upper trace) and flexor (lower trace) musculature of the wrist is recorded in a patient with a diagnosis of Parkinson´s disease.

3.3. EMG analysis

The analysis of MUAPs can be performed on a qualitative or quantitative basis. At least 20 samples from each studied muscle is widely accepted as representative [5].

3.3.1. Qualitative analysis

Visual recognition only provides limited information, detecting alterations in few components of MUAPs. The effectiveness of this method depends on the experience of the performer, as the accuracy in measurements is limited by the presence of background noise and depends on collaboration from the patients. To perform qualitative MUAP analysis, the number of phases of a single MUAP and recruitment during voluntary activity are visually analyzed from the MUAPs.

3.3.2. Semi-quantitative analysis

The classical method consists of manual measurement of duration, amplitude, and number of phases of individual MUAPs; and then comparison of these data with a set of normal values for the studied muscle and age group.

3.3.3. Quantitative analysis

The parametric method establishes a comparison between sample mean values and reference intervals (standard deviation), while the nonparametric method considers both extremes of the samples ("outliers"). Both methods offer different sensitivities. The combination of outliers and mean values may be the optimal way to detect abnormalities in a sample [28,29].

The principal measurements during a voluntary contraction include:

- *Count of "turns"*: consists of the number of turns recorded in one second. It generally reflects the number of active MUAPs, their complexity and frequency of discharge. A "turn" was traditionally defined as any amplitude change signal of 100 uV [30]. It is important to take in account that a turn may correspond to a peak within an MUAP, an interaction between superimposed MUAPs, as well as background noise.
- *Mean amplitude between turns (A/T)* and the *number of turns divided by the mean amplitude between turns (T^2/A)* are indicators for identifying neuropathies and myopathies, and also establishing severity [30,31].
- *Upper centil amplitude* defines the upper limit of the peak-to-peak amplitude; the spikes with amplitude that exceeds by 1% are identified. This parameter is normal or decreased in some myopathies, whereas it is normal or increased in neuropathies [30,32].
- *Activity parameter* measures the 'fullness' of the interference pattern, and is the sum of the duration of specific segments [30,32].
- *Number of small segments (NSS)* quantifies the small inflexions of MUAPs, including the smallest segment between subsequent turns. NSS increases with the number of MUAP discharges, but reaches a constant value at higher MUAP discharge rates. This parameter has been shown as increased in myopathic and normal or decreased in neurpathic conditions [30].
- *Spectral analysis (SA)* traditionally consists of a fast Fourier transformation of the EMG signals; the output displays the range and amplitude of the component frequencies. SA is been used extensively in the study of muscle fatigue. The diagnostic value varies according to different power frequencies [33,34].
- *Automatic decomposition electromyography* comprises the extraction of MUAPs from EMG interference pattern employing digital filtering; the decomposition and analysis of validated MUAPs. Measured parameters include duration, amplitude, rise time, area, ratio, area/amplitude, number of phases, turns and fire rates [35-37].
- *Computer-aided MU nerve estimation:* high density multichannel EMG recording provides the spatio-temporal information for MUAPs. This technique allows the assessment of the number of functioning MUs [38].

3.4. EMG recording in peripheral nerve stimulation

Electroneurography (ENG) assesses the function and integrity of peripheral motor nerve structures by means of sEMG recording after electrical stimulation. ENG contributes to localize, typify (axonal or demyelinating nature), and establish the course and the severity of the lesion, and is temperature sensitive [39]. On the other hand, magnetic stimulation is also a tool for the electrical stimulation of peripheral nerves and spinal roots [40].

The summation of all underlying individual muscle fiber action potentials after electrical stimulation of a peripheral nerve is called compound muscle action potential (CMAP). Abnormalities of its components are useful in the diagnostic evaluation of neurological disorders (fig 5).

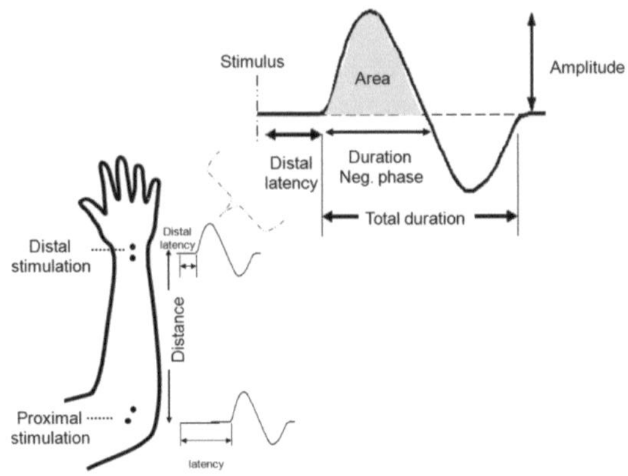

Figure 5. Parameters of a schematic CMAP assessed in motor nerve conduction study.

Special recording techniques are required when significantly different CMAP amplitude is recorded between two nerve segments in order to rule out the presence of anatomical variants [41-44].

On the other hand, the proximal segment of the peripheral motor nerve system can be assessed by means of determination of late responses: H-waves (elicited by subthreshold activation of muscle spindle afferents) and F-waves (elicited by supramaximal antidromic activation of motor neurons) (fig 6). Nevertheless, sensibility and specificity are limited in both tests [44,45].

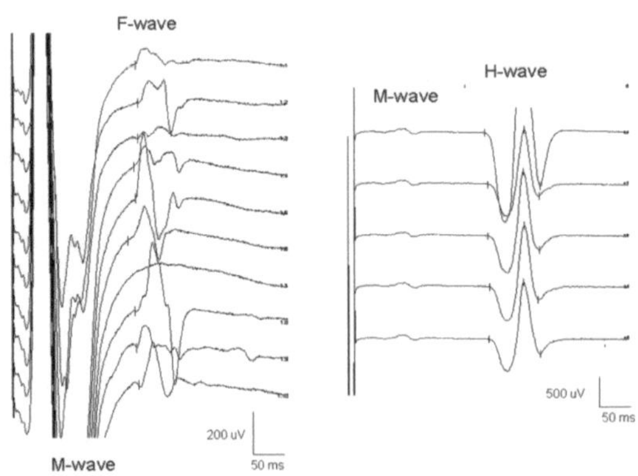

Figure 6. Late responses. Left: F-wave evoked from supramaximal stimulation of median nerve at the wrist, recording in abductor pollicis brevis muscle. Right: H-wave recorded over the soleus muscle from submaximal stimulation of tibial nerve in the popliteal fossa.

The integrity of some cranial nerves can be assessed by specific tests [46]:

- Electrical elicited Blink Reflex allows the evaluation of the trigeminal-facial reflex arc by means of stimulating the first division of the trigeminal nerve (fig 7).

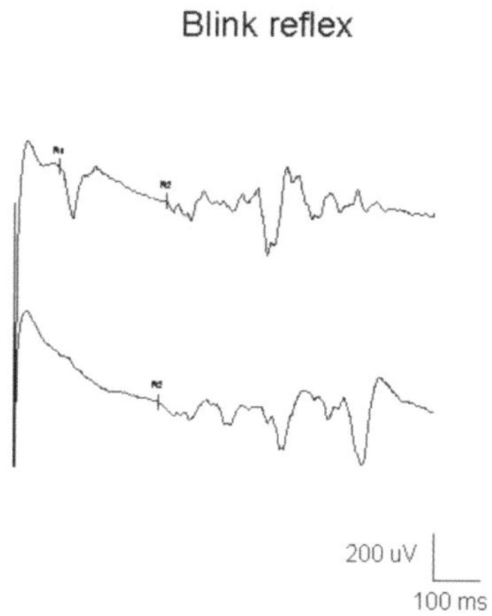

Figure 7. Blink reflex. Normal ipsilateral early (R1) with ipsilateral late (R2) responses, and contralateral R2 response recorded over both orbicularis oculi muscles, by left supraorbital nerve stimulation.

- Masseter reflex is elicited by a brisk tap to the lower jaw and allows assessment of the motor component of the trigeminal nerve.

However, motor nerve conduction studies have some limitations. First, selectivity is lacking in the assessment of small muscles and some nerves are not accessible. Second, the greater the intensity of the stimulation, the greater the chance of the stimulus being perceived as painful by the patient, especially during proximal stimulation in the assessment of root and plexus. In addition, stimulation is more difficult in patients who are obese, edemic, or have unusually thick or calloused skin. Third, variability due to examiner and side differences also exists [47].

Several parameters of a CMAP can be measured:

Latency refers the time from the stimulus to the initial negative deflection from baseline. In peripheral motor nerve stimulation, the latency obtained from the stimulation of the most distal segment of the nerve is named "distal latency (DL)". DL reveals nerve conduction time from the stimulus site to the NMJ, the time delay across the NMJ, and the depolarization time across the muscle and reflects only the conduction of the fastest conducting motor fibers. Pathological conditions with delayed CMAPs include:

- Demyelinating diseases [48].

- Axonal degeneration with primary damage of the largest and fastest myelinated fibers [44,49].

Amplitude is commonly measured from baseline to negative peak. It is proportional to the distance from the recording electrode to the muscle fiber. CMAP amplitude reflects only those depolarized fibers nearest to the recording electrode, and is the most studied outcome measurement.

Abnormalities of CMAP amplitude can be observed in:

- Axonal neuropathies: characterized by axon loss, can show CMAPs of reduced amplitude. In chronic axonal neuropathies, CMAP amplitude reflects the functioning muscle mass [44,45].
- NMJ disorders: amplitude of CMAPs is a fundamental parameter in the assessment of the integrity of neuromuscular transmission by means of repetitive nerve stimulation (RNS). This technique consists of applying repetitive stimulation at low and high rates, and determining the decreasing or increasing CMAP responses that in conjunction with the CMAP at baseline, allows a diagnosis of pre- or postsynaptic NMJ disorders to be established [49] (Fig. 8).

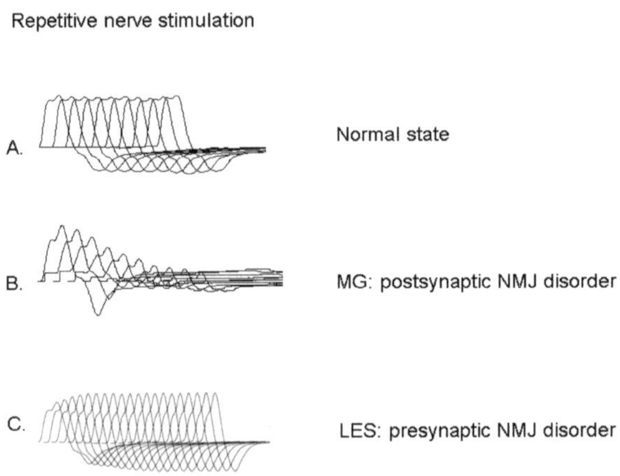

Figure 8. Repetitive stimulation of ulnar nerve: recording over the abductor digiti minimi muscle. A. In normal subjects, compound muscle action potential (CMAP) amplitude remains very stable. B. In a miastenia gravis (MG) patient, CMAP amplitude is normal at rest but decreases during low-rate repeated stimulation at 3 Hz. C. In a patient with Lambert–Eaton syndrome (LES), the initial CMAP amplitude is reduced. During high-rate repeated stimulation at 20 Hz, CMAP amplitude dramatically increases. NMJ: neuromuscular junction.

- Demyelinating lesions: Impediment to the conduction of the action potential without axonal degeneration is named conduction block (CB). No absolute expert agreement has been established in the definition criteria of CB [49]. Nevertheless, a decay of proximal CMAP amplitude/area of at least 50% has been observed in patients with nerve CB in some studies, and has even been proposed as criteria for CB. [51-53].

Duration is measured from the initial deflection from baseline to the first baseline crossing, but can also be measured from the initial to the terminal deflection back to baseline. It is a parameter that indicates the synchrony of the activated muscle fibers. It increases in conditions that result in slowing of some motor nerve fibers but not others (e.g., in a demyelinating lesion) [44,54].

Area is conventionally measured between the baseline and the negative peak and represents a combination of the amplitude and the duration; the calculation is performed by computerized software. Therefore, CMAP area reflects also the number and synchrony of the muscle fibers activated close to the recording electrode. "Temporal dispersion" results from the spatial distribution of the scattered motor end-plates of a MU, and depends on the individual distance and time of conduction along the muscle fibers. This phenomenon is observed with more proximal stimulation, while the distance from the recording electrodes increases [55].

Motor conduction Velocity (MCV) obtained from standard recording techniques reflects only the conduction of the fastest conducting fibers. The determination of true motor conduction velocity must not include the NMJ transmission and muscle depolarization times. Conduction velocity along the studied segment is usually calculated with the following formula: (distance between the proximal and distal stimulation sites) divided by (proximal latency - distal latency) [44]. MCV is dependent on internode distance and also on the total fiber diameter (axon plus myelin), since MCV increases proportionally with myelin thickness [56]. MCV increases progressively during the first 5 years of life, in relation to physiological maturation of myelinization process. Otherwise, there is a progressive and slight decrease of MCV in relation with increase of age over 20-30 years [44,57,58].

MCV is an important parameter in the determination of demyelinating disease. In hereditary demyelinating neuropathies, a uniformly slowed MCV has been shown; whereas in acquired demyelinating neuropathies, slowed MCV is observed in a patchy way [44]. In reinnervation process, the slowing in conduction velocity results from the regenerating nerve fibers that contain thinner axons and myelin sheaths and shorter internodal lengths [59].

3.5. EMG recording in cortical stimulation

Motor evoked potential (MEP) is defined as an EMG response obtained by means of activation of the corticospinal tract by means of stimulation to the motor cortex. Transcranial Magnetic Stimulation (TMS), a painless (unlike Transcranial Electrical Stimulation) method is widely used with this aim [60].

The following components of MEP elicited by single pulse TMS, are measured to evaluate the integrity of corticospinal pathways:

Latency refers to the time between the delivery of a TMS pulse over the scalp (area corresponding to the primary motor cortex – M1) and the appearance of MEP at the periphery. MEP latency is mainly reflective of the efficiency of conduction between the stimulated motor cortical area and the peripheral target muscle [61].

Central motor conduction time (CCT) can be obtained by two methods of calculation. The CCT calculated by subtracting the CMAP latency obtained by stimulation of the spinal (cervical or lumbar) motor root from the latency of MEP [62] includes the time for central motor conduction, the synaptic delay at the spinal level and time from the proximal root to the intervertebral foramen. More precise central conduction time can be calculated by use of F-wave latency [60]. On the other hand, CCT is significantly influenced by the motor system maturation [63], and partially dependent upon the subject height. A significant interside difference indicates a lateralized prolonged CCT even if still within normal values (Fig 9).

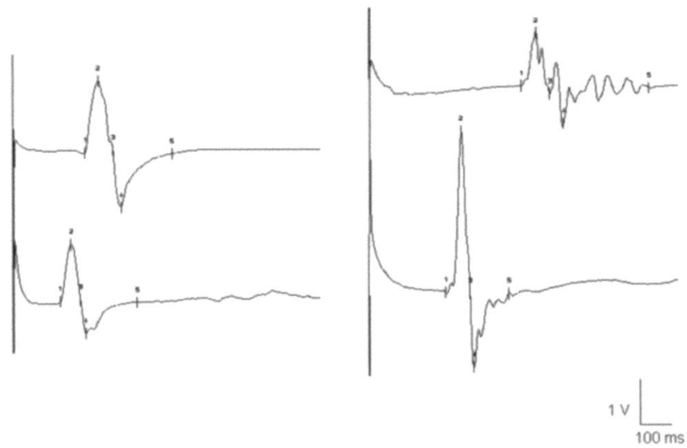

Figure 9. Left: MEP recorded from abductor pollicis brevis muscle. The top trace shows the MEP evoked by single pulse TMS over the corresponding M1. The lower trace shows the MEP elicited by ipsilateral cervical (motor root) stimulation. Right: MEP recorded from extensor digitorum brevis muscle. The top trace shows the MEP induced by cortical stimulation. The lower trace shows the MEP elicited by ipsilateral lumbar stimulation.

Amplitude is often measured from peak-to-peak amplitude. MEP amplitude can also be measured from baseline EMG activity to the first positive or negative deflection. Amplitude of MEP reflects the integrity and excitability of motor cortex, corticospinal tract, nerve roots and peripheral motor pathway to the muscles [64]. Dispersion of the alpha-motoneuron response to the descending volley in the corticospinal tract, leads to a broad range of normal values. The triple stimulation technique (TST) provides a more precise assessment of corticospinal tract conduction by suppressing desynchronization of MEPs. The TST involves three stimuli (transcranial, distal and proximal on the peripheral nerve) timed to produce two collisions. The TMS descending impulses collide with the antidromic impulses from the distal stimulus. Proximal stimulation on the nerve evokes orthodromic impulses, which cancel out any uncollided impulses from the distal stimulus. The response from the third stimulus therefore reflects the number of peripheral neurons activated from TMS [65].

Lengthening of MEP latency and CCT suggests impairment of the white matter fibers, while abnormalities of MEP amplitude or absence of responses are more suggestive of loss of neurons or axons. TMS has the potential to facilitate early diagnosis of myelopathy by detecting signals of demyelination of the pyramidal tract [66,67], plexus entrapment and injuries [62]. Moreover, MEP abnormalities may be useful objective markers of progression of amyotrophic lateral sclerosis (ALS) [68], and effective parameters in spinal pathology for deciding the timing of the surgical intervention [69].

TMS can however be performed using single pulse or pair pulse paradigm in order to explorer the reactivity of the motor cortex. Since motor threshold (MT) is believed to reflect membrane examine of corticospinal neurons, motor neurons in the spinal cord, NMJs and muscle [70], it is used as benchmark for the intensity of TMS. MT is usually defined by the lowest intensity of stimulation required to generate 50% probability of MEPs of more than 50 μV [60].

Silent period (SP) is defined as the period of EMG suppression; normally it refers to the time from the end of the MEP to the return of voluntary EMG activity, after a single suprathreshold TMS pulse applied to the M1 corresponding to the active target muscle. The first 50–60 ms of the SP has been supposedly contributed to spinal inhibition and the late part originates most likely in the motor cortex, termed *cortical silent period* [71]. Abnormalities of SP have been shown in patients with various movement disorders [72,73]. In patients with a diagnosis of ALS, shortened PS has been observed [74].

Transcallosal conduction (TC): Application of a single suprathreshold TMS pulse to the M1 can suppress tonic voluntary EMG activity in ipsilateral hand muscles, by transcallosal inhibition. Delayed or absent TC suggests lesions of the corpus callous [75]. In addition, application of single stimuli to both motor cortexes at a short interval, allows assessment of the interhemispheric interactions and also the TC [76].

Short interval intracortical inhibition (SICI) can be accessed by combining a subthreshold (60–80% of resting MT) conditioning (first) stimulus with a suprathreshold (second) test stimulus over M1, at short inter-stimulus intervals of 1-6 ms [77]. Significantly reduced SICI has been observed in patients with dystonia and Parkinson's disease [78,79].

Intracortical facilitation (ICF) reflects the excitatory phenomenon occurring in the M1, and is elicited by applying a conditioning subthreshold TMS pulse and a suprathreshold test stimulus over M1 with inter-stimulus intervals between 6 and 20 ms [80]. Significantly enhanced ICF has been recorded from amputated limbs in patients with neuropathic pain [81].

In addiction to the study of the pathophysiology of diverse neurological diseases, paired-pulse TMS has been widely used to explore the effects of central nervous system (CNS)-active drugs on the motor cortex [70].

3.6. EMG recording in Intraoperative neuromonitoring

Intraoperative neuromonitoring includes mapping and true monitoring techniques. Mapping techniques are used intermittently during surgery for functional identification and preservation of anatomically ambiguous nervous tissue. On the other hand, true monitoring techniques permit a continuous assessment of the functional integrity of neural pathways [82].

In posterior fossa and brainstem surgeries, mapping the floor of the fourth ventricle allows the surgeon to find a safe entry to the brainstem, and therefore, helps to identify and preserve cranial nerves and their motor nuclei. Traditionally, Intraoperative monitoring of the facial nerve has been employed in operations for acoustic tumors to reduce the risk of neural damage. To date, EMG recording of the activity of selective cranial nerve muscles is currently included in the intraoperative set during surgical manipulation of the brainstem. [83,84].

During brain surgery, neurophysiological mapping techniques have been employed in the identification of eloquent areas such as the motor areas. In addition, these techniques have been introduced in surgery for deep-seated gliomas, insular tumors and lesions involving the cerebral peduncle [82,84]. The goal is an aggressive resection of such lesions to the greatest extent as possible, to improve the patient's survival chance and the postoperative life quality. With this aim, monopolar or bipolar stimulation of cortical and subcortical areas is applied carefully. Visual detection of the elicited movement of the limb contralateral to the operative side is usually employed during the mapping of motor areas. However, it is difficult to detect visually a subtle twitch over an entire contralateral limb at once, specially during awake surgery (because of the specific patient positioning). EMG recording is more sensitive than the visual detection of muscle twitch. EMG signals precede the visually observed motor activity, since the applied stimulation may weakly activate motor pathways enough to elicit EMG responses and yet not recruit a sufficiently large pool of motor neurons to produce visible muscle movement. Moreover, multichannel EMG recording has three important advantages: First, it facilitates the monitoring of the face, upper and lower extremities simultaneously, detecting motor responses that may not be observed during gross inspection (Fig.10). This advantage is particularly important during mapping of subcortical pathways. Second, EMG recording also improves the ability to detect subclinical ictal events (EMG activity elicited by stimulation that persists after the end of the stimulation). In addition, EMG—complementary to electrocorticography— allows the early detection of spreading muscle activation over a limb as a sign of seizure. The immediate removal of stimulation diminishes the likelihood of the progression of a seizure. Third, the sensitivity of EMG recording allows the application of lower intensity and duration of stimuli during mapping procedures [85-87].

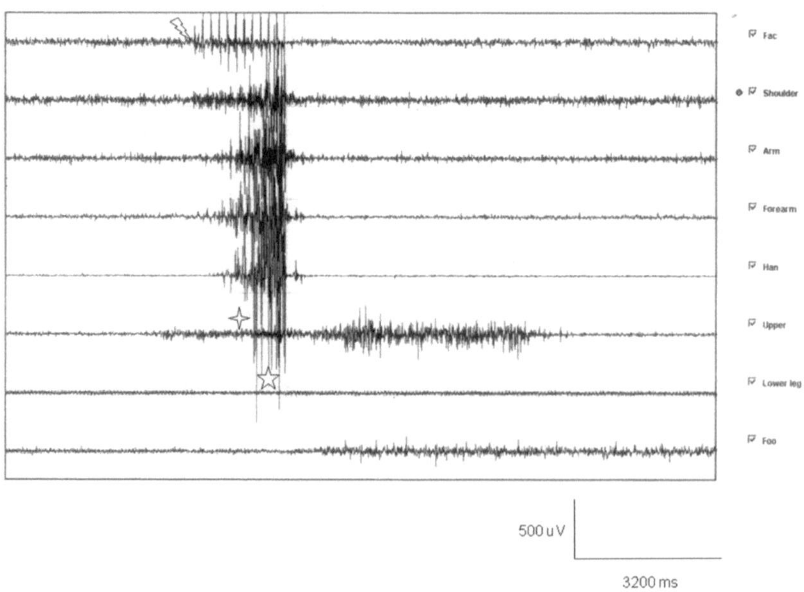

Figure 10. Multichannel EMG recording during mapping for glioma surgery. Stimuli artifact. ( ) Muscle activity ( ) recorded preceding visual muscle twitch ( ).

EMG as a monitoring technique has a high sensitivity but a low specificity. To date, some limitations of EMG recording have been overcome using multimodality intraoperative monitoring, including motor evoked potentials, somatosensory evoked potentials and some reflex responses (H- reflex, blink reflex, etc). Transcranial MEP elicited by transcranial multipulse electric stimulation of the motor cortex (TcMEP) are currently the most effective means of continuous monitoring of the functional integrity of corticospinal and corticobulbar pathways in diverse surgical procedures [82,84].

During spinal procedures, free running EMG (frEMG) and stimulus-triggered EMG (stEMG) are basic monitoring tools to assess the functional integrity of nerve roots, plexus and peripheral nerves. Train activity or neurotonic discharges recorded by means of spontaneous EMG indicate excessive direct or indirect nerve contact during manipulation; therefore, adjustment should be made to avoid nerve injury. Recently, frEMG or stEMG have been included in the intraoperative set applied during minimally invasive surgeries such as transpsoas approaches. On the other hand, stEMG have been used to control the correct pedicular screw placement during orthopedic surgery [88]. Unlike the CMAPs recorded in neurophysiological laboratories, intraoperative CMAP are typically elicited using submaximal stimulation and are recorded as highly complex polyphasic responses with variable onset latencies and amplitudes. Stimulus threshold however can provide some information about the proximity to the nerve root [89].

TMS is likewise an advantageous optional technique in planning brain surgery, based on non-invasive mapping. TMS mapping consists of locating where the largest MEP responses can be measured by using suprathreshold single stimuli applied to the assumed area (M1) of the optimal stimulation site [90]. There is some evidences of the reliability of this planning method in correlation with the gold standard "direct cortical stimulation" described previously [91,92]. Interestingly, a recent report has provided the first result of the reliability of TMS, in the assessment of the plasticity changes of the involved M1 concurrent with multistage surgery, in a patient with a diagnosis of low grade glioma. However, further studies should confirm the power of this non-invasive mapping technique, in regard to patient-specific variation, and especially to functional anatomy [93].

4. Conclusion

Virtually all primary neuromuscular diseases result in changes in the electric activity recorded from the muscle fibers. The pattern of abnormalities can usually mark the underlying pathology as neuropathic (e.g. disorders affecting the CNS, nerve roots, plexuses and peripheral nerves), myopathic, or NMJ disorder, etc. EMG recording allows measurement of the severity of the injury, and provides prognostic information.

In the field of intraoperative neuromonitoring, to date, EMG recording – despite its low specificity - continues to be a valuable tool included in a multimodal monitoring set during diverse neurosurgical and orthopedic procedures.

Acknowledgements

We thank the Service of Clinical Neurophysiology, University Hospital "Marqués de Valdecilla", Spain; and Faranak Farzan Ph.D for their collaboration in the elaboration of this chapter.

Author details

Yunfen Wu*, María Ángeles Martínez Martínez and Pedro Orizaola Balaguer

*Address all correspondence to: yfenwufriendship@hotmail.com

Clinical Neurophysiology department, University Hospital "Marqués de Valdecilla", Spain

References

[1] Enoka RM. Morphological features and activation patterns of motor units. J Clin Neurophysiol 1995; 12(6) 538–559.

[2] Buchthal. Electromyography in the evaluation of muscle diseases. Methods in Clinical Neurophysiology 1991; 2 25-45.

[3] Delgado TE, Bucheit WA, Rosenholtz HR, Chrissian S. Intraoperative monitoring of facila muscle evoked responses obtained by intracranial stimulation of the facila nerve: a more accurate technique for facila nerve dissection. Neurosurgery 1979; 4(5) 418-421.

[4] Merletti R, Farina D. Analysis of intramuscular electromyogram signals. Philos Transact A Math Phys Eng Sci 2009; 367(1887): 357-68. http://www4.fct.unesp.br/docentes/fisio/augusto/artigos% 20cient% EDficos/2009% 20% 20Analyssis% 20of% 20intramuscular% 20electromyogram% 20signals.full.pdf (accessed 24 October 2012).

[5] Podnar S, Mrkaić M. Size of motor unit potential sample. Muscle Nerve. 2003; 27(2) 196-201.

[6] Reinstein L, Twardzik FG, Mech KF Jr. Pneumothorax: a complication of needle electromyography of the supraspinatus muscle. Arch Phys Med Rehabil 1987; 68(9) 561-562.

[7] Quan D, Bird SJ. Nerve Conduction Studies and Electromyography in the Evaluation of Peripheral Nerve Injuries. The University of Pennsylvania Orthopaedic Journal 1999; 12 45–51.

[8] Rutkove SB. Effects of temperature on neuromuscular electrophysiology. Muscle Nerve 2001; 24(7) 867-882.

[9] Pullman SL, Goodin DS, Marquinez AI, Tabbal S, Rubin M. Clinical utility of surface EMG: report of the therapeutics and technology assessment subcommittee of the American Academy of Neurology. Neurology 2000; 55(2) 171-177.

[10] Sacoo G, Buchthal F, Rosenfalck P. Motor unit potentials at different ages. Arch Neurol 1962; 6 366-373.

[11] Liguori R, Fuglsang-Frederiksen A, Nix W, Fawcett PR, Andersen K. Electromyography in myopathy. Neurophysiol Clin 1997; 27(3) 200-203.

[12] Izzo KL, Aravabhumi S. Clinical electromyography. Principles and practice. Clin Podiatr Med Surg 1990; 7(1) 179-194.

[13] Uncini A, Lange DJ, Lovelace RE, Solomon M, Hays AP. Long-duration polyphasic motor unit potentials in myopathies: a quantitative study with pathological correlation. Muscle Nerve 1990; 13(3) 263-267.

[14] Daube JR, Rubin DI. Needle electromyography. Muscle Nerve 2009; 39(2) 244-270.

[15] Lateva ZC, McGill KC. Satellite potentials of motor unit action potentials in normal muscles: a new hypothesis for their origin. Clin Neurophysiol 1999; 110(9) 1625-1633.

[16] Farrugia ME, Weir AI, Cleary M, Cooper S, Metcalfe R, Mallik A. Concentric and single fiber needle electrodes yield comparable jitter results in myasthenia gravis. Muscle Nerve 2009; 39(5) 579-585.

[17] Benatar M, Hammad M, Doss-Riney H. Concentric-needle single-fiber electromyography for the diagnosis of myasthenia gravis. Muscle Nerve 2006; 34(2)163-168.

[18] Tanhehco JL. Single-fiber electromyography. Phys Med Rehabil Clin N Am 2003; 14(2) 207-229.

[19] Nandedkar SD, Barkhaus PE, Sanders DB, Stålberg EV. Analysis of amplitude and area of concentric needle EMG motor unit action potentials. Electroencephalogr Clin Neurophysiol 1988; 69(6) 561-567.

[20] McNeil CJ, Doherty TJ, Stashuk DW, Rice CL. Motor unit number estimates in the tibialis anterior muscle of young, old, and very old men. Muscle Nerve 2005; 31(4) 461-467.

[21] Barnes WS. The relationship of Motor-unit activation to isokinetic muscular contraction at different contractile velocities. Phys Ther 1980; 60(9) 1152-1158.

[22] Ounjian M, Roy RR, Eldred E, Garfinkel A, Payne JR, Armstrong A, Toga AW, Edgerton VR. Neurol Clin. Physiological and developmental implications of motor unit anatomy. J Neurobiol 1991; 22(5) 547-559.

[23] Preston DC, Shapiro BE. Needle electromyography. Fundamentals, normal and abnormal patterns. Neurol Clin 2002; 20(2) 361-396.

[24] Daube JR. AAEM minimonograph #11: Needle examination in clinical electromyography Muscle Nerve 1991; 14(8) 685-700.

[25] Grimaldi G, Manto M. Neurological tremor: sensors, signal processing and emerging applications. Sensors (Basel) 2010; 10(2) : 1399-1422. http://www.ncbi.nlm.nih.gov/pmc/articles/PMC3244020/pdf/sensors-10-01399.pdf (accessed 23 October 2012).

[26] Kojovic M, Cordivari C, Bhatia K. Myoclonic disorders: a practical approach for diagnosis and treatment. Ther Adv Neurol Disord 2011; 4(1) 47-62.

[27] Piboolnurak P, Yu QP, Pullman SL. Clinical and neurophysiologic spectrum of orthostatic tremor: case series of 26 subjects. Mov Disord 2005; 20(11) 1455-1461.

[28] Podnar S. Comparison of parametric and nonparametric reference data in motor unit potential analysis. Muscle Nerve 2008; 38(5) 1412-1419.

[29] Stålberg E, Bischoff C, Falck B. Outliers, a way to detect abnormality in quantitative EMG. Muscle Nerve 1994; 17(4) 392-329.

[30] Abel EW, Zacharia PC, Forster A, Farrow TL. Neural network analysis of the EMG interference pattern. Med Eng Phys 1996; 18(1) 12-17.

[31] Stålberg E, Chu J, Bril V, Nandedkar S, Stålberg S, Ericsson M. Automatic analysis of the EMG interference pattern. Electroencephalogr Clin Neurophysiol 1983; 56(6) 672-681.

[32] Nandedkar SD, Sanders DB, Stålberg EV. Simulation and analysis of the electromyographic interference pattern in normal muscle. Part II: Activity, upper centile amplitude, and number of small segments. Muscle Nerve 1986; 9(6) 486-490.

[33] Yaar I, Niles L. EMG interference pattern power spectrum analysis in neuro-muscular disorders. Electromyogr Clin Neurophysiol 1989; 29(7-8) 473-484.

[34] Rønager J, Christensen H, Fuglsang-Frederiksen A. Power spectrum analysis of the EMG pattern in normal and diseased muscles. J Neurol Sci 1989; 94(1-3) 283-294.

[35] McGill KC, Cummins KL, Dorfman LJ. Automatic decomposition of the clinical electromyogram. IEEE Trans Biomed Eng 1985; 32(7) 470-477.

[36] Le Fever RS, Xenakis AP, De Luca CJ. A procedure for decomposing the myoelectric signal into its constituent action potential. Part II: execution and test for accuracy. IEEE Trans Biomed Eng 1982; 29 158-164.

[37] Doherty TJ, Stashuk DW. Decomposition-based quantitative electromyography: methods and initial normative data in five muscles. Muscle Nerve 2003; 28(2) 204-211.

[38] Nandedkar SD, Barkhaus PE, Charles A. Multi-motor unit action potential analysis (MMA). Muscle Nerve 1995; 18(10) 1155-1166.

[39] Rutkove SB. Effects of temperature on neuromuscular electrophysiology. Muscle Nerve 2001; 24(7) 867-882.

[40] Abdeen MA, Stuchly MA. Modeling of magnetic field stimulation of bent neurons. IEEE Trans Biomed Eng. 1994; 41(11) 1092-5.

[41] Pyun SB, Kwon HK. The effect of anatomical variation of the sural nerve on nerve conduction studies. Am J Phys Med Rehabil 2008; 87(6) 438-442.

[42] Beheiry EE. Anatomical variations of the median nerve distribution and communication in the arm. Folia Morphol (Warsz) 2004; 63(3) 313-318.

[43] Rayegani SM, Daneshtalab E, Bahrami MH, Eliaspour D, Raeissadat SA, Rezaei S, Babaee M. Prevalence of accessory deep peroneal nerve in referred patients to an electrodiagnostic medicine clinic. J Brachial Plex Peripher Nerve Inj 2011; 6(1) 3.

[44] Falck B, Stålberg E. Motor nerve conduction studies: measurement principles and interpretation of findings. J Clin Neurophysiol 1995; 12(3) 254-279.

[45] Fisher MA. F response latencies and durations in upper motor neuron syndromes. Electromyogr Clin Neurophysiol 1986; 26(5-6) 327-332.

[46] Hopf HC. Topodiagnostic value of brain stem reflexes. Muscle Nerve 1994; 17(5) 475-484.

[47] Kimura J. Long and short of nerve conduction measures: reproducibility for sequential assessments. J Neurol Neurosurg Psychiatry 2001; 71(4) 427-430.

[48] Logigian EL, Kelly JJ Jr, Adelman LS. Nerve conduction and biopsy correlation in over 100 consecutive patients with suspected polyneuropathy. Muscle Nerve 1994; 17(9) 1010-1020.

[49] Zivković SA, Shipe C. Use of repetitive nerve stimulation in the evaluation of neuromuscular junction disorders. Am J Electroneurodiagnostic Technol 2005; 45(4) 248-261.

[50] Franssen H, van den Bergh PY. Nerve conduction studies in polyneuropathy: practical physiology and patterns of abnormality. Acta Neurol Belg 2006; 106(2) 73-81

[51] Feasby TE, Brown WF, Gilbert JJ, Hahn AF. The pathological basis of conduction block in human neuropathies. J Neurol Neurosurg Psychiatry 1985; 48(3) 239-244.

[52] Olney RK, Lewis RA, Putnam TD, Campellone JV Jr; American Association of Electrodiagnostic Medicine. Consensus criteria for the diagnosis of multifocal motor neuropathy. Muscle Nerve 2003; 27(1) 117-121.

[53] Rhee EK, England JD, Sumner AJ. A computer simulation of conduction block: effects produced by actual block versus interphase cancellation. Ann Neurol 1990; 28(2) 146-156.

[54] Isose S, Kuwabara S, Kokubun N, Sato Y, Mori M, Shibuya K, Sekiguchi Y, Nasu S, Fujimaki Y, Noto Y, Sawai S, Kanai K, Hirata K, Misawa S; Tokyo Metropolitan Neu-

romuscular Electrodiagnosis Study Group. Utility of the distal compound muscle action potential duration for diagnosis of demyelinating neuropathies. J Peripher Nerv Syst 2009; 14(3)151-158.

[55] Olney RK, Budingen HJ, Miller RG. The effects of temporal dispersion on compound muscle action potential area in human peripheral nerve. Muscle Nerve 1987; 10 728-733.

[56] Smith RS, Koles ZJ. Myelinated nerve fibers: computed effect of myelin thickness on conduction velocity. Am J Physiol 1970; 219(5) 1256-1258.

[57] García A, Calleja J, Antolín FM, Berciano J. Peripheral motor and sensory nerve conduction studies in normal infants and children. Clin Neurophysiol 2000; 111(3) 513-520.

[58] Hakamada S, Kumagai T, Watanabe T, Koike Y, Hara K, and Miyazaki S. The conduction velocity of slower and the fastest fibres in infancy and childhood. J Neurol Neurosurg Psychiatry 1982; 45(9) 851–853.

[59] Waxman SG. Determinants of conduction velocity in myelinated nerve fibers. Muscle Nerve 1980; 3(2)141-150.

[60] Rossini PM, Barker AT, Berardelli A, Caramia MD, Caruso G, Cracco RQ, Dimitrijević MR, Hallett M, Katayama Y, Lücking CH, et al. Non-invasive electrical and magnetic stimulation of the brain, spinal cord and roots: basic principles and procedures for clinical application: report of an IFCN committee. Electroencephalogr Clin Neurophysiol 1994; 91(2) 79-92.

[61] Hess CW, Mills KR, Murray NM. Responses in small hand muscles from magnetic stimulation of the human brain. J. Physiol 1987; 388 397-419.

[62] Rayegani SM, Hollisaz MT, Hafezi R, Nassirzadeh S. Application of magnetic motor stimulation for measuring conduction time across the lower part of the brachial plexus. J Brachial Plex Peripher Nerve Inj 2008; 3 7.

[63] Muller K, Homberg V, Lenard HG. Magnetic stimulation of motor cortex and nerve roots in children. Maturation of cortico-motoneuronal projections. Electroencephalogr Clin Neurophysiol 1991; 81: 63-70

[64] Morita H, Olivier E, Baumgarten J, Petersen NT, Christensen LO, Nielsen JB (2000) Differential changes in corticospinal and Ia input to tibialis anterior and soleus motor neurones during voluntary contraction in man. Acta Physiol Scand 170(1) 65–76.

[65] Magistris MR, Rösler KM, Truffert A, Myers P. Transcranial stimulation excites virtually all motor neurons supplying the target muscle. A demonstration and a method improving the study of motor evoked potentials. Brain 1998; 121 437-450.

[66] Chen R, Cros D, Curra A, et al. The clinical diagnostic utility of transcranial magnetic stimulation: report of an IFCN committee. Clin Neurophysiol 2008; 119(3) 504–532.

[67] Ogino H, Tada K, Okada K, et al. Canal diameter, anteroposterior compression ratio and spondylotic myelopathy of the cervical spine. Spine 1983; 8 1–15.

[68] Floyd AG, Yu QP, Piboolnurak P, Tang MX, Fang Y, Smith WA, Yim J, Rowland LP, Mitsumoto H, Pullman SL. Transcranial magnetic stimulation in ALS: utility of central motor conduction tests. Neurology 2009; 72(6) 498-504.

[69] Nakamae T, Tanaka N, Nakanishi K, Fujimoto Y, Sasaki H, Kamei N, Hamasaki T, Yamada K, Yamamoto R, Izumi B, Ochi M. Quantitative assessment of myelopathy patients using motor evoked potentials produced by transcranial magnetic stimulation. Eur Spine J 2010; 19(5) 685-690.

[70] Ziemann U, Lönnecker S, Steinhoff BJ, Paulus W. Effects of antiepileptic drugs on motor cortex excitability in humans: a transcranial magnetic stimulation study. Ann Neurol 1996; 40(3) 367-378.

[71] Chen R, Lozano AM, Ashby P. Mechanism of the silent period following transcranial magnetic stimulation. Evidence from epidural recordings. Exp Brain Res 1999; 128(4) 539-542.

[72] Rona S, Berardelli A, Vacca L, Inghilleri M, Manfredi M. Alterations of motor cortical inhibition in patients with dystonia. Mov Disord 1998; 13 118–124.

[73] Berardelli A, Rona S, Inghilleri M, Manfredi M. Cortical inhibition in Parkinson's disease. A study with paired magnetic stimulation. Brain 1996; 119 (Pt 1) 71-17.

[74] Caramia MD, Palmieri MG, Desiato MT, Iani C, Scalise A, Telera S, Bernardi G. Pharmacologic reversal of cortical hyperexcitability in patients with ALS. Neurology 2000; 54(1) 58-64.

[75] Meyer BU, Röricht S, Gräfin von Einsiedel H, Kruggel F, Weindl A. Inhibitory and excitatory interhemispheric transfers between motor cortical areas in normal humans and patients with abnormalities of the corpus callosum. Brain 1995; 118 (Pt 2) 429-440.

[76] Ferbert A, Priori A, Rothwell JC, Day BL, Colebatch JG, Marsden CD. Interhemispheric inhibition of the human motor cortex. J Physiol 1992; 453 525-546.

[77] Kujirai T, Caramia MD, Rothwell JC, et al. Corticocortical inhibition in human motor cortex. J Physiol 1993; 471 501–519.

[78] Ridding MC, Sheean G, Rothwell JC, Inzelberg R, Kujirai T. Changes in the balance between motor cortical excitation and inhibition in focal, task specific dystonia. J Neurol Neurosurg Psychiatry 1995; 59(5) 493-438.

[79] Ridding MC, Inzelberg R, Rothwell JC. Changes in excitability of motor cortical circuitry in patients with Parkinson's disease. Ann Neurol 1995; 37(2) 181-188.

[80] Ziemann U, Rothwell JC, Ridding MC. Interaction between intracortical inhibition and facilitation in human motor cortex. J Physiol 1996; 496(Pt 3) 873–881.

[81] Schwenkreis P, Witscher K, Janssen F, Dertwinkel R, Zenz M, Malin JP, Tegenthoff M. Changes of cortical excitability in patients with upper limb amputation. Neurosci Lett 2000; 293(2) 143-146.

[82] Sala F, Lanteri P. Brain surgery in motor areas: the invaluable assistance of intraoperative neurophysiological monitoring. J Neurosurg Sci 2003; 47 79-88.

[83] Moller, A.R. Monitoring and mapping the cranial nerves and the brainstem, In: Deletis, V, and Shils, J.L., eds.: Neurophysiology in Neurosurgery: A Modern Intraoperative Approach, Chapter 13, pp 283-310, Amsterdam, 2002, Academic Press.

[84] Sala F, Manganotti P, Tramontano V, Bricolo A, Gerosa M. Monitoring of motor pathways during brain stem surgery: what we have achieved and what we still miss? Neurophysiol Clin 2007; 37(6) 399-406.

[85] Szelényi A, Bello L, Duffau H, Fava E, Feigl GC, Galanda M, Neuloh G, Signorelli F, Sala F; Workgroup for Intraoperative Management in Low-Grade Glioma Surgery within the European Low-Grade Glioma Network. Intraoperative electrical stimulation in awake craniotomy: methodological aspects of current practice. Neurosurg Focus 2010; 28(2) E7.

[86] González-Hidalgo M, Saldaña CJ, Alonso-Lera P, Gómez-Bustamante G. The usefulness of electromyographical monitoring with intraoperative brain mapping during motor lesionectomy. Rev Neurol 2009; 16-30; 48(12) 620-624.

[87] Yingling CD, Ojemann S, Dodson B, Harrington MJ, Berger MS. Identification of motor pathways during tumor surgery facilitated by multichannel electromyographic recording. J Neurosurg 1999; 91(6) 922-927.

[88] Gonzalez AA, Jeyanandarajan D, Hansen C, Zada G, Hsieh PC: Intraoperative neurophysiological monitoring during spine surgery: a review. Neurosurg Focus 2009; 27(4) E6.

[89] Holland NR. Intraoperative electromyography. J Clin Neurophysiol 2002; 19(5) 444-453.

[90] Wilson SA, Thickbroom GW, Mastaglia FL. Transcranial magnetic stimulation mapping of the motor cortex in normal subjects. The representation of two intrinsic hand muscles. J Neurol Sci 1993; 118(2)134-144.

[91] Forster MT, Hattingen E, Senft C, Gasser T, Seifert V, Szelényi A. Navigated transcranial magnetic stimulation and functional magnetic resonance imaging: advanced adjuncts in preoperative planning for central region tumors. Neurosurgery 2011; 68(5) 1317-1324.

[92] Picht T, Schmidt S, Brandt S, Frey D, Hannula H, Neuvonen T, Karhu J, Vajkoczy P, Suess O. Preoperative functional mapping for rolandic brain tumor surgery: comparison of navigated transcranial magnetic stimulation to direct cortical stimulation. Neurosurgery 2011; 69(3) 581-588.

[93] Takahashi S, Jussen D, Vajkoczy P, Picht T. Plastic relocation of motor cortex in a patient with LGG (low grade glioma) confirmed by NBS (navigated brain stimulation). Acta Neurochir (Wien) 2012 Sep 4.

Chapter 2

Characteristics of the F-Wave and H-Reflex in Patients with Cerebrovascular Diseases: A New Method to Evaluate Neurological Findings and Effects of Continuous Stretching of the Affected Arm

Toshiaki Suzuki, Tetsuji Fujiwara, Makiko Tani and Eiichi Saitoh

Additional information is available at the end of the chapter

http://dx.doi.org/10.5772/55887

1. Introduction

The F-wave is a result of the backfire of α-motoneurons following an antidromic invasion of propagated impulses across the axon hillock (Kimura, 1974). Its occurrence reflects excitability changes in the spinal motor neurons, as reported in patients with spasticity (Odusote & Eisen, 1979) and in healthy subjects with isometric contraction (Suzuki, Fujiwara & Takeda, 1993). In our previous study that investigated the nervous system of hemiplegic patients, excitability of spinal neural function was evaluated using F-wave data of patients with cerebrovascular disease (CVD) (Suzuki, Fujiwara & Takeda, 1993). We also reported that the persistence and amplitude ratio of F/M in patients with CVD were affected by the grade of muscle tonus, tendon reflex, or voluntary movement. Persistence reportedly depends on the number of neuromuscular units activated, while the amplitude ratio of F/M depends on their excitability (Eisen and Odusote, 1979). Therefore, we concluded that F-wave measurement was an effective neurological test for evaluating muscle tonus and voluntary movements.

Generally, current stimulus intensity required to generate an F-wave is 20% more than that required to generate a supramaximal M-wave because only the F-wave appears in healthy subjects; the H-reflex that is elicited by electrical stimulation of a peripheral mixed nerve, especially muscle spindle Ia fibers, does not appear in healthy subjects. However, we observed that the H-reflex could be evoked with supramaximal stimulation, a test for measuring the F-wave in CVD patients with hypertonus and hyperreflexia. As a result, the H-reflex can be mistaken for an F-wave during F-wave measurement using supramaximal stimulation.

We hypothesized that evaluation of F-wave and H-reflex patterns resulting from increased stimulus intensity in CVD patients could be a potential new method for the neurological evaluation of the affected arm or leg. In this report, we investigated the excitability of spinal neural function by evaluating H-reflex and F-wave patterns resulting from increased stimulus intensity during muscle relaxation in healthy subjects and CVD patients. The results were analyzed in terms of the characteristic appearance of the H-reflex and F-wave in the healthy subjects and the relationship between the neurological findings of CVD and the characteristic appearance of the H-reflex and F-wave in the CVD patients.

In the field of rehabilitation medicine, muscle stretching is generally used to increase range of motion and improve muscle tonus. The effects of leg muscle stretching have been previously evaluated using H-reflex data (Angel et al., 1963 and Nielsen et al., 1993), and the results showed that the H-reflex following passive stretching was decreased to a lesser extent in spastic patients than in healthy subjects. However, in that study, the calf muscles and not the arm muscles were stretched; moreover, the periods of continuous stretching were different.Therefore, we also investigated the effects of continuous stretching of the affected arm for 1 min by evaluating H-reflex and F-wave characteristics in different stretched arm positions in the CVD patients.

2. Characteristics of H-reflex and F-wave patterns resulting from increased stimulus intensity during muscle relaxation

The H-reflex and F-wave of the affected arm were examined under conditions of increased stimulus intensity during muscle relaxation in 31 patients (17 male and 14 female) with hemiplegia caused by CVD. The mean patient age was 56 years (range: 30–82 years). Eighteen patients had cerebral infarction (7 with right and 11 with left hemiplegia) and 13 had cerebral hemorrhage (7 with right and 6 with left). The control group included 30 healthy subjects with a mean age of 56.2 years (range: 28–80 years). Written informed consent was obtained from all subjects. The experiments were conducted in accordance with the Declaration of Helsinki, and no conflicts of interest were declared by the authors.

Examination was performed in a supine, relaxed position. H-reflex and F-wave data under conditions of increased stimulus intensity following median nerve stimulation at the wrist were recorded at the opponens pollicis muscle, which was in a relaxed state, of the affected arm of the CVD patients or the right arm of the healthy subjects (Fig 1). The stimulus frequency was 0.5 Hz and the stimulus duration was 0.2 ms. H-reflex and F-wave patterns that resulted from increased stimulus intensity were divided into 4 types (types 1–4).

http://dx.doi.org/10.5772/55887

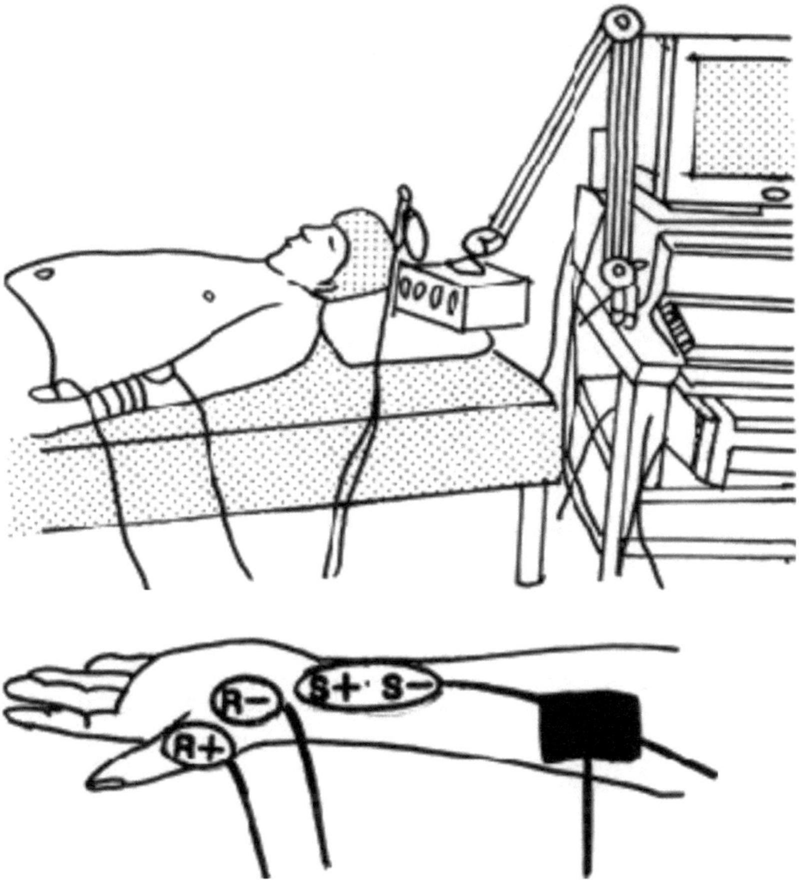

R+: Recording Electrode (+), R–: Recording Electrode (–)
S+: Stimulating Electrode (+), S–: Stimulating Electrode (–)

Figure 1. Measurement of the H-reflex and F-wave

In type 1, the F-wave appeared with increased stimulus intensity, but there was no H-reflex (Fig 2). The F-wave pattern for the upper arm, especially the distal portion in healthy subjects, roughly indicated a type 1 pattern. In type 2, the H-reflex and F-wave both appeared with increased stimulus intensity, but the F-wave followed the disappearance of the H-reflex (Fig 3). In type 3, the H-reflex and F-wave both appeared with increased stimulus intensity, but the F-wave appeared during the H-reflex (Fig 4). In type 4, only the H-reflex appeared with increased stimulus intensity; there was no F-wave (Fig 5).

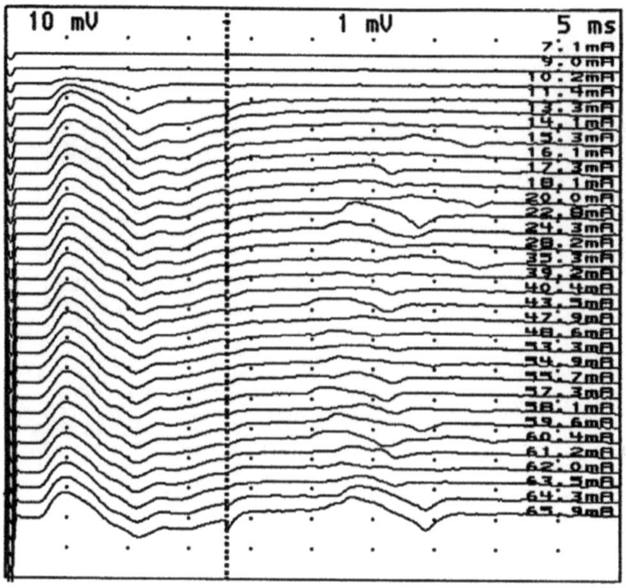

Figure 2. H-reflex and F-wave patterns resulting from increased stimulus intensity (Type 1) The F-wave appeared with increased stimulus intensity, but there was no H-reflex.

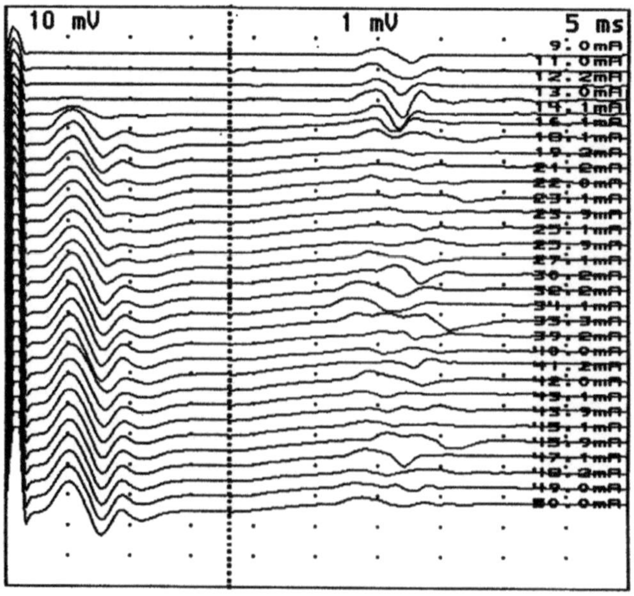

Figure 3. H-reflex and F-wave patterns resulting from increased stimulus intensity (Type 2) The H-reflex and F-wave both appeared with increased stimulus intensity, but the F-wave followed the disappearance of the H-reflex.

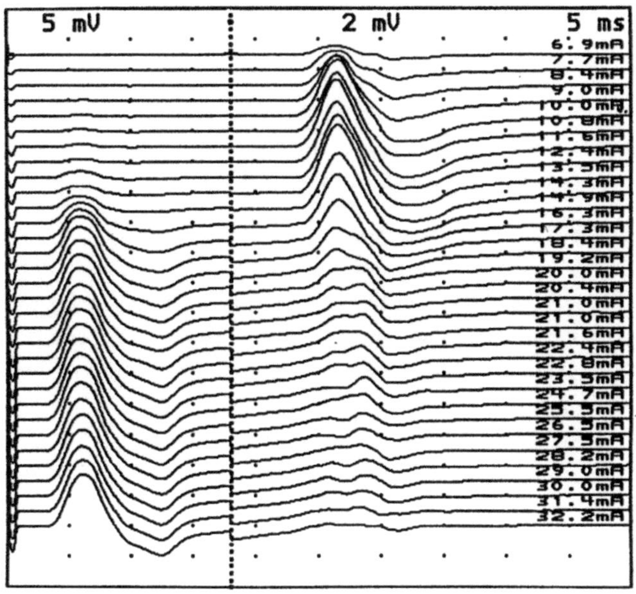

Figure 4. H-reflex and F-wave patterns resulting from increased stimulus intensity (Type 3) The H-reflex and F-wave both appeared with increased stimulus intensity, but the F-wave appeared during the H-reflex.

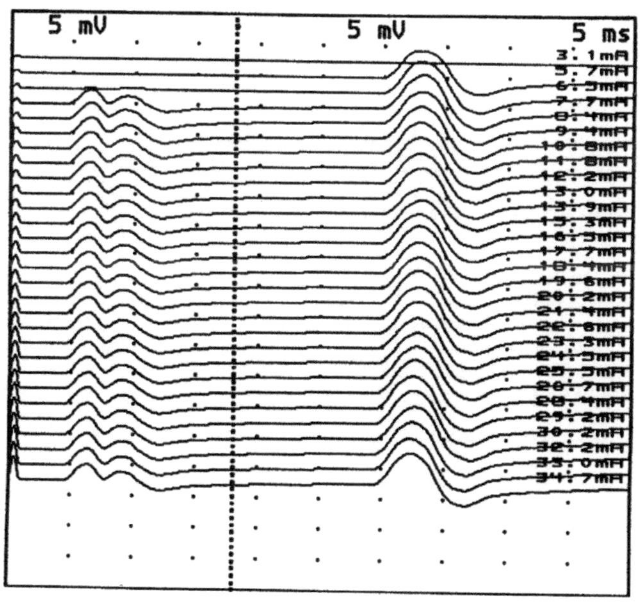

Figure 5. H-reflex and F-wave patterns resulting from increased stimulus intensity (Type 4) Only the H-reflex appeared with increased stimulus intensity, but there was no F-wave.

Neurological findings, including muscle tonus and tendon reflex, were also evaluated. Findings of muscle tonus and tendon reflex were classified into increased (markedly, moderately, and slightly), normal, and decreased.

The results were analyzed in terms of the characteristic appearance of the H-reflex and F-wave in the healthy subjects and the relationship between the neurological findings of CVD and the characteristic appearance of the H-reflex and F-wave in the CVD patients.

H-reflex and F-wave patterns resulting from increased stimulus intensity were type 1 in all healthy subjects. The relationship between H-reflex and F-wave patterns resulting from increased stimulus intensity and the neurological signs of CVD is shown in Tables 1 and 2. H-reflex and F-wave patterns resulting from increased stimulus intensity in patients with markedly increased muscle tonus and tendon reflex were most frequently type 4 patterns, those in patients with moderately increased muscle tonus and tendon reflex were type 2 or 3 patterns, those in patients with slightly increased muscle tonus and tendon reflex were type 1 or 2 patterns, and those in patients with normal or decreased muscle tonus and tendon reflex were type 1 patterns.

		Increased		Normal	Decreased
	Markedly	**Moderately**	**Slightly**		
Type 1	0	0	2	5	3
Type 2	0	4	4	0	0
Type 3	2	4	1	0	0
Type 4	5	1	0	0	0

The number of subjects was 31 (Type 1: 10, Type 2: 8, Type 3: 7, Type 4: 6)

Table 1. The relationship between H-reflex and F-wave patterns resulting from increased stimulus intensity and muscle tonus

		Increased		Normal	Decreased
	Markedly	**Moderately**	**Slightly**		
Type 1	0	0	1	6	3
Type 2	0	3	5	0	0
Type 3	2	4	1	0	0
Type 4	4	2	0	0	0

The number of subjects was 31(Type 1: 10, Type 2: 8, Type 3: 7, Type 4: 6)

Table 2. The relationship between H-reflex and F-wave patterns resulting from increased stimulus intensity and tendon reflex

These results indicated that the H-reflex, and not the F-wave, appeared with supramaximal stimulation in patients with a relative increase in excitability of spinal neural function. Furthermore, the neurological signs of muscle tonus and tendon reflex affected H-reflex and F-wave patterns in the CVD patients. These H-reflex and F-wave patterns were therefore used for the neurological evaluation of the CVD patients.

3. Characteristics of the H-reflex and F-wave in different stretched arm positions in the CVD patients

3.1. The effects of continuous stretching of the affected arm (the H-reflex study)

Ten hemiplegic patients (4 male and 6 female) with hypertonus caused by CVD were tested. The mean patient age was 53.2 years (range: 34–63 years). There were 5 patients with cerebral hemorrhage (2 with right and 3 with left hemiplegia) and 5 with cerebral infarction (2 with right and 3 with left hemiplegia). The cortical location of the lesion, as verified by brain computed tomography, was temporal in 4 patients, parietal in 2, and temporo-occipital in 2. The lesion was located in the brain stem in the remaining 2 patients. Patients were divided into 3 groups on the basis of the extent of increase in muscle tonus: one group with slightly increased muscle tonus (2 patients), one with moderately increased muscle tonus (6 patients), and one with markedly increased muscle tonus (2 patients).

The H-reflexes before, during, and 0, 2, 4, 6, 8, and 10 min after continuous stretching of the abductor pollicis brevis (APB) muscle of the affected side were recorded following stimulation of the median nerve at the wrist. The intensity of the constant stimulation current was 1.2 times greater than that of the minimum current required to evoke an M-wave with a stimulus frequency of 0.5 Hz and duration of 0.2 ms. Stimulation was performed 30 times in each trial. The H-reflex was analyzed for persistence, amplitude ratio of H/M, and latency, which was determined as the mean of measurable H-reflexes. Stretching comprised continuous stretching of the affected arm with shoulder joint abduction, elbow joint extension, wrist joint dorsiflexion, and finger extension for 1 min (Fig 6). Using this data, we analyzed H-reflex characteristics resulting from continuous stretching of the affected arm as well as the relationship between the effects of continuous stretching and neurological findings in the CVD patients.

Persistence and amplitude ratio of H/M were significantly lower ($p < 0.05$) after stretching than before stretching; these characteristics gradually recovered after continuous stretching. Figure 7 shows the amplitude ratio of H/M before, during, and after continuous stretching. A typical H-reflex is shown in Figure 8. There was no significant difference in latency. Persistence and amplitude ratio of H/M during continuous stretching were lower than those before and after stretching in the patients with moderately increased muscle tonus. The amplitude ratio of H/M before, during, and after continuous stretching in patients with moderately increased muscle tonus is shown in Figure 9. On the other hand, H-reflex characteristics were the same before, during, and after continuous stretching in the patients with slightly or markedly increased muscle tonus (Fig 10). Latency was the same before, during, and after continuous stretching in all patients, irrespective of slightly, moderately, or markedly increased muscle tonus.

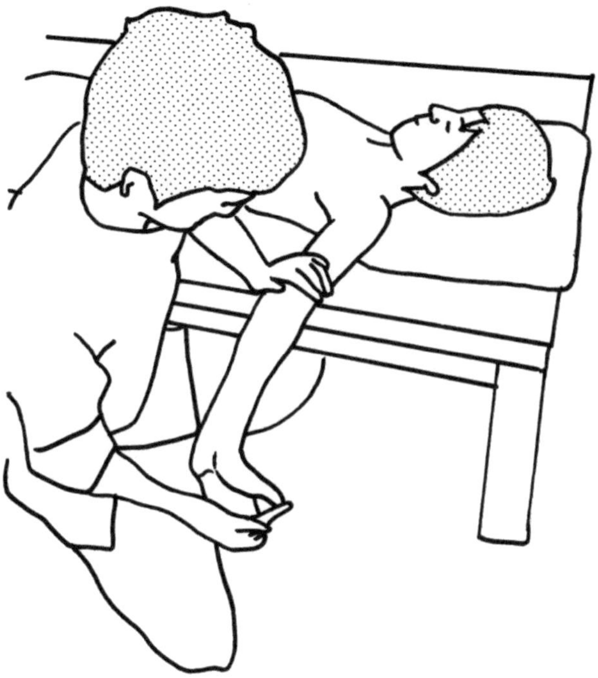

Figure 6. Continuous stretching of the affected arm with shoulder joint abduction, elbow joint extension, wrist joint dorsiflexion, and finger extension for 1 min

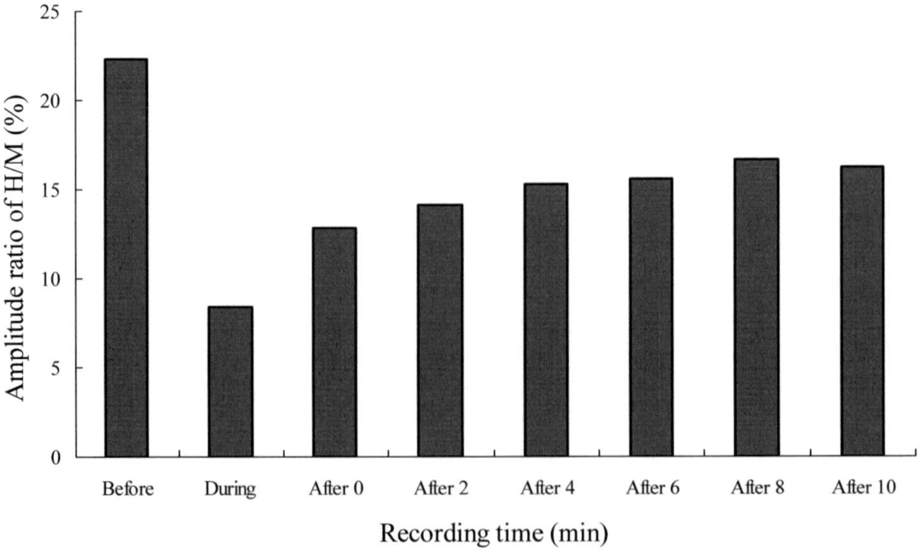

Figure 7. Characteristics of the amplitude ratio of H/M before, during, and after continuous stretching The amplitude ratio of H/M during ($p < 0.05$) and after stretching was lower than that before stretching, and it gradually increased after stretching.

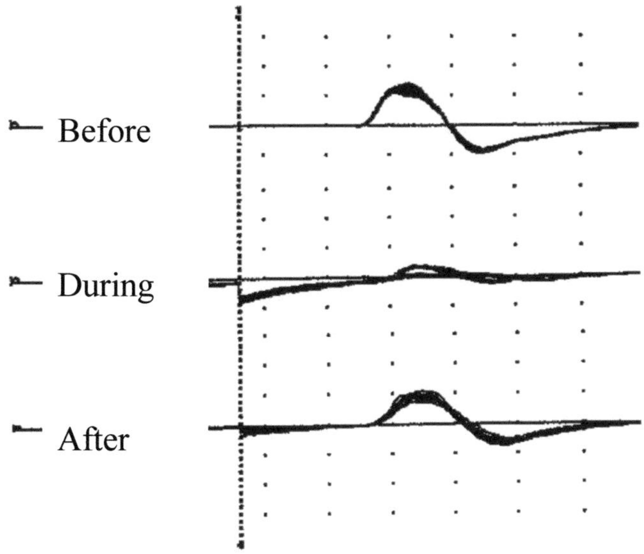

Figure 8. A typical H-reflex pattern before, during, and after continuous stretching (Left hemiplegia, 59-year-old male) The amplitude of the H-reflex during and after stretching was lower than that before stretching. The amplitude gain was 5 mV (M wave) and 1 mV (H-reflex). Gain of latency was 5 ms.

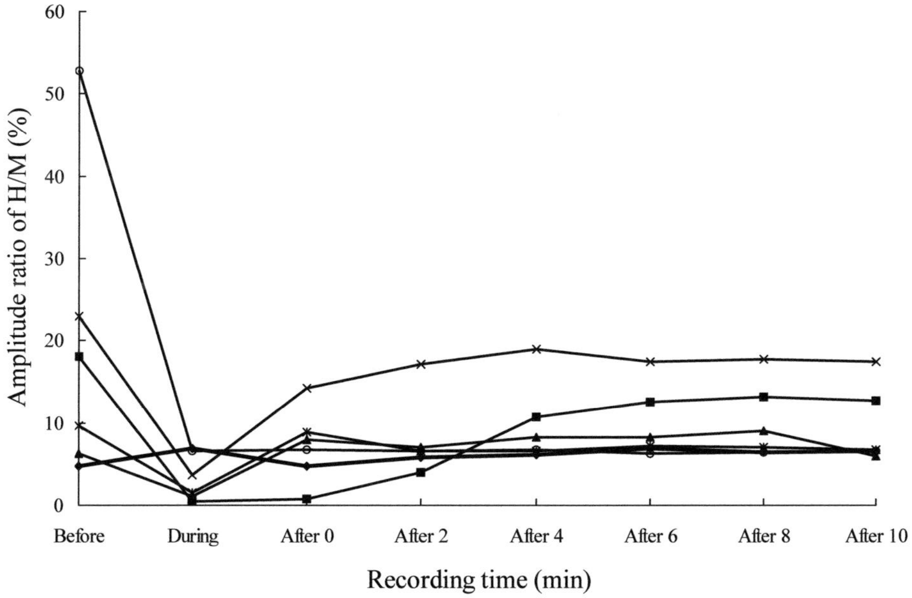

Figure 9. Characteristics of the amplitude ratio of H/M before, during, and after continuous stretching in patients with moderately increased muscle tonus The amplitude ratio of H/M during stretching was lower, while that after stretching gradually increased.

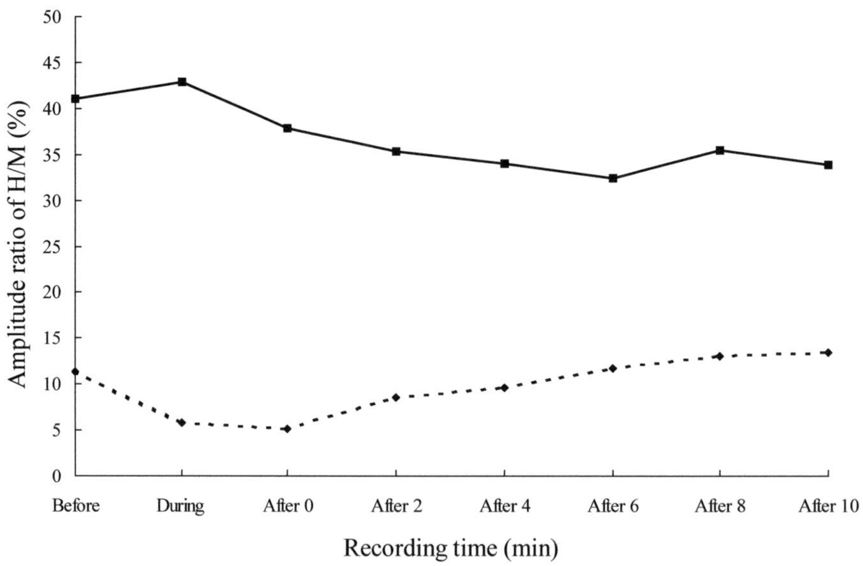

Figure 10. Characteristics of the amplitude ratio of H/M before, during, and after continuous stretching in patients with slightly and markedly increased muscle tonus The figure shows typical data in patients with slightly (dash line) and markedly (solid line) increased muscle tonus. The amplitude ratio of H/M before, during, and after stretching remained the same.

Generally, the H-reflex is suppressed during passive stretching in healthy subjects, although the mechanism has not been clarified. Depression was thought to be caused by a decrease in the number of afferent fibers fired from the Golgi tendon organs and muscle spindle during passive stretching (Paillard, 1959 and Mark et al., 1968). The increase in the H-reflex following passive stretching, caused by excitability of cortical and spinal neural function, was greater in spastic patients than in healthy subjects (Angel et al., 1963, Niesen et al., 1993, and Hashizume et al., 1985). However, our results demonstrate that H-reflexes during 1 min of continuous stretching of the affected arm were significantly decreased compared with those before continuous stretching, especially in the CVD patients with moderately increased muscle tonus. There are 3 differences between the results of other studies and our results. First is the duration of stretching, which was considerably shorter (1 min) in our study than in the other studies. It is well known that in healthy subjects, excitability of spinal neural function during continuous stretching is decreased because of the inhibitory neurons from the Ib afferents. These Ib afferents from the Golgi tendon organs, which fire in response to muscle tension, are reportedly influenced by corticospinal fibers (Lundberg et al., 1978). Excitability of spinal neural function during muscle stretching showed a greater increase in the spastic CVD patients than in the healthy subjects because Ib afferent inhibitory neurons are not fired under short stretching durations. Therefore, CVD patients require longer durations of continuous stretching of the affected hypertonic muscle to fire the Ib inhibitory neurons. The second difference lies in the stretched muscle. In the other studies, affected calf muscles were stretched, whereas in our study, the arm muscles were stretched. Therefore, differences in stretched muscle also influence excitability of spinal neural function. The last difference concerns the method used. We speculate that differences in the method of muscle stretching also affect the excitability of spinal neural function. Clinically, continuous stretching of the arm involves the simultaneous stretching of several joints, particularly according to the Bobath concept. Therefore, the affected muscle tonus is changed by muscle contraction and muscle stretching in remote parts of the body.

Patients with moderately increased muscle tonus were more affected by these stretch conditions in our study. Excitability of spinal neural function during 1 min of continuous stretching was inhibited in the patients with moderately increased muscle tonus, whereas that in the patients with slightly or markedly increased muscle tonus was less affected. Therefore, it is important to examine neurological findings using continuous stretching as one of the rehabilitation treatments.

3.2. F-wave characteristics in different stretched positions of the affected arm in CVD patients

The subjects were 20 hemiparesis patients with moderate hypertonus (modified Ashworth scale score of 2 or 3) caused by CVD. Their mean age was 49.5 years. There were 10 patients with cerebral hemorrhage (5 with right and 5 with left) and 10 with cerebral infarction (5 with right and 5 with left). Computed tomography or magnetic resonance imaging confirmed the cortical lesions to be located in the temporal region in 5 patients, parietal region in 3, temporo-occipital region in 3, and brain stem in 5. The muscle tonus of the affected arm, especially the distal part, was moderately increased according to a modified Ashworth scale score of 2 or 3. The F-wave was recorded at the APB during continuous stretching for 1 min after stimulation of the median nerve at the wrist. The first trial was a relaxation trial, followed by continuous stretching of the affected arm for 1 min in the following positions: stretched position with shoulder joint abduction (trial 2, Fig 11), stretched position with shoulder joint abduction and elbow joint extension (trial 3, Fig 12), and stretched position with shoulder joint abduction, elbow joint extension, and wrist joint extension (trial 4, Fig 6). The intensity of the constant stimulation current was 1.2 times greater than that of the minimum current required to evoke a maximal M-wave with a stimulus frequency of 0.5 Hz and duration of 0.2 ms. Stimulation was performed 30 times in each trial. The F-wave was analyzed for persistence, amplitude ratio of F/M, and latency, which were the mean values of the measurable F-waves. Using this data, F-wave characteristics during continuous stretching (trials 2–4) were compared with those during relaxation (trial 1) in the CVD patients with moderately increased muscle hypertonus.

The following results were analyzed: 1) relationship between F-wave characteristics in trial 1 and trial 2, 2) relationship between F-wave characteristics in trial 1 and trial 3, and 3) relationship between F-wave characteristics in trial 1 and trial 4.

With regard to the relationship between F-wave characteristics in trial 1 and trial 2, persistence, amplitude ratio of F/M, and latency were the same in trial 1 and 2.

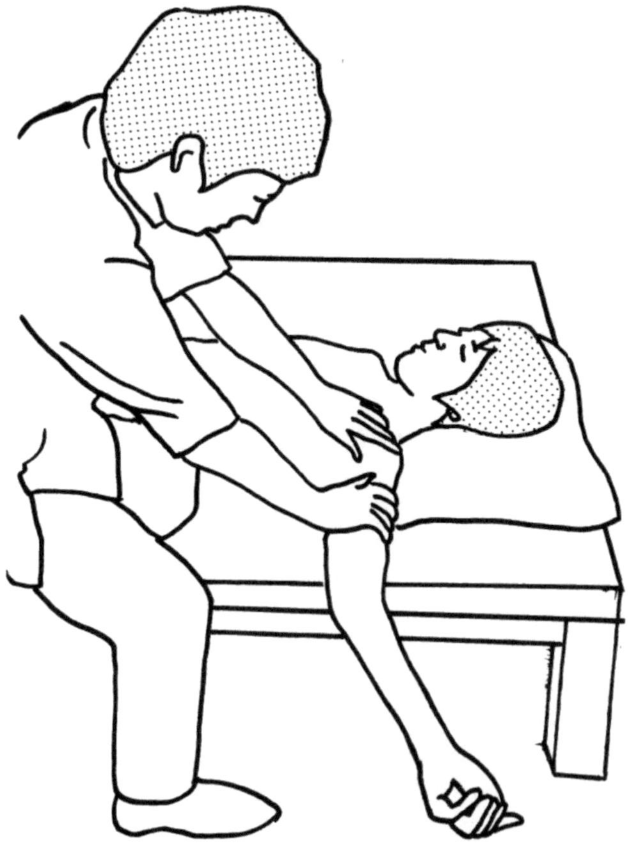

Figure 11. Continuous stretching of the affected arm with shoulder joint abduction for 1 min

http://dx.doi.org/10.5772/55887

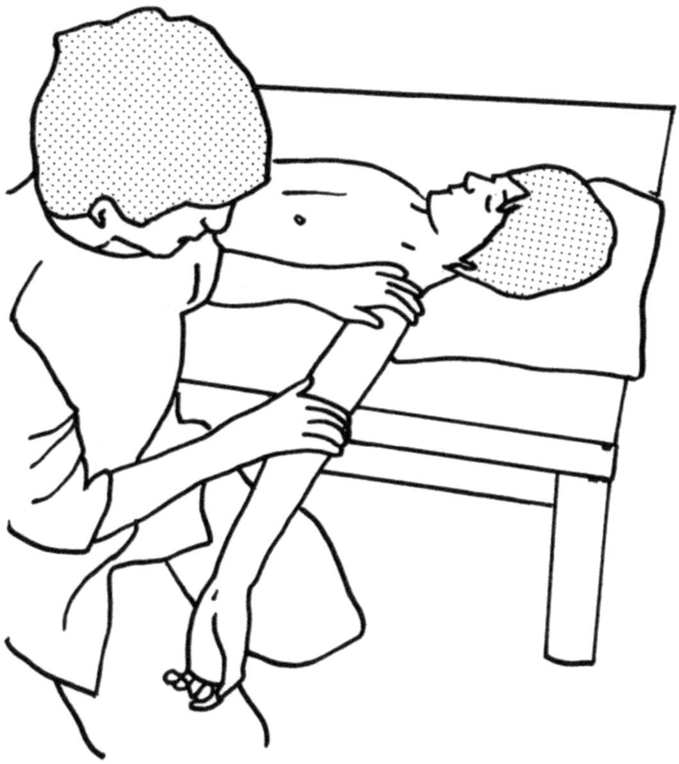

Figure 12. Continuous stretching of the affected arm with shoulder joint abduction and elbow joint extension for 1 min

With regard to the relationship between F-wave characteristics in trial 1 and trial 3, persistence and amplitude ratio of F/M were significantly lower in trial 3 than in trial 1 ($p < 0.05$; Table 3 and Fig 13). No significant difference was noticed in latency between trials 1 and 3.

	trial 1	trial 3	t-test
Persistence (%)	100 ± 0.00	91.0 ± 41.8	p < 0.05
Amplitude ratio of F/M (%)	10.8 ± 3.5	2.71 ± 3.53	p < 0.05
Latency (ms)	25.3 ± 2.28	25.6 ± 3.17	NS

NS: Not Significant

Persistence and amplitude ratio of F/M in trial 3 were significantly lower than those in trial 1.

Table 3. F-wave characteristics in trials 1 and 3

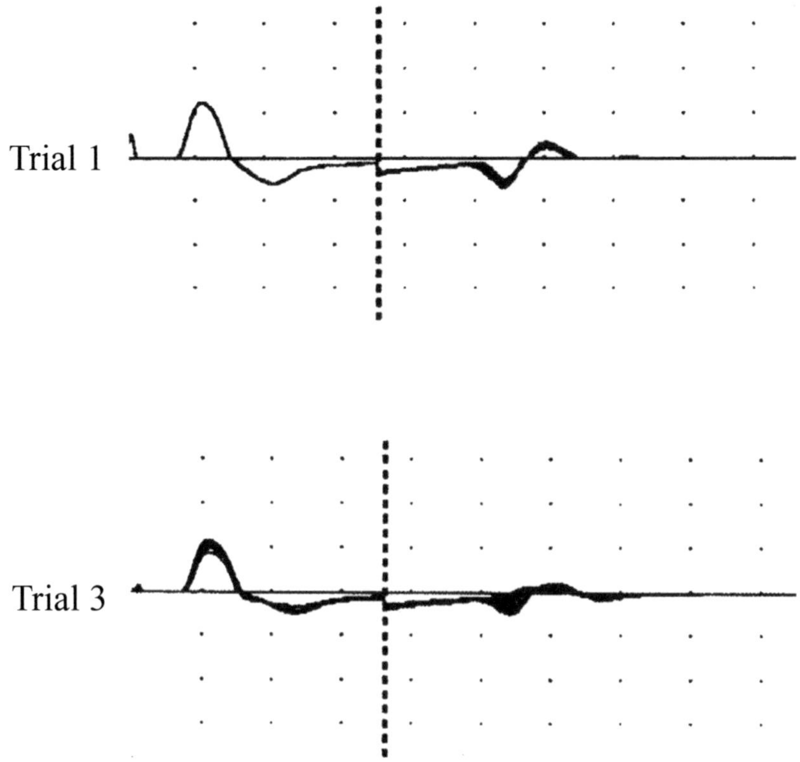

Figure 13. A typical F-wave in trial 1 and 3 Amplitude of the F-wave in trial 3 was significantly lower than that in trial 1. The amplitude gain was 5 mV/D (M-wave) and 2 mV/D (F-wave). The latency gain was 5 ms/D for both the M-wave and F-wave.

With regard to the relationship between F-wave characteristics in trial 1 and trial 4, persistence and amplitude ratio of F/M were significantly lower in trial 4 than in trial 1 ($p < 0.05$; Table 4 and Fig 14). No significant difference was noticed in latency between trials 1 and 4.

	trial 1	trial 4	t-test
Persistence (%)	100 ± 0.00	82.5 ± 21.8	p < 0.05
Amplitude ratio of F/M (%)	7.34 ± 3.5	4.26 ± 3.78	p < 0.05
Latency (ms)	24.5 ± 2.58	24.5 ± 2.58	NS

NS: Not Significant

Persistence and amplitude ratio of F/M in trial 4 were significantly lower than those in trial 1.

Table 4. F-wave characteristics in trials 1 and 4

http://dx.doi.org/10.5772/55887

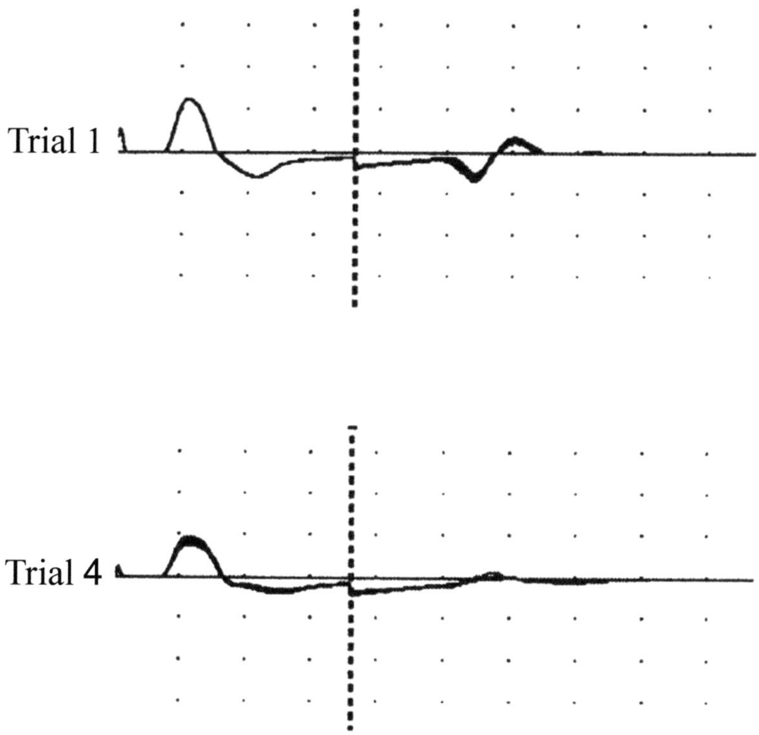

Figure 14. A typical F-wave in trials 1 and 4 The F-wave amplitude in trial 4 was significantly lower than that in trial 1. The amplitude gain was 5 mV/D (M-wave) and 2 mV/D (F-wave). The latency gain was 5 ms/D for both the M-wave and F-wave.

Furthermore, persistence and amplitude ratio of F/M of F-waves generated by the APB were significantly lower during 1 min of stretching in all positions than during relaxation (no stretched position) in the CVD patients with moderate hypertonus. All stretching positions decreased the excitability of spinal neural function.

The method of stretching the affected arm involved the simultaneous stretching of several muscles rather than just one muscle. The period of continuous stretching in our study was shorter (1 min) than that in the other studies (10 min, 30 min; Odeen, 1981).

Continuous stretching of the proximal shoulder and elbow of the affected arm is believed to decrease excitability of spinal neural function due to Ib inhibitory neuron afferents (Mark et al., 1968) and central nervous function (Staines WR et al., 1997). We hypothesize that decreasing excitability of proximal spinal and central neural function can decrease excitability of distal spinal neural function in patients with hemiparesis accompanied by moderate hypertonus caused by CVD.

Our study suggests that excitability of distal spinal neural function in the APB of the affected arm decreases during continuous stretching of the proximal muscle and shoulder and elbow joints or all the shoulder, elbow, and wrist joints.

4. Conclusions

Summary of this study report

1. We examined H-reflex and F-wave data resulting from increased stimulus intensity in the affected arm in patients with CVD. The results suggested that the characteristic appearance of the H-reflex and F-wave resulting from increased stimulus intensity reflects the neurological findings of CVD and can be used to evaluate excitability of spinal neural function in patients with CVD.

2. To investigate excitability of spinal neural function during stretching in CVD patients, H-reflex data was obtained before, during, and after 1 min of continuous stretching of the APB of the affected arm after stimulation of the median nerve. Persistence, amplitude, and amplitude ratio of H/M were lower during stretching than before and after stretching in the patients with moderately increased muscle tonus, whereas these characteristics were the same before, during, and after continuous stretching in the patients with slightly and markedly increased muscle tonus. These results suggested that excitability of spinal neural function during 1 min of continuous stretching of the affected arm was inhibited in CVD patients with moderately increased muscle tonus.

3. F-wave data was obtained from the APB during relaxation (trial 1) and continuous stretching of the affected arm for 1 min in different positions in patients with CVD: stretched position with shoulder abduction (trial 2), stretched position with shoulder abduction and elbow extension (trial 3), and stretched position with shoulder abduction, elbow extension, and wrist extension (trial 4). Persistence and amplitude ratio of F/M were the same in trial 2 and trial 1 and significantly lower in trials 3 and 4 than in trial 1. These results suggested that excitability of spinal neural function in the APB of the affected arm was decreased during continuous stretching of the proximal muscle and shoulder and elbow joints or all the shoulder, elbow, and wrist joints in patients with hemiparesis accompanied by moderate hypertonus caused by CVD.

Acknowledgements

We would like to thank Mr. Onuma T. for his assistance in this study.

Author details

Toshiaki Suzuki[1], Tetsuji Fujiwara[2], Makiko Tani[1] and Eiichi Saitoh[3]

1 Graduate School of Kansai University of Health Sciences, Japan

2 Kyoto University, Japan

3 Fujita Health University, Japan

References

[1] Angel RW & Hofmann WW (1963). The H-reflex in normal, spastic, and rigid subjects. *Archives of Neurology*, Jun 1963), 0003-9942, 9, 591-596.

[2] Eisen A & Odusote K (1979). Amplitude of the F-wave: A potential means of documenting spasticity. *Neurology*, Sep 1979), 0028-3878, 29, 1306-1309.

[3] Fisher MA (1983). F response analysis of motor disorders of central origin. *J. Neurolo. Sci.*, Dec 1983), 0002-2510X, 62(1-3), 13-22.

[4] Hashizume M, Koike Y, Hayashi F, Sakurai N, & Sobue I (1985). The inhibition of H-reflexes by passive static and sinusoidal stretch in normal subjects and spastic patients (In Japanese). *Clinical Neurology*, Aug 1985), 0000-9918X, 25(8), 911-919.

[5] Kimura J (1974). F-wave velocity in the central segment of the median and ulnar nerves. A study in normal subjects and in patients with Charcot-Marie-Tooth disease. *Neurology*, Jun 1974), 0028-3878, 24(6), 539-546.

[6] Lundberg A, Malmgren K, & Schomburg ED (1978). Role of joint afferents in motor control exemplified by effects on reflex pathways from Ib afferents. *Journal of Physiology*, Nov 1978), 0022-3751, 284, 327-343.

[7] Mark RF, Coquery JM, & Paillard J (1968). Autogenetic reflex effects of slow or steady stretch of the calf muscles in man. *Experimental Brain Research*, 0014-4819, 6(2), 130-145.

[8] Nielsen J, Petersen N, Ballegaard M, Biering-Sørensen F, & Kiehn O (1993). H-reflexes are less depressed following muscle stretch in spastic spinal cord injured patients than in healthy subjects. *Experimental Brain Research*, 0014-4819, 97(1), 173-176.

[9] Odéen I & Knutsson E (1981). Evaluation of the effects of muscle stretch and weight load in patients with spastic paraplegia. *Scand J Rehabili Med*, 0036-5505, 13(4), 117-121.

[10] Odusote K & Eisen A (1979). An electrophysiological quantitation of the cubital tunnel syndrome. *The Canadian Journal of Neurological Sciences*, Nov 1979), 0317-1671, 6(4), 403-410.

[11] Paillard J (1959). Functional organization of afferent innervation of muscle studied in man by monosynaptic testing. *American Journal of Physical Medicine*, Dec 1959), 0002-9491, 38, 239-247.

[12] Staines WR, Brook JD, Cheng J, Misiaszek JE, & MacKay WA (1997). Movement-induced gain modulation of somatosensory potentials and soleus H-reflexes evoked from the leg. I. Kinaesthetic task demands. *Exp Brain Res*, (Jun 1997), Jun 1997), 0014-4819, 115(1), 147-155.

[13] Suzuki T, Fujiwara T, & Takeda I (1993). Excitability of the spinal motor neuron pool and F-wave during isometric ipsilateral and contralateral contraction. *Physiotherapy Theory and Practice*, 0959-3985, 9, 19-24.

[14] Suzuki T, Fujiwara T, & Takeda I (1993). Characteristics of F-wave during relaxation in patients with CVD (In Japanese). PT journal, 0915-0552, 27, 277-281.

Chapter 3

Different Types of Fibrillation Potentials in Human Needle EMG

Juhani Partanen

Additional information is available at the end of the chapter

http://dx.doi.org/10.5772/55352

1. Introduction

Rhythmic fibrillation potentials are the hallmark of denervated muscle fibres in needle EMG of a striated muscle (Conrad et al. 1972, Heckmann & Ludin 1982). They are readily activated by the insertion of an EMG needle electrode (Kugelberg & Petersén 1949). Irregular fibrillation potentials may also be present (Buchthal & Rosenfalck 1966, Purves & Sakmann 1974). There is, however, an obvious difficulty to discriminate between true irregular fibrillation potentials of a denervated muscle and end plate spikes, which occur in a normal muscle. This may lead to the conclusion that only rhythmic fibrillation potentials matter (Stöhr 1977). We have pointed out that fibrillation potentials, whether regular or irregular, have longer minimum interpotential intervals than end plate spikes (Partanen & Danner 1982). During long sequences, the mean interval between successive end plate spikes and rhythmic fibrillation potential tends to increase, whereas irregular fibrillations do not show this type of "self-inhibition" (Partanen & Danner 1982, Partanen & Nousiainen 1983). The aim of this chapter is to describe fibrillation potentials of different categories in either completely or partially denervated human limb muscles, or after a muscle injury. We also compare the characteristics of fibrillation potentials to neurally driven sequences, such as "myokymic" fibrillation potentials and end plate spikes (Brown & Varkey 1981, Partanen & Nousiainen 1983, Partanen 1999). "Myokymic" fibrillation potentials are a rare phenomenon of innervated muscle fibres. They have not been described earlier and are readily confused with end plate spikes. The term "myokymic" fibrillations is descriptive. The pathophysiology of "myokymic fibrillation" is different from true myokymia of whole motor units (see Willison 1982, Stålberg & Trontelj 1982).

2. Material and methods

Spontaneous activity was recorded with concentric needle electrodes (DISA 13L58) and a 4-channel Disa 1500 EMG machine interfaced with a 4-channel Teac R 61 D cassette recorder. Amplification was set at 50 µV/div, and high-pass and low-pass filters at 20 and 2000 Hz, respectively. 94 sequences of spontaneous activity were divided into the following categories by audiovisual analysis: random fibrillations, slightly irregular fibrillations with occasional pauses, regular fibrillations (Partanen & Danner 1982), "myokymic" fibrillations, and end plate spikes (Partanen 1999). 10- or 20-second samples of the given sequences were digitized (sampling frequency 10 kHz) and analyzed in a Hewlett Packard 340 computer for interpotential intervals and wave forms.

"Myokymic" discharges of partially denervated muscles usually exhibited short sequences and they were found to be either "fibrillation-like" or "motor unit potential-like". These sequences were occasionally studied with another EMG needle inserted a few millimeters from the primary electrode in parallel with the muscle fibres. In "fibrillation-like" myokymic discharges it was difficult to find a synchronous discharge of the same muscle fibre in the second EMG channel whereas in "motor unit potential-like" sequences a synchronous discharge was readily observed indicating a sum potential of several muscle fibres of the motor unit. In such a case the sequence was omitted.

The raw EMG data were processed with an automatic analysis system (Partanen 1999). The rise rate, computed using a simple "low pass differentiator" (Usui & Admiror 1982) with a user definable threshold level was applied for potential recognition. Each potential recognized as belonging to the given sequence was marked with a cursor. Thereafter the sequence was checked visually on a large screen, potential by potential in order to correct possible misclassifications of the automatic program. In case of uncertainty, caused, for example, by superimposition of potentials the data were discarded and a new sample of the given sequence was taken from the tape and the procedure was repeated.

Subsequently the analysis program computed the number of intervals, mean, standard deviation, median, minimum, maximum, and interval range of the intervals, as well as the amplitude, and the spike duration of the averaged potential. The initial positive deflection of the potential could also be measured. In order to assess the regularity of firing, also the mean consecutive difference (MCD) (Stålberg et al. 1971) and the average proportional consecutive interval difference (APCID) (Conrad et al. 1972) were calculated.

The different potential categories were analyzed using Student´s unpaired t-test.

3. Results

Figures 1-3 show the typical firing pattern of different spontaneous fibrillation categories. Random and slightly irregular fibrillations with pauses could usually be recorded for several minutes. In many cases we collected several samples of a sequence, one of which was chosen for the analysis. This was possible because these fibrillation sequences were persistent with the same firing pattern. Also a sequence of rhythmic fibrillation potentials had to proceed several seconds in order to be accepted. Rhythmic fibrillations were usually elicited by needle insertion and they showed a gradual shift of interpotential intervals during the recording time (Conrad et al. 1972). A short-lasting burst of insertion activity was not accepted. Slightly irregular fibrillations with pauses did not show a gradual shift in the basal interval, nor were they affected by needle insertion.

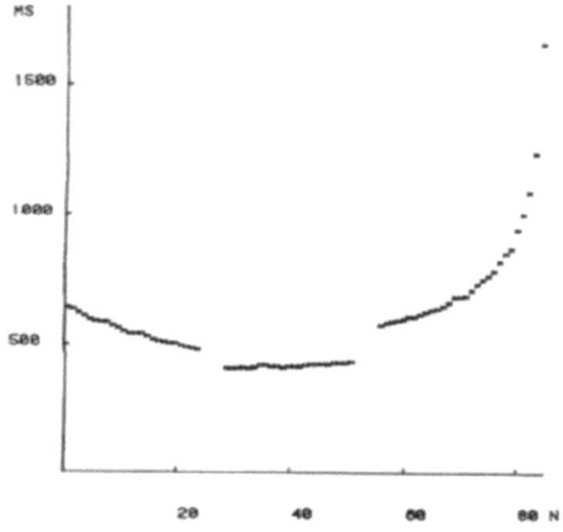

Figure 1. A regular sequence of fibrillation potentials. Interruptions in line indicate interruptions in recording. On the vertical axis is the interpotential interval of fibrillation potentials. On the horizontal axis is the number of successive intervals. There are 20 intervals per division. From Partanen, J.V. & Danner, R. (1982), Author´s own work.

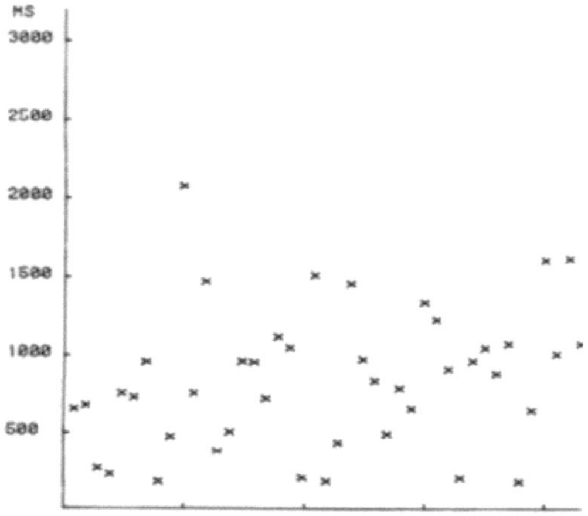

Figure 2. Randomly occurring fibrillations 33 days after muscle biopsy. Vertical axis is the interpotential interval. Horizontal axis is the number of successive intervals; there are 10 intervals per division. From Partanen, J.V. & Danner, R. (1982), Author´s own work.

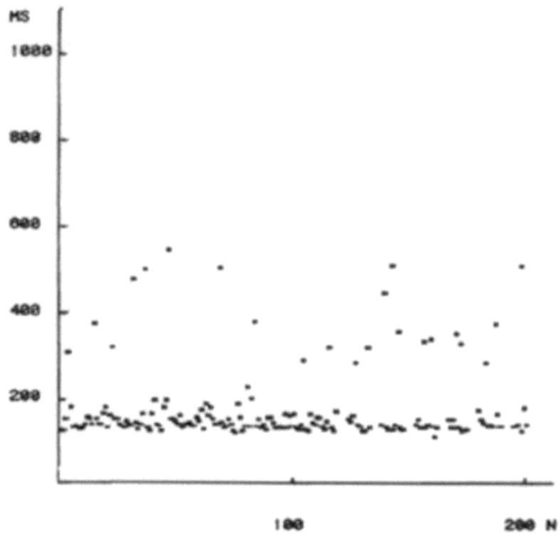

Figure 3. Slightly irregular fibrillations with occasional pauses (long intervals); 51 days after muscle biopsy. Note the slight irregularity in the basal (short) intervals. From Partanen, J.V. & Danner, R. (1982), Author´s own work.

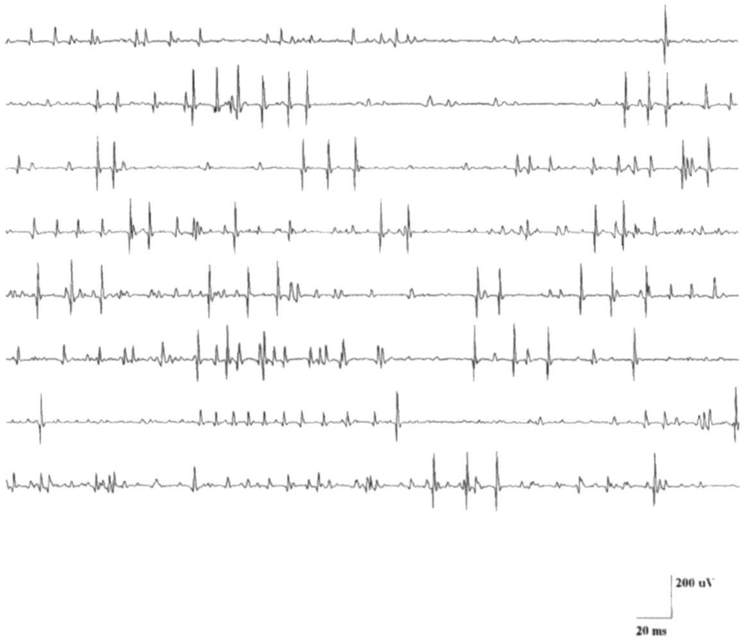

Figure 4. "Myokymic" fibrillations. Note the doublets and triplets and short rapid bursts of potentials.

"Myokymic" fibrillations were found in chronically partially denervated muscles, polymyositis and after chemotherapy. The duration of the bursts was short. There were also single fibrillation potentials, doublets and triplets and independent potentials from several different muscle fibres (Fig. 4). The bursts were spontaneous, not elicited by needle insertion. End plate spikes were found when the needle insertion hit an "active spot" of the muscle (Fig. 5-6). They were most readily found at the end plate zone, but they were not confined to it (Partanen, 1999). In several instances we could simultaneously record two unsynchronous foci of end plate spikes at completely different sites of a normal muscle.

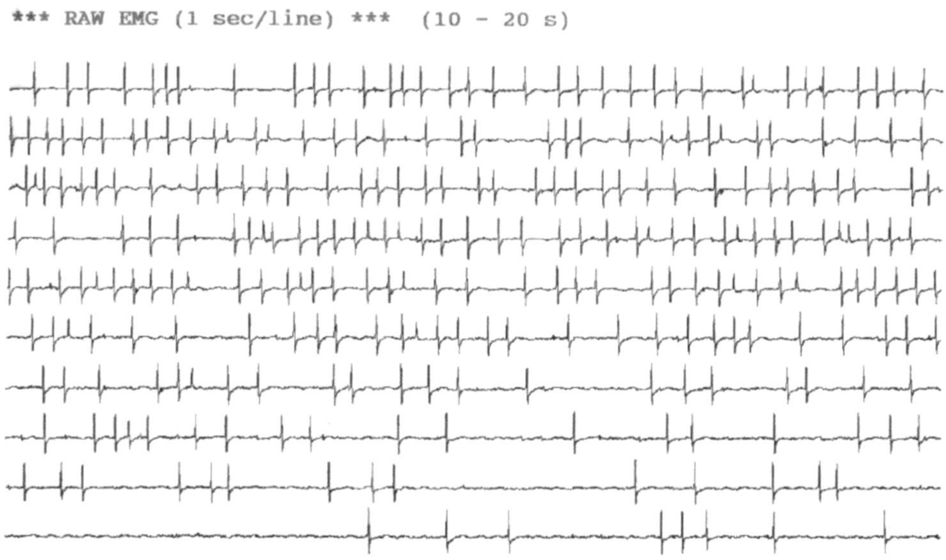

Figure 5. A sequence of end plate spikes. Observe the gradual slowing of the firing frequency.

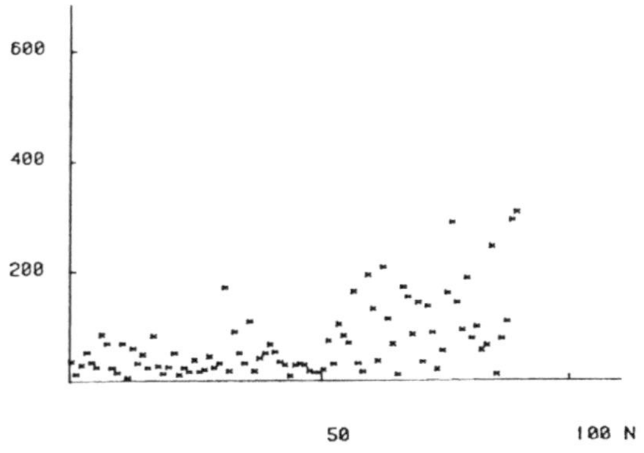

Figure 6. The firing pattern of a single sequence of end plate spikes (about 10 s, 78 intervals) recorded from the gastrocnemius muscle. Horizontal axis: number of successive intervals. Vertical axis: interpotential interval in ms. Note the variability in interpotential intervals, numerous short intervals and the gradual increase of the mean interval. APCID 176.4 ms, MCD 48.0 ms and the minimum and maximum intervals 9 ms and 292 ms, respectively. From Partanen, J. & Nousiainen, U. (1983), Author´s own work.

We also performed an analysis of the initial positivity on 39 different end plate spikes and 33 different fibrillation potentials. 14 out of the 39 end plate spikes had an initial positive deflection, with the mean duration 0.5 ms, SD 0.17, and range 0.3-0.9 ms. The rest had a negative onset. All 33 fibrillation potentials had an initial positive deflection, with mean duration 1.6 ms, SD 0.4, and range 0.6-2.4 ms. Thus, when an initial positive deflection was observed in end plate spikes, it was significantly (t= 9.9; p<0.001) shorter than that of fibrillation potentials. The 95 % confidence interval for difference was 0.8 to 1.2 ms.

Table 1 presents the mean characteristics in different fibrillation potential categories and the significance of difference of the variables compared to end plate spikes. Table 2 presents the differences between variables of different fibrillation categories.

	Fibrillations						**Neurally driven sequences**			
	Random		**With pauses**		**Regular**		**"Myokymic"**		**End plate spikes**	
N	41		13		13		12		15	
Intervals (ms)	mean	SE	mean	SE	mean	SE	mean	SE	mean	SE
mean	510***	43	223	37	556*	191	142	37	130	42
median	387***	37	209*	39	548*	190	104	30	95	31
minimum	159***	14	148***	25	513***	186	25*	5	12	3
maximum	1406***	127	412	49	637	199	736	204	578	163
					Regularity					
APCID	151	7	52*	6	5***	1	128*	14	175	13
MCD	358***	42	47	7	13*	5	111	36	116	42
					Potential					
Ampl (μV)	145	13	120	14	117	19	169	36	128	14
Spike duration (ms)	2.3	0.1	3.1	0.4	2.4	0.1	2.5	0.2	2.8	0.4

*** p ≤ 0.001

** p ≤ 0.01

* p ≤ 0.05 compared to end plate spikes

Table 1. Interval, regularity and potential variables of different spontaneous activity categories. "With pauses": slightly irregular fibrillation potentials with pauses.

	Random/With pauses	Random/Regular	With pauses/Regular
	Interval		
Min	NS	NS	NS
Max	***	**	NS
Mean	***	NS	NS
APCID	***	***	***
MCD	***	***	***
Amplitude	NS	NS	NS
Spike duration	NS	NS	NS

*** $p \leq 0.001$, ** $p \leq 0.01$, * $p \leq 0.05$

Table 2. The significance of differences between various fibrillation categories. "With pauses": slightly irregular fibrillation potentials with pauses.

4. Discussion

4.1. Firing patterns of fibrillation potentials

Denny-Brown & Pennybacker (1938) described the periodic contractions of denervated muscle fibres as true fibrillations and differentiated fibrillation from fasciculations and myokymia. Jasper & Ballem (1949) found positive sharp waves, often in combination with fibrillation potentials and claimed that they may represent local potentials set up at the needle point by the injury. They stated that positive sharp waves do not occur in a normal muscle. Kugelberg & Petersén (1949) also described positive sharp waves, "synchronized activity" in totally denervated muscles as well as fibrillation potentials of both constant frequency (regular fibrillations) and "repetitive fibrillary activity", i.e. slightly irregular fibrillations with pauses (see Results). It was claimed that only rhythmic, regular fibrillation potentials have clinical significance (Stöhr 1977). However, also irregular fibrillations do exist, and in fact there are several types of them. Irregular fibrillations do not usually change their firing pattern during the time of an EMG recording. The incidence of irregular fibrillations reported in literature is very variable. Heckmann & Ludin (1982) pointed out that even in totally denervated muscle irregularly firing potentials may be found (in canine muscle), and Buchthal & Rosenfalck (1966) stated that half of the fibrillation potentials whose discharge pattern was examined appeared irregular. In fact, the period of time after nerve or muscle injury seems to be essential. Approximately half of fibrillation sequences were irregular 30 days after muscle injury, while in more recent injuries the sequences were mainly regular (Partanen & Danner 1982). My experience in clinical ENMG work is that irregular fibrillations are most common 1 – 3 months after axonal injury and in extreme cases only a number of irregular fibrillation sequences may be present with no regular fibrillations at all (unpublished personal observation). There may also be mixed forms of fibrillations, with mainly regular rhythm but sudden changes of the interval (Partanen & Danner 1982, Conrad et al. 1972).

4.2. End plate spikes

Jasper and Ballem (1949) were the first to describe end plate spikes in clinical EMG: "Action potentials comparable to those described by Snodgrass and Sperry (mammalian muscle action potentials of less than a millisecond) were sometimes seen from limb muscles were thought to have been derived from nerve filaments since they were usually associated with particularly acute pain (as though the needle tip were penetrating a nerve) and were of the same form as those obtained when the needle was deliberately inserted in nerve". Kugelberg & Petersén (1949) described end plate spikes as "protracted irregular activity". "Such discharge was mostly irregular, might be ordinary motor unit potentials as in fasciculation or little amplitude and duration as in fibrillation. The activity in question cannot be voluntarily controlled. It does not disappear in relaxation, nor does it increase in frequency on slight voluntary contraction. A slight pressure or bending of the needle may increase the frequency while a discharge is going on, start new ones or reactivate potentials which had stopped".

Jones et al. (1955) further studied the origin of end plate spikes as "nerve potentials" with iron marks at sites of their appearance and found most of these iron dots close to peripheral intramuscular nerve twigs. Buchthal & Rosenfalck (1966) observed that miniature end plate potentials (MEPPS) were often associated with end plate spikes, "spontaneous diphasic potentials". They conjectured that these potentials originated in the muscle fibres, "several synchronized miniature potentials attaining an amplitude sufficient to elicit a propagated response". Finally, Brown & Varkey (1981) proved "nerve potentials" to be postsynaptic potentials, recorded from muscle fibres. End plate spikes show very irregular firing pattern with numerous short intervals less than 30 ms and gradual slowing of the firing (Partanen 1999).

The prevailing hypothesis concerning end plate spikes states that they are elicited by nerve irritation caused by the needle electrode and recorded postsynaptically by the same needle electrode (Brown & Varkey 1981). However, injury potentials of peripheral motor nerve fibres present a different firing pattern (Wall et al. 1974, Macefield 1998). Thus there is an obvious discrepancy between the sustained firing pattern of end plate spikes and experimentally observed real firing patterns of injured or irritated motor axons. Firing of end plate spikes differs also from abnormal firing patterns of motor nerve fibres or motor units (see Willison, 1982, Stålberg & Trontelj 1982). On the other hand, there is evidence that end plate spikes actually represent action potentials of intrafusal muscle fibres and beta motor units (Partanen & Nousiainen 1983, Partanen 1999, Partanen et al. 2010). The propagation patterns of intrafusal nuclear bag and nuclear chain muscle fibres (Barker at al. 1978) are similar to those of end plate spikes (Partanen & Palmu 2009, Partanen 2012).

4.3. Wave form of fibrillation potentials and end plate spikes

It was emphasized that end plate spikes, ("spontaneous diphasic potentials"), which have a negative onset at the end plate zone, may show positive onset phase as fibrillation potentials do when they are propagated outside the end plate zone and thus the form of the potential is indistinguishable from that of a fibrillation potential (Buchthal & Rosenfalck 1966). We note that there is a distinct difference between the wave forms of end plate spikes and fibrillation potentials. The former show either a negative onset or a short positive onset, whereas fibrillation potentials show a positive onset which always is longer than that of end plate spikes (see Results). However, the amplitude and spike duration of fibrillation potentials and end plate spikes are similar (Table 1). We have observed fibrillation potentials with negative onset, (mainly as "negative sharp waves", obviously cannula-recorded positive sharp waves with inverted polarity), but these are rare and do not happen to be present in the material collected for this work. This fact is not in concert with the data published earlier, which state that a considerable number of fibrillation potentials may have a negative onset (Buchthal & Rosenfalck 1966, Heckmann & Ludin 1982). In any case fibrillation potentials and end plate spikes may be distinguished both by the firing pattern and the wave form at the onset of the potential (Fig. 7).

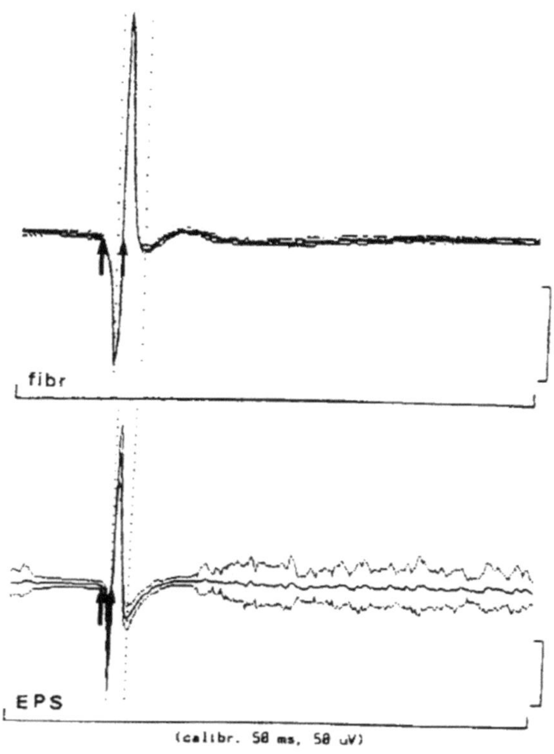

Figure 7. The positive deflection before the main spike component (pair of arrows) is shorter in averaged end plate spike (EPS) than in averaged fibrillation potential (fibr). The averaged mean potential is shown with ± 1 SD curves. From Partanen, J. (1999), Author´s own work.

The formation of the shape of end-plate spikes was extensively studied by Dumitru (2000) according to the needle irritation hypothesis of peripheral nerve branch or nerve terminal (tip or shaft irritation of the terminal nerve). He explained the formation of biphasic and triphasic form of an end plate spike and considered that triphasic end plate spikes are rather common. However, he could not differentiate the shape of triphasic end plate spikes from that of triphasic fibrillation potentials. The spreading of an ectopic nerve irritation potential to the other nerve branches of the motor unit was not considered. Ectopic nerve action potential will spread to both directions from its place of origin, and thus a motor unit or fasciculation potential should be formed instead of an end plate spike. Dumitru (2000) also describes the formation of "atypical" biphasic/monophasic end plate spike configuration (resembling positive sharp waves). First, the electrode may completely compress the muscle fibre, preventing action potential propagation past the electrode ("sealed end effect"). Second, a "compressed end" may occur; following crushing or compression of tissue, the membrane retains no functional sodium channels and, therefore, can only sustain a passive current flow, but not an active current flow. However, Pickett & Schmidley (1980) explained end plate spikes with positive sharp wave form, "sputtering positive potentials" elegantly. These potentials represented cannula-recorded potentials of the concentric needle electrode and changed their form from positive waves to usual end plate spikes when the electrode was withdrawn. Sputtering positive potentials could not be recorded with a monopolar needle electrode.

4.4. Origin of regular and irregular fibrillation potentials

Based on the pattern of discharges, two classes of spontaneously active fibres were found in experimental study of rat diaphragm: rhythmically discharging fibres, and fibres in which action potentials occur at irregular intervals (Purves & Sakmann 1974). The majority of the sites of origin in both regular and irregular fibres were at the former end plate zone; however, there was no region along the length that could not be a site of origin. Regularly occurring action potentials were associated with oscillations of the membrane potential. Irregularly discharging fibres were brought to threshold by discrete non-propagated depolarizations called fibrillatory origin potentials (f.o.p.s.) (Purves & Sakmann 1974). F.o.p.s. are generated at the T-tubuli, since detubulation with glycerol abolishes the spontaneous activity (Smith & Thesleff 1976). Thus, the integrity of the transverse tubular system is a prerequisite for the presence of irregular spontaneous activity. It was also observed, that these discrete depolarizations are caused by regenerative increase in the Na conductance of the membrane, similar to that associated with the normal action potential (Purves & Sakmann 1974, Smith & Thesleff 1976).

We may presume that in humans, fibrillations with regular rhythm also derive from the membrane potential oscillations of denervated muscle fibres (Thesleff 1982a) or the denervated part of a muscle fibre, as in muscular injury (Partanen & Danner 1982). Irregular fibrillations are accordingly caused by f.o.p.s reaching the firing threshold of an action potential. Immediately after a f.o.p. there is a period during which the probability of a second f.o.p. occurring is very low (Purves & Sakmann 1974). In denervated muscle fibres there are newly synthesized potassium channels, and they produce a longer duration of the hyperpolarization of the intracellular action potential compared to normal tissue. This hyperpolarization may last up to 100 ms and more (Thesleff 1982a, Dumitru 2000). Thus the refractory period after which a second action potential may occur is increased in denervated muscle fibres, compared to normal muscle fibres. Thus slightly irregular fibrillations with pauses may be fired by a muscle fibre eliciting a large number of f.o.p.s., which mainly reactivate the fibre immediately after the refractory period of a spontaneous potential. An occasional failure of a f.o.p. to occur may be seen as a pause in the fibrillation sequence. We have rarely observed a slightly irregular fibrillation sequence even without pauses, evidently representing a muscle fibre with a large number of f.o.p.s. On the other hand, random fibrillations may be associated with very infrequently occurring f.o.p.s. In any case, regular fibrillations are the first to be present also in experimental studies and irregular fibrillations arise later on (Purves & Sakmann 1974, Smith & Thesleff 1976).

4.5. "Myokymic" fibrillations

"Myokymic" fibrillations have not been categorized as an entity of its own earlier. They may be distinguished from true myokymia by the single fibre potential pattern. True myokymia exhibits a motor unit potential pattern, and was not studied in the present work. The high firing frequency of "myokymic" fibrillations shows that these potentials are not elicited by denervated muscle fibres with a prolonged refractory period. We attribute these potentials to spontaneous large acetylcholine release (giant or slow-rising MEPPs) to the synaptic cleft. This type of transmitter release may occur spontaneously in regenerating nerve terminals or after botulin toxin injection or application of 4-aminoquinoline, without any motor nerve action potential and depolarization of the motor nerve terminal (Thesleff 1982b, Sellin et al. 1996). Evidently large spontaneous transmitter release may cause a short burst of postsynaptic potentials of a single muscle fibre, recorded as "myokymic" fibrillations. It is conceivable that no antidromic spreading of the potential to the rest of motor unit takes place without depolarization of the nerve terminal, as in peripherally originating fasciculation potentials (see Stålberg & Trontelj 1982).

"Myokymic" fibrillations and end plate spikes can be distinguished by their firing pattern. "Myokymic" fibrillations fire in short high-frequency bursts, doublets and triplets and they may be found at any region in the muscle. Needle insertion does not activate them. End plate spikes show sustained firing with a very irregular rhythm with numerous short but also long intervals, and the mean interval lengthens if the needle is not moved. End plate spikes are found in the active spots of the muscle being studied, often associated with miniature end plate potentials and pain (Wiederholt 1970).

5. Comments

It is of utmost importance that a clinical neurophysiologist performing ENMG studies recognizes different types of spontaneous activity. Confusing end plate spikes with fibrillation potentials may cause false positive findings of axonal damage. Even the difference between rhythmic and irregular fibrillation potentials may be difficult to grasp and there are differences between individual examiners in this respect (Trillenberg & Spencer 2010). False classification of potentials is a frequent error, especially among resident-level examiners (Kendall & Werner 2006). We studied parameters by which it could be possible to distinguish between different types of fibrillation potentials: rhythmic, random, and slightly irregular fibrillations with pauses, "myokymic" fibrillations, and end plate spikes. The most effective differentiating variables in this respect proved to be the minimum interval, APCID and MCD. Interval analysis of the activity of a single motor unit also shows an entirely different discharge pattern compared to spontaneous potentials (Conrad et al. 1972). The functionality to calculate these variables for sequences of spontaneous EMG potentials should be included in future ENMG devices. The lack of tools for editing and interval analysis of EMG potential sequences can be considered to be a major shortcoming in the present ENMG machines.

Author details

Juhani Partanen*

University Hospital of Helsinki, Department of Clinical Neurophysiology, Helsinki, Finland

References

[1] Barker, D, Bessou, P, Jankowska, E, Pagès, B, & Stacey, M. J. (1978). Identification of intrafusal muscle fibres activated by single fusimotor axons and injected with fluorescent dye in cat tenuissimus spindles. *J Physiol*, , 275, 149-165.

[2] Brown, W. F, & Varkey, G. P. (1981). The origin of spontaneous electrical activity at the end-plate zone. *Ann Neurol*, , 10, 557-560.

[3] Buchthal, F, & Rosenfalck, P. (1966). Spontaneous electrical activity of human muscle. *Electroenceph Clin Neurophysiol*, , 20, 321-336.

[4] Conrad, B, Sindermann, F, & Prochazka, V. J. (1972). Interval analysis of repetitive denervation potentials of human skeletal muscle. *J Neurol Neurosurg Psychiat*, , 35, 834-840.

[5] Denny-brown, D, & Pennybacker, J. B. (1938). Fibrillation and fascicultation in voluntary muscle. *Brain*, , 61, 311-334.

[6] Dumitru, D. (2000). Physiologic basis of potentials recorded in electromyography. *Muscle & Nerve*, , 23, 1667-1685.

[7] Heckmann, R, & Ludin, H. P. (1982). Differentiation of spontaneous activity from normal and denervated skeletal muscle. *J Neurol Neurosurg Psychiat*, , 45, 331-336.

[8] Jasper, H, & Ballem, G. (1949). Unipolar electromyograms of normal and denervated muscle. *J Neurophysiol*, , 12, 231-244.

[9] Jones, R. V, Lambert, E. H, & Sayre, G. P. (1955). Source of a type of "insertion activity" in electromyography with evaluation of a histologic method of localization. *Arch Phys Med*, , 36, 301-310.

[10] Kendall, R, & Werner, R. A. (2006). Interrater reliability of the needle examination in lumbosacral radiculopathy. *Muscle & Nerve*, , 34, 238-241.

[11] Kugelberg, E, & Petersén, I. (1949). Insertion activity" in electromyography. *J Neurol Neurosurg Psychiat*, , 12, 268-273.

[12] Macefield, V. G. (1998). Spontaneous and evoked ectopic discharges recorded from single human axons. *Muscle & Nerve*, , 21, 461-468.

[13] Partanen, J. V, & Danner, R. (1982). Fibrillation potentials after muscle injury in humans. *Muscle & Nerve*, , 5, S70-S73.

[14] Partanen, J. V, & Nousiainen, U. (1983). End-plate spikes in electromyography are fusimotor unit potentials. *Neurology*, Cleveland, 33, 1039-1043.

[15] Partanen, J. (1999). End plate spikes in the human electromyogram. Revision of the fusimotor theory. *J Physiol (Paris)*, , 93, 155-166.

[16] Partanen, J. V, & Palmu, K. (2009). Different ways of propagation of human end plate spikes in electromyography. *Muscle & Nerve*, , 40, 720-721.

[17] Partanen, J. V, Ojala, T. A, & Arokoski, J. (2010). Myofascial syndrome and pain: A neurophysiological approach. *Pathophysiology*, , 17, 19-28.

[18] Partanen, J. (2011). Electromyography in myofascial syndrome. In Schwartz M (ed): EMG methods for evaluating muscle and nerve function. Intech Open, 2011 www.intechopen.com,, 55-64.

[19] Pickett, J. B, & Schmidley, J. W. Sputtering positive potentials in the EMG: An artefact resembling positive waves. *Neurology*, , 30, 215-218.

[20] Purves, D, & Sakmann, B. (1974). Membrane properties underlying spontaneous activity of denervated muscle fibres. *J Physiol*, , 239, 125-153.

[21] Sellin, L. C, Molgó, J, Törnquist, K, Hansson, B, & Thesleff, S. (1996). On the possible origin of "giant or slow-rising" miniature end-plate potentials at the neuromuscular junction. *Pflügers Arch- Eur J Physiol*, , 431, 325-334.

[22] Smith, J. W, & Thesleff, S. (1976). Spontaneous activity in denervated mouse diaphragm muscle. *J Physiol*, , 257, 171-186.

[23] Stöhr, M. (1977). Benign fibrillation potentials in normal muscle and their correlation with endplate and denervation potentials. *J Neurol Neurosurg Psychiat*, , 40, 765-768.

[24] Stålberg, E, Ekstedt, J, & Broman, A. (1971). The electromyographic jitter in normal human muscles. *Electroenceph Clin Neurophysiol*, , 31, 429-438.

[25] Stålberg E & Trontelj JV(1982). Abnormal discharges generated within the motor unit as observed with single-fiber electromyography. In: *Abnormal nerves and muscles as impulse generators,* Culp, W. J. & Ochoa, J. Oxford University Press, New York, 443-474.

[26] Thesleff, S. (1982a). Fibrillation in denervated mammalian muscle. In: *Abnormal nerves and muscles as impulse generators,* Culp, W. J. & Ochoa, J. Oxford University Press, New York, 678-694.

[27] Thesleff, S. (1982b). Spontaneous transmitter release in experimental neuromuscular disorders of the rat. *Muscle & Nerve,* , 5, S12-S16.

[28] Trillenberg, P, & Spencer, A. (2010). How precisely can the regularity of spontaneous activity be recognized acoustically? *Clin Neurophysiol,* , 121, 1969-1971.

[29] Usui, S, & Admiror, I. (1982). Digital low-pass differentiation for biological signal processing. *IEEE Trans Biomed Eng,* , 29, 686-693.

[30] Wall, P. D, Waxman, S, & Basbaum, A. I. (1974). Ongoing activity in peripheral nerve: injury discharge. *Exp Neurol,* , 45, 576-589.

[31] Wiederholt, W. C. (1970). End-plate noise" in electromyography. *Neurology,* , 20, 214-224.

[32] Willison, R. G. (1982). Spontaneous discharges in motor nerve fibers. In: *Abnormal nerves and muscles as impulse generators,* Culp, W. J. & Ochoa, J. Oxford University Press, New York, 383-392.

Chapter 4

Experimental and Simulated EMG Responses in the Study of the Human Spinal Cord

Rinaldo André Mezzarane, Leonardo Abdala Elias,
Fernando Henrique Magalhães,
Vitor Martins Chaud and André Fabio Kohn

Additional information is available at the end of the chapter

http://dx.doi.org/10.5772/54870

1. Introduction

Advances in the study of human spinal cord neurophysiology have been strongly based on the analysis of the electrical activity of muscles (electromyogram - EMG). The EMG measured over the skin reflects the general behavior of motor units (MUs) and hence of spinal motoneurons (MNs). It can be used, for instance, to infer changes in the behavior of neuronal circuits within the spinal cord during the performance of a motor task or in response to peripheral and/or descending inputs.

In the beginning of the 20th century, Paul Hoffmann introduced a non-invasive technique – the H-reflex – that helped to pave the way for subsequent investigations into the mechanisms of stretch reflex regulation [1]. The neuronal organization of the spinal cord is now better understood thanks to studies of reflex modulation in response to different conditionings and motor contexts, e.g., electrical or mechanical stimulation of sensory afferent pathways, magnetic or electric activation of descending tracts (DTs), passive movement of limbs and joints, voluntary isometric contractions and performance of motor tasks.

Reflexes play a fundamental functional role in motor control, as they are involved in the coordination of voluntary movements and maintenance of postural stability. This justifies the high contingent of fibers from peripheral (cutaneous, muscle and joint afferents), segmental (propriospinal interneurons), and supra-segmental (descending tracts) origins that synapse on different spinal cord elements (synaptic terminals, interneurons and MNs). This also highlights the important integrative function of the spinal cord, contrasting with the naive notion that it is only a relay station, or a pathway that simply transfers information from the brain to the muscle fibers.

Despite the relative limitations of non-invasive techniques employed in humans, it is currently possible to establish a parallel between the findings from animal preparations (such as cat) and experiments in humans (e.g., [2, 3]). In addition to the use of animal models as aids for understanding human data, another source of information comes from new multi-scale computer simulators of neuronal circuitry and muscle control [4, 5]. Moreover, with the development of these simulators, supported by anatomical and biophysical data from animal experiments, it is also possible to reinforce hypotheses formulated to explain experimental results obtained from humans (e.g., [5]).

The aim of the present chapter is to provide some conceptual and methodological background for researchers and clinicians who intend to use EMG to study human spinal cord neurophysiology. Here we will discuss different methods frequently used in the study of human neurophysiology based on surface EMG. These will be illustrated by results from both experimental studies and simulations performed in a multi-scale model of the spinal cord and leg muscles. Additionally, a brief account will be given of some processing techniques of surface EMG that are used to quantify spinal cord excitability and effects of inhibitory pathways. The methods explored in the chapter have been used in both healthy subjects and patients with a variety of neuromuscular disorders.

2. Brief review and basic methodological considerations

This brief review presents a few basic concepts related to electrical muscle activity recorded with electrodes over the skin. Methodological aspects that might influence the interpretation of experimental results are discussed. Further details concerning these basic aspects can be found elsewhere [6, 7].

2.1. Some important definitions

In the preceding section we have referred to EMG as the electrical muscle activity recorded with surface electrodes. This electrical activity is the result of the depolarization of a number of muscle fibers. A group of muscle fibers innervated by the same spinal cord MN is called a muscle unit while the MN and the muscle unit it innervates is the motor unit (MU). During voluntary muscle activation, the number of recruited muscle fibers contributing to the EMG depends on the net excitatory drive from the brain and peripheral sensory afferents arriving onto the spinal MNs. During a mild voluntary contraction only a small fraction of MUs is recruited. As the excitatory command is increased, two distinct mechanisms take place: the MUs previously recruited increase their firing rate (rate coding) and new MUs with higher firing threshold are recruited (population coding). These basics may be found in many references, such as [8].

The activity of a single MU is easily recorded with needle electrodes inserted into the muscle (the most common is the concentric needle electrode). However, during low-intensity contraction, surface electrodes can also record activity of superficial MUs [9] as can be seen in the upper trace in Figure 1. For increased levels of voluntary contraction additional MUs are recruited (see middle trace in Figure 1). For high-intensity contraction the EMG recording tends to show a filled random pattern due to the superposition of a greater number of MU action potentials (MUAPs) known as interference pattern (bottom trace in Figure 1). Thus, the interference pattern of the EMG is associated with the asynchronous firing of different MUs. When the conditioning of an interference pattern EMG is used to infer spinal cord processes, the experimental control of the level of activity is crucial. When the strength of descending commands changes, different populations of MNs and interneurons (INs) are recruited, leading to different conditioned EMG responses.

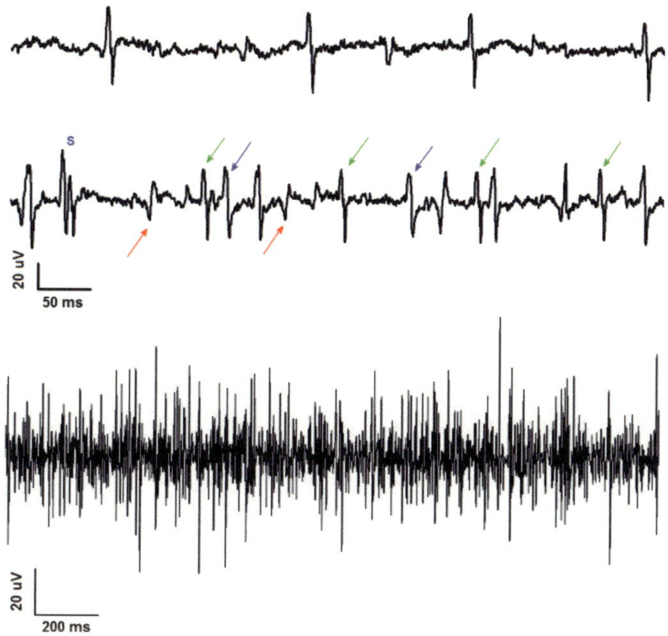

Figure 1. Surface EMG recordings from soleus (SO) muscle during a weak contraction (unpublished data). Upper panel: EMG recording during a very weak contraction in which only one MU is recruited. Middle panel: when the subject was told to slightly increase the voluntary contraction, the MU previously recruited increased its firing rate (see the green arrows) and other MUs with different firing rates were recruited (red and blue arrows). The letter "S" indicates a sum of at least two distinct MUAPs. Lower panel: Interference pattern of EMG.

2.2. Acquisition

Some technical aspects need to be considered for an accurate recording of the EMG signal. Here we are going to briefly discuss filtering, sampling rate and electrode positioning.

The spectral composition of a signal has implications on the choice of the band-pass filter cutoff frequencies used before the analog-to-digital conversion as well as for the selection of a suitable sampling frequency (SF). Figure 2 shows the power spectrum of an EMG recorded with surface (upper panel) and needle (lower panel) electrodes during a sustained contraction. It is interesting to note the dramatic difference in the spectra of both recordings (note the different calibrations of the abscissa). For the surface EMG, band-pass filter cutoff frequencies from 10Hz to 500Hz would be appropriate and a SF of at least 1kHz would be used; however, in the second example, the 500Hz cutoff frequency (see the red area in the lower panel of Figure 2) would be clearly inappropriate due to the significant contributions of high-frequency spectral components of the signal. Therefore, when using needle EMG, the high-frequency cutoff should be higher, e.g., 5kHz-10kHz and sampling done at 20kHz-40kHz.

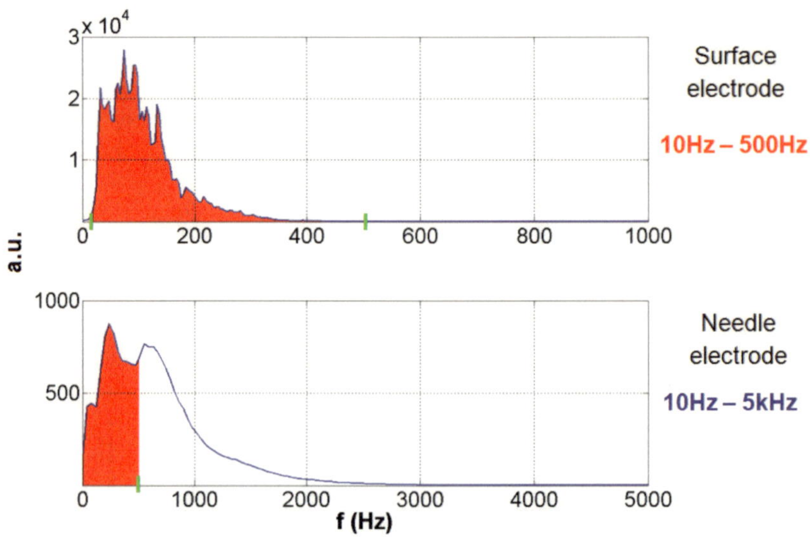

Figure 2. Power spectra of EMG signals from the SO muscle recorded with surface (upper panel) and needle (lower panel) electrodes (unpublished data). They show the frequency content (in Hz) of each signal. The green marks in the abscissa (small vertical lines) comprise the frequencies of the band-pass filter used for surface EMG. The corresponding frequency ranges are indicated in red (upper panel) and in blue (lower panel) for surface and needle recordings, respectively. It is clear in the lower panel that if we used the same frequency range of surface EMG for needle EMG a considerable amount of information would be lost (see the red area delimited by the green marks).

The choice of a suitable frequency range for the band-pass filter to be applied to the surface EMG signal needs to be done with caution according to the objectives of the study. A wrong choice of filter parameters may cause information loss and misleading interpretations of the results. For instance, if the focus is to investigate slow variations of the surface EMG signal during stepping or gait (e.g., EMG envelope), a frequency band of 10-300Hz could be adequate [10]. However, using the same recording technique to evaluate reflex components (e.g., H-reflex), the high cutoff frequency should be raised to 1kHz (with a SF of at least 2kHz) for better reproduction of the phasic EMG signal generated [10].

Generally, in surface EMG, the electrodes are located on the skin above the belly of the muscle of interest, in a region between the tendon and the innervation zone [11]. The electric currents generated by depolarization of the muscle fibers travel through the connective tissues, fat, vessels, skin (all of which comprises the volume conductor), reaching the region underneath the electrodes. The volume conductor has the property of a low-pass filter [12] and the signals reach the electrodes placed over the skin with a slower time course and decreased amplitude. On the other hand, a needle electrode is much closer to the source of the electrical activity than a surface electrode and hence it does not suffer the low-pass filtering and amplitude attenuation caused by volume conduction [6, 12]. This explains why the needle EMG signals have better signal-to-noise ratios and why their power spectra have components at higher frequencies (see the lower panel in Figure 2).

The main advantage of invasive techniques such as needle or wire EMG is its high selectivity (one or very few MUs can be recorded with a high signal-to-noise ratio). Conversely, this may be a disadvantage when the purpose is to evaluate a larger number of MUs to obtain a more comprehensive view of muscle activation. In this case, surface EMG is more indicated. The main shortcomings of surface EMG are that (1) not all muscles are superficial and (2) the possibility of interference from nearby muscles' electrical activities on the EMG signal recorded from the desired muscle. These recorded interferences are attenuated or perhaps distorted versions of the electrical activities from the nearby muscles and are known as crosstalk [13, 14]. The crosstalk effect can sometimes be minimized by a careful placement of the electrodes.

The distance between electrodes is a key factor to increase or decrease the relative selectivity of the EMG recording. Figure 3 shows an example in which the EMG activity is recorded with an array of three electrodes. When the potential difference is calculated between the more distant pair of electrodes (E1 – E3) the recording is less selective than when the electrodes are closer to each other (E1 – E2).

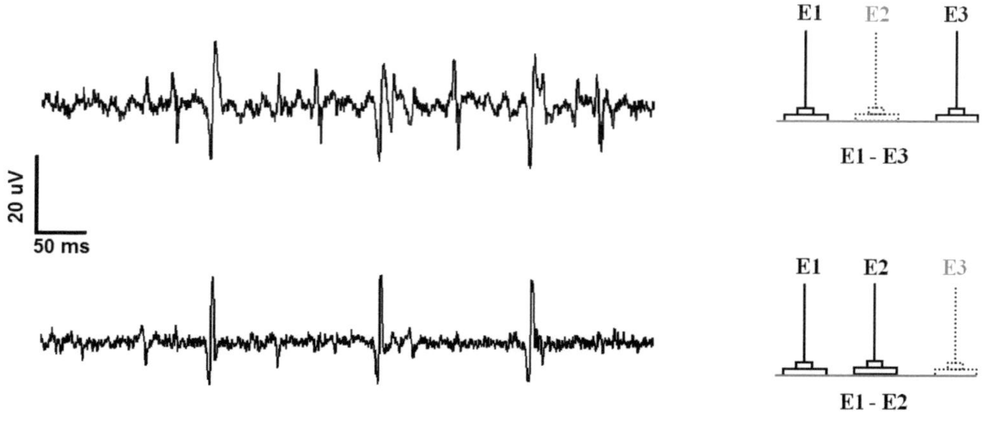

Figure 3. Surface EMG showing the effect of the distance between electrodes (unpublished data). Upper panel: EMG recorded with a distance of 2.5cm between electrodes (E1-E3). The lower panel shows the same recording with inter-electrode distance of 1cm (E1-E2).

3. Conditioning of the constant ("asynchronous") muscle activity

The EMG interference pattern is useful to help understanding the conditioning effects coming from a variety of sources. These conditionings fundamentally act on the modulation of muscle activity and are context-dependent [15]. Therefore, it is possible to study the effects of a variety of inhibitory and excitatory pathways on MNs by means of EMG signal conditioning, and hence extract information on spinal cord neurophysiology.

The voluntary activity of the SO muscle (sustained low-level isometric contraction) can be modulated by the activation of the primary (Ia) afferents from the antagonist muscle spindles [15, 16]. The diagram depicted in Figure 4 shows surface transcutaneous electrical stimulation (1ms rectangular pulse) applied to the common peroneal nerve (CPN) that supplies the tibialis anterior (TA) muscle. The conditioning stimulus substantially reduces the SO muscle activity via reciprocal inhibition (RI) [16]. A typical example of the resulting EMG signals is shown in Figure 5.

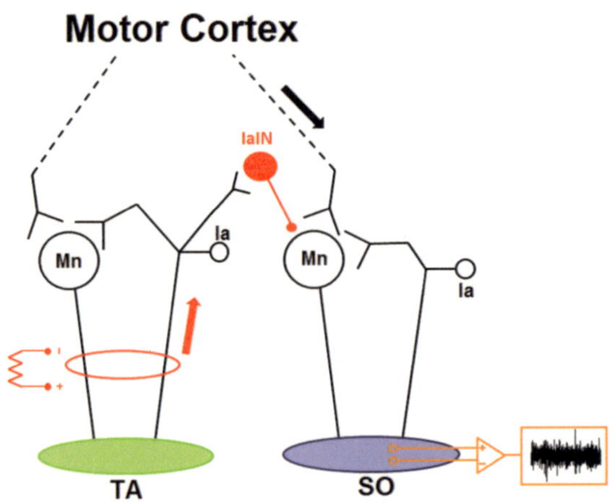

Figure 4. Schematic showing the pathway of reciprocal inhibition (RI). The black arrow indicates the descending drive from the motor cortex to the SO muscle that generates the interference pattern shown in the oscilloscope (small rectangle in orange color). The EMG activity can be conditioned by an electrical stimulus applied to the nerve that supplies the antagonist muscle (TA). The action potentials in the Ia afferents (red arrow) activate the inhibitory Ia IN (IaIN) that generates an inhibitory post-synaptic potential (IPSP) in the membrane of the MN. Hence, after the conditioning electrical stimulus, some MNs will stop firing and the EMG interference pattern will show a transitory decrease in the amplitude (see also Figure 5).

Looking at one or a few sweeps of conditioned-EMG signals (left panel of Figure 5), it is not possible to determine if the inhibition is present. Note that the low voluntary muscle activity produced a very sparse MU firing in the recordings (upper traces) shown on the left panel of Figure 5. When the sweeps (a total of 50) are superimposed (lowermost signal at the left panel of Figure 5), the inhibition becomes clear (see the red horizontal bar below). Thus, several tenths (or even hundreds) of stimuli are necessary to allow the detection/quantification of the effect of RI on the SO MNs [1]. However, to quantify the amount of inhibition, additional signal processing of the EMG signal is needed: (1) subtraction of the DC level, (2) computation of the absolute value of each EMG sample, also called EMG rectification, (3) computation of the ensemble average of the several rectified conditioned-EMG signals (or sweeps). The number of sweeps to be averaged depends on the strength of the conditioning effect and the level of voluntary muscle contraction [16]. These procedures will be illustrated based on the superimposed sweeps shown at the right uppermost panel of Figure 5. The results of step (2) above are shown in the middle panel at the right of Figure 5. The bottommost trace of the right panel of Figure 5 is the ensemble average of the traces displayed just above it (step 3).

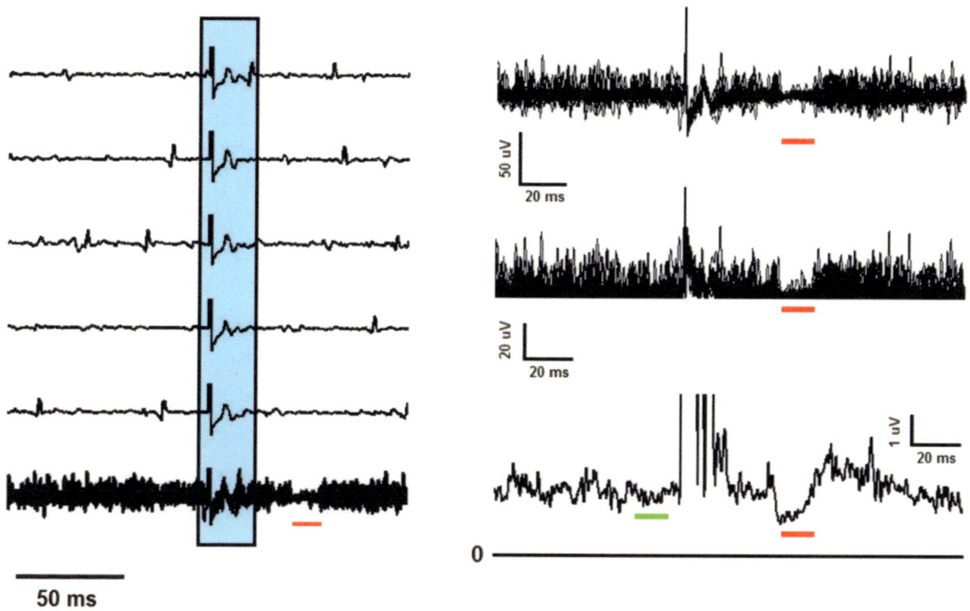

Figure 5. Left panel: EMG recordings of the SO showing the muscle activity before and after the delivery of an electrical stimulus to the CPN nerve (unpublished data). The traces show sparse MU firings. The rectangle in blue encompasses the stimulus artifact followed by a crosstalked activity from the antagonist (TA) muscle. An interesting observation is that the inhibition is not quite clear by the examination of a single recording. The bottom trace shows all the 50 recordings superimposed. A clear reduction in muscle activity ~40ms after the electrical stimulation is indicated by a red bar. Right panel: same traces superimposed (upper trace). All the EMG recordings were rectified (superimposed traces in the middle) and averaged (bottom trace). The red bar indicates the reduction in muscle activity due to RI induced by the procedure depicted in the schematic of Figure 4.

The inhibitory period indicated by the red bar under the averaged trace of Figure 5 can then be quantified either by the peak (lowest point of the recording), the mean or the RMS [7] and normalized with respect to a similar computation of the pre-stimulus period (green bar). In an alternative approach, RMS values in each sweep at the right-top corresponding to the time windows defined by the green (control) and red (inhibited) bars are computed and averaged. This yields a mean RMS value in the control period and a mean RMS value in the time interval associated with the effect of the RI. To allow comparisons between subjects one may adopt the ratio of the latter to the former as an index of the level of RI.

Besides changing the excitability of MNs, pathways converging to the spinal cord may also affect the excitability of several spinal cord elements by acting on presynaptic terminals (e.g., the Ia-MN synapse). Presynaptic effects will be discussed later.

4. Conditioning of the evoked phasic ("synchronous") muscle activity

So far, we have discussed the case of asynchronous voluntary activity of MUs that generates the EMG interference pattern. Another way to assess spinal cord processes is by means of reflex-generated compound muscle action potentials (CMAP).

A variety of reflexes (stretch reflex, cutaneous reflex, H-reflex, etc) has been studied at rest, during locomotion and during the performance of a number of motor tasks in an attempt to better understand how the central nervous system (CNS) integrates the descending signals with those coming from the periphery [1]. Ascending signals from the periphery are incorporated into motor plans in order to continuously update the CNS and generate suitable commands to muscles that will work in concert to produce a functionally relevant motor output. At the spinal cord level, the afferent influx coming from muscles, joints and skin help to sculpt motor behavior by playing a significant role in the modulation of the excitability of different reflex pathways [1].

The stretch reflex pathway is one of special interest and will be the focus of this topic. The excitability of this pathway (or parts of it) can be assessed by means of either electrical stimulation of peripheral nerve (H-reflex, F-wave and V-wave) or mechanical stimulation of the tendon (T-reflex). In what follows we will discuss the methodology of these techniques as well as their modulation in response to a variety of conditionings.

4.1. The H-reflex

The H-reflex was first described in 1918 by Paul Hoffmann [17] and is the electrical homologous of the stretch reflex. It is elicited by a transcutaneous electrical stimulation (rectangular pulse with 1ms duration) applied to a mixed nerve that synchronously activates afferent fibers from muscle spindles (see the arrow showing the orthodromic sensory activation in Figure 6). The evoked afferent volley generates excitatory post-synaptic potentials (EPSPs) in α-MNs (hereafter referred to as MNs) that may fire action potentials if they surpass the firing threshold. These EPSPs seem to be generated mainly by the monosynaptic Ia-MN excitatory pathway but they are also influenced by oligosynaptic pathways [18]. The action potentials originating from the MNs lead to the generation of a CMAP recorded with surface EMG electrodes at the homonymous muscle. The evoked CMAP is termed H-reflex and is different from the interference pattern of EMG described in the preceding text (see sections 2 and 3), which is characterized by the asynchronous firing of MUs. The technique of H-reflex has been widely used to assess the excitability of the stretch reflex pathway and infer spinal cord mechanisms contributing towards motor control [1, 19]. In the lower limbs, the SO muscle has often been used because its electrically-elicited reflex response is relatively easy to obtain.The muscle afferents of group I (Ia and Ib) and II are also depicted in the schematic of Figure 6. However, for low intensity stimulation, group I muscle afferents (mainly Ia) are primarily activated [20].

The presence of a stable M-wave (direct motor response, see below) is desired in most studies to assure (by indirect means) a constant stimulation (see the arrow showing the orthodromic motor activation in Figure 6). Thus, any changes in H-reflex amplitude would be related to neurophysiological factors and not to alterations in stimulus efficacy, which would change the M-wave as well [21].

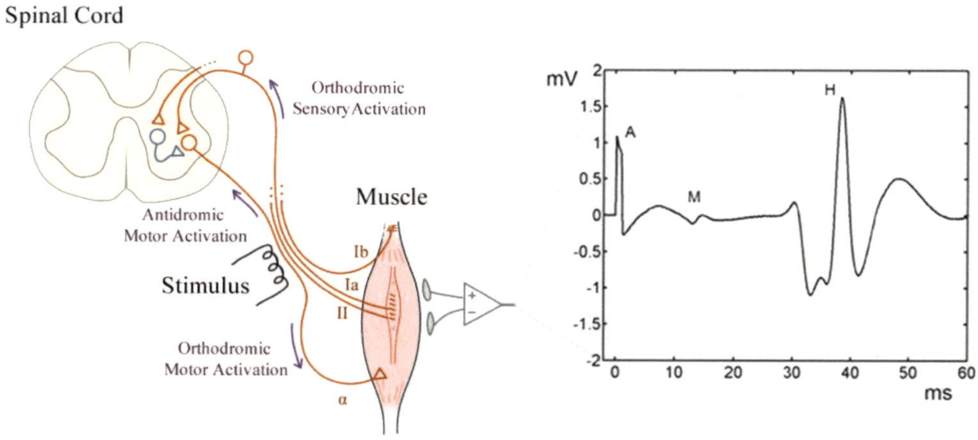

Figure 6. Schematic of the stretch reflex pathway and the mixed nerve stimulation that generates orthodromic and antidromic nerve activity (only the monosynaptic pathway from the Ia is shown). EMG trace showing an H-reflex and M-wave elicited by a transcutaneous electrical stimulus (1ms duration) applied through electrodes located over the skin at the popliteal fossa. The stimulus activates Ia afferent and motor axons from the mixed nerve (PTN) that supplies the SO muscle. The resulting H-reflex and M-wave are recorded with surface electrodes (see the schematic on the left). **A**: Stimulus artifact indicating when the stimulus was delivered; **M**: M-wave; **H**: H-reflex.

4.1.1. *Recruitment order of reflexively activated motoneurons*

With the increase of the stimulus intensity, a larger number of Ia afferents are activated leading to reflex recruitment of more MNs. The MNs in the spinal cord are synaptically recruited according to the size principle [22], i.e., the small size MUs (with low threshold for synaptic input) are recruited first. Therefore, H-reflexes of low amplitude reflect the activation of small MUs (see Figure 7). Higher amplitudes of H-reflex correspond to the activation of intermediated sized MUs along with the small ones. The increment in H-reflex amplitude reaches a limit that is not only related to the number of MNs within the pool, but also to the phenomenon of "annihilation", i.e., action potentials in the efferent axon generated reflexively collide with the antidromic volley due to the firing of the distal part of the efferent axon by the electrical stimulus (Figure 8). Therefore, those motor axons that were activated by the transcutaneous electrical stimulation generate antidromic spikes (shown in Figure 6 as the "antidromic motor activation") that prevent the action potentials of reflex origin from reaching the muscle (see Figure 8). As the axonal conduction velocity of efferents is lower than the afferents, there is enough time for the collision to take place in the efferent axons. The action potentials generated in the efferent axons also propagate toward the muscle (orthodromic motor activation in Figure 6 and red arrows in Figure 8) and will generate a shorter latency response (M-wave). The stimulus intensity that generates the lowest amplitude M-wave is termed motor threshold (MT). The direct motor response (M-wave) increases monotonically with stimulus intensity until its maximum (M_{MAX}), as there is no annihilation in the distal part of the motor axons (distal to the stimulation point; see Figure 8). A supramaximal stimulus intensity will discharge 100% of the efferent axons, yielding the M_{MAX} and blocking the generation of any H-reflex response due to the antidromic motor volley (see Figure 7).

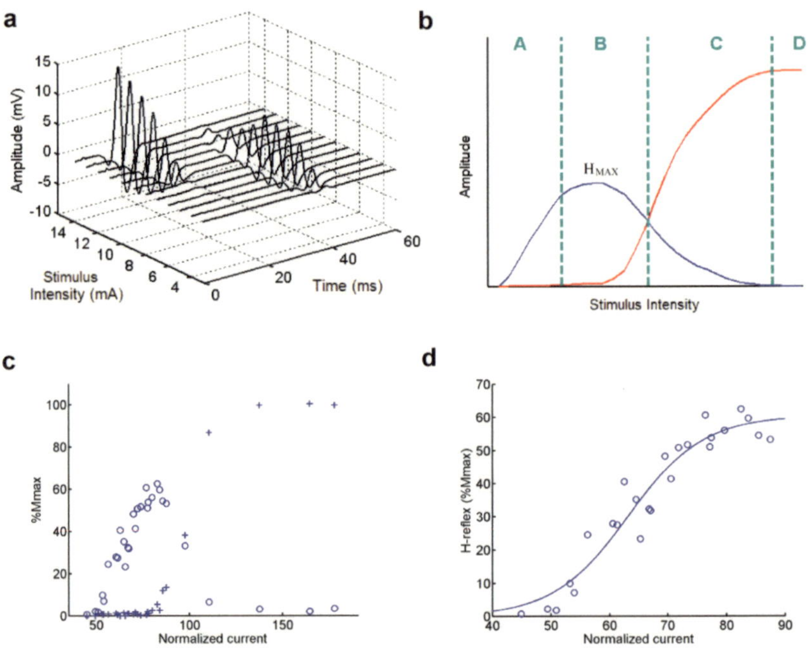

Figure 7. a) EMG traces recorded from the SO muscle showing changes in H-reflex and M-wave amplitudes as a function of stimulus intensity (unpublished data). Note the extinction of the H-reflex when the M_{MAX} is present in the recording (under the maximal stimulus intensity). **b)** Schematic recruitment curve with the peak-to-peak values of H-reflexes (blue) and M-waves (red) along the stimulus intensity. The regions A-D delimited by the green dashed vertical lines contain, respectively: the ascending limb of recruitment curve; motor threshold and H_{MAX}; descending limb of the curve; M_{MAX}. **c)** Recruitment curve obtained from the SO muscle of one representative subject. Data based on [10]. The circles and crosses represent the peak-to-peak amplitude values of the H-reflex and M-wave, respectively. **d)** Same data from **c** showing a sigmoidal fit to the ascending limb of the H-reflex recruitment curve. Data based on [9], but figures are unpublished.

http://dx.doi.org/10.5772/54870

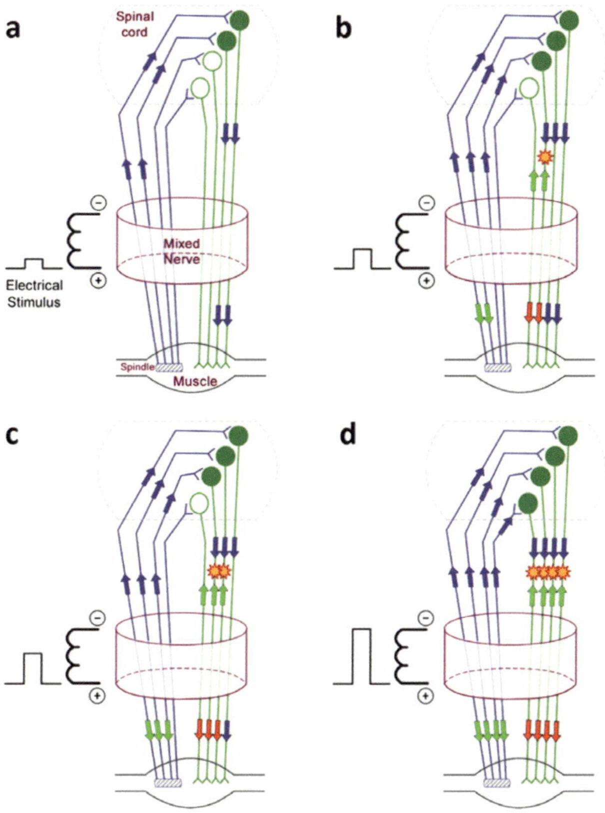

Figure 8. Schematics illustrating the recruitment of sensory and motor fibers by transcutaneous electrical stimulus. The stimulus intensity increases from **a** to **d** (see also the corresponding A-D regions in Figure 7) but the duration is always the same, 1ms. Note the bidirectional propagation of potentials (toward the spinal cord and muscle) in **b-d**. The blue arrows indicate the afferent volley (travelling across the blue axons) and the action potentials reflexively evoked in the motor axons (green cells) that will generate the H-reflex. The red arrows represent the orthodromic motor activation (see also Figure 6) that will generate the M-wave. The green arrows represent the antidromic volleys in either sensory or motor axons. The green arrows in the motor axons will cause a collision (indicated by a yellow star) with the reflexively evoked volley (blue arrows) in the efferent fibers. **a)** For low intensity stimulus the smallest MUs (filled circles) are recruited according to the size principle and no collision is observed. At this point only the H-reflex (without M-wave) is present in the EMG recording (see also Figure 7). **b)** With the increased intensity of electrical stimulation (1ms rectangular pulse), a few motor axons discharge action potentials that propagate antidromically leading to the annihilation of spikes. At this point the H-reflex is accompanied by an M-wave in the EMG recording. The M-wave has a shorter latency than the H-reflex because it is a direct response, i.e., it does not travel to the spinal cord and back to the muscle (red arrows reach the muscle before the blue ones). **c)** The stimulus intensity is much higher and the collision occurs in a larger number of efferent axons, despite the number of afferents recruited by the electrical stimulation being the same (or even higher) than in situation **b**. At this point the H-reflex amplitude is lower than the M-wave (C region of Figure 7b). **d)** The supramaximal intensity recruits 100% of the sensory and motor fibers inducing 100% of annihilation. No H-reflex is identified in the EMG recording and the M-wave reaches its maximal amplitude (M_{MAX}) (D region of Figure 7b).

In this scenario, the H-reflex will never reflect the activation of all the MNs within the pool, even if the stimulus intensity is increased. Instead, this reflex response reaches a maximum (H_{MAX}) as a result of a balance between mechanisms that tend to change the reflex amplitude when the stimulus is increased. The main mechanism that increases H-reflex amplitude (assuming the subject is in a relaxed and controlled state) is the larger number of Ia axons activated by the higher intensity stimulus. The main mechanism that decreases the H-reflex amplitude in response to a stimulus intensity increase is the above mentioned collision of action potentials in the efferent axons. Other mechanisms that may also contribute to decrease the H-reflex amplitude for a higher stimulus amplitude include (1) the activation of Ib afferents (see schematic in Figure 6) [20], (2) the activation of large-diameter cutaneous afferents, (3) the firing of Renshaw cells in response to the synchronous antidromic (or orthodromic) firing of MNs in the pool [19, 23]. These longer latency mechanisms have their putative effect on H-reflex amplitude because the later phases of the H-reflex waveform (after its rise) have been associated with the longer latency oligosynaptic pathways that excite the MNs [18]. For stimulus intensities above that corresponding to H_{MAX} (from the beginning of the descending phase of the recruitment curve, Figure 7b and c), the larger the number of efferents undergoing collision the lower the amplitude of the H-reflex (see Figure 7 and Figure 8).

It is always recommended keeping the amplitude of the test H-reflex in the ascending limb of the recruitment curve, where there is no (or very few) collision in the motor axons. The best fit for the ascending limb of the curve is a sigmoid (Figure 7d) [24]. This fitting is important to define some parameters that can be extracted from the curve, such as slope, current threshold and H_{MAX} [10] (see ahead). It is also highly recommended using a test H-reflex amplitude within the range of 20-30%M_{MAX} [25] because at this amplitude reflexes are more responsive to conditioning.

4.1.2. H-reflex amplitude and ongoing EMG activity under different conditions

The H-reflex can be evoked in different conditions: at rest, during voluntary muscle contraction, in upright stance, during rhythmic movements of different limbs, during walking, running, and so on [1, 10, 26]. Usually, H-reflex evoked during contraction of the homonymous muscle shows higher amplitude compared to H-reflex evoked at rest [1, 21] (Figure 9). This happens because the MNs that were not fired by the afferent volley caused by the electrical stimulus might reach the firing threshold during contraction due to the summation of EPSPs generated by the activation of DTs. Figure 9 shows an example of H-reflex obtained at rest and during tonic voluntary isometric contraction of the SO muscle. When the level of voluntary contraction increases (more MUs are recruited), the size of the H-reflex increases in parallel [26]. Therefore, care should be taken when the objective is to study the modulation of the H-reflex during motor activity as its amplitude depends on the excitability of the MNs in the pool [21]. In practical terms, it is crucial to maintain a constant level of muscle activity throughout the experiment [1, 21].

During a sustained voluntary contraction there is a momentary silence in the muscle activity (silent period) following the H-reflex, as seen in the EMG recording of Figure 10. The silent period is mainly ascribed to the after-hyperpolarization (AHP) of the MNs after the synchronous reflex activation, since the EPSPs caused by descending commands cannot ellicit another spike in the MN during its refractory period (which is related to the AHP). After this period, the constant descending drive causes the MNs to reach the firing threshold almost at the same

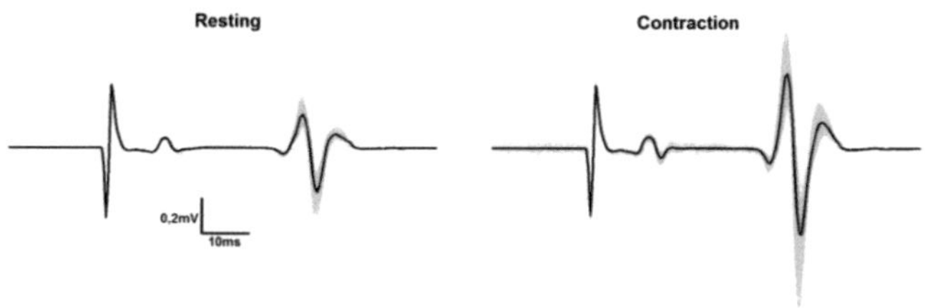

Figure 9. EMG recordings from the SO muscle showing the H-reflexes elicited in two different conditions, at rest and during isometric voluntary contraction (unpublished data). The black trace represents the averaged response.

time, i.e., when the refractory period ceases. This generates a rebound effect that can be seen in the EMG recordings of Figure 10. Other mechanisms might be involved in the generation of the silent period such as recurrent inhibition from Renshaw cells [27, 28]. This silent period has been shown to be useful, e.g. for the quantification of the degree of crosstalk between two muscles [14] and for the study of involuntary sustained muscle contraction after a train of stimuli [29].

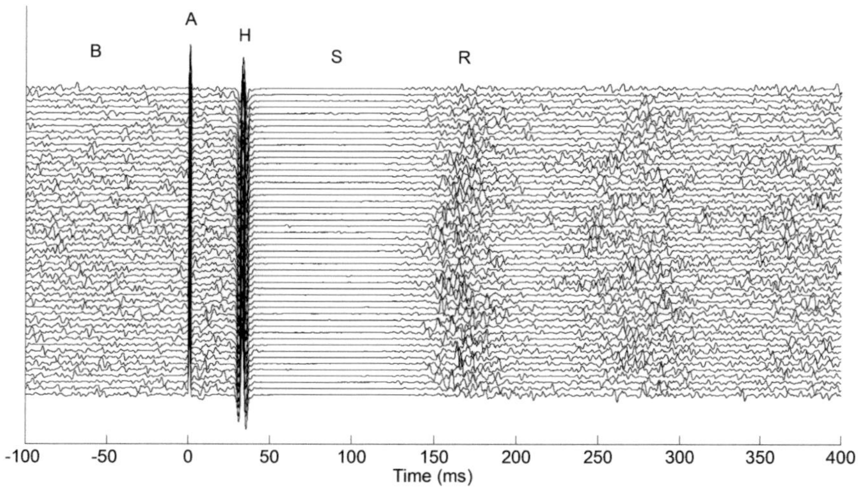

Figure 10. EMG recordings (unpublished data; $n = 50$) from the SO muscle during upright stance showing 100ms of background muscle activity (B) prior to the delivery of a stimulus to the PTN (A) to generate an H-reflex (H). Following the H-reflex, a clear silent period (S) of ~100ms is noticed. A rebound effect (R) can also be seen in the interval between 150 and 200ms.

Not only tonic voluntary contraction induces changes in reflex excitability. There are pre- and post-synaptic influences that affect H-reflex amplitude from a variety of sources. Presynaptic inhibition (PSI) is perhaps one of the most important mechanisms of reflex modulation [30]. By means of PSI the CNS can regulate the excitability of the stretch reflex pathway in different motor contexts. For instance, it is generally accepted that PSI increases from the standing position to walking and even more during running [26].

Even in motor tasks involving rhythmic movements of limbs that mimic patterns of locomotor movements (e.g., arm swing during walking) modulation of reflex responses can be observed. It has been suggested that arm cycling in an ergometer decreases reflex amplitude of the SO muscle by increasing the level of PSI [31]. This result has been used as an evidence for the existence of a neuronal linkage between upper and lower limbs responsible for coordinated actions during locomotion [10]. An example of reduced amplitude H-reflex is shown in Figure 11.

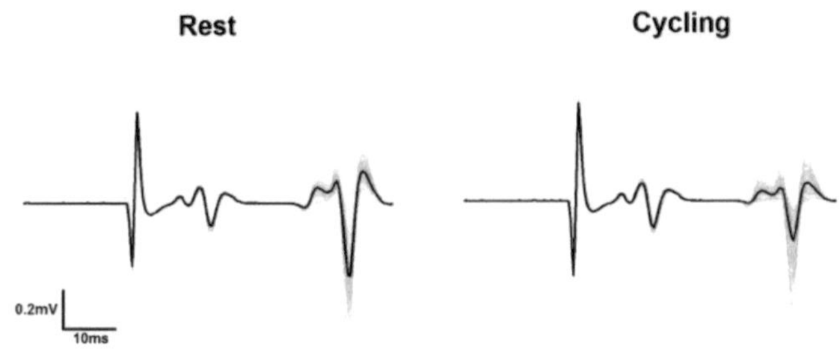

Figure 11. Comparison of H-reflex amplitude from the SO muscle at rest and during arm cycling. The constant amplit tude of the M-wave indicates that there were no changes in stimulus efficacy. The black trace represents the averaged response. Data based on [32], but figures are unpublished.

It is also possible to explore a wider range of MUs by examining the behavior of the H-reflex evoked at different stimulus intensities during the performance of a motor task. Therefore, instead of comparing test reflex responses of a given amplitude (just like those shown in Figure 11) that would represent a single point in the recruitment curve (hence, a limited fraction of active MUs within the pool), the whole recruitment curve can be analyzed (Figure 12). Several parameters may then be extracted from the recruitment curve and compared across conditions [10, 24] and the input-output relations of the system under study can be properly examined. Figure 12 shows an example of changes in the SO recruitment curve during rhythmic arm movements using a stepping ergometer. One can notice a reduction in H_{MAX} values as well as a right shifting of the curve, indicating changes in the threshold of reflex response (see the right panel of Figure 12). It is also possible to investigate changes in the recruitment gain by comparing the slope of the ascending curve between conditions. Note that no significant changes occurred in the M-wave curve (crosses), indicating that the stimulus efficacy was constant for both conditions.

In an attempt to better describe mechanisms responsible for reflex modulation, protocols based on conditioning stimulation have been developed. For example, it is possible to assess the level of PSI under different conditions [33, 34]. The technique (illustrated in Figure 13a) consists in applying a conditioning electrical stimulus to the CPN (1ms rectangular pulse) and a test stimulus to the PTN with a conditioning-to-test (CT) interval of 100ms [35] (compare gray and red traces in the upper panel of Figure 13b). The reflex response conditioned by the CPN

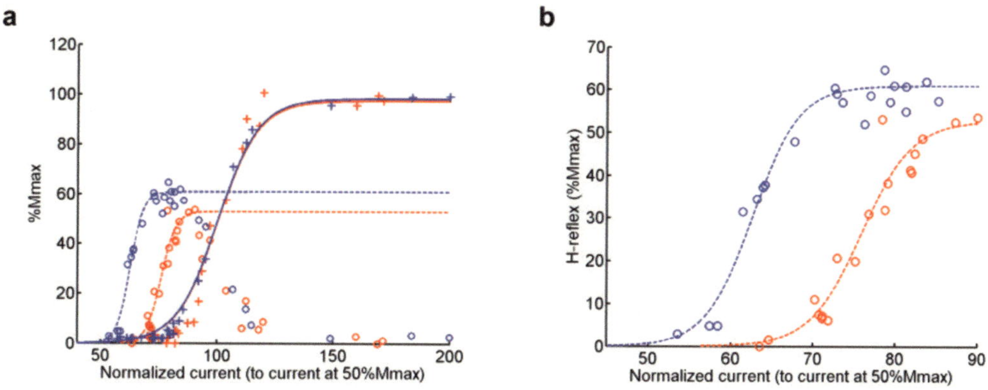

Figure 12. Recruitment curves obtained in two distinct conditions, at rest (blue) and during rhythmic arm movement (red). **a)** It is possible to note a decrease in H_{MAX} amplitude along with a right shift of the red curve. Note that the M-wave recruitment was very similar in both conditions. **b)** A closer inspection reveals a slight change in recruitment gain as indicated by the steeper slope of the blue curve compared to the red one. A clear change in H-reflex threshold can also be observed. Data based on [10], but figures are unpublished.

stimulus will have a lower amplitude as compared to the H-reflex elicited without conditioning due to the PSI effect. This procedure has been widely used in many research laboratories to investigate changes in the degree of PSI in different conditions.

Another pre-synaptic mechanism that affects H-reflex amplitude is post-activation depression (or homosynaptic depression - HD), which consists in a frequency-dependent reduction of reflex amplitude, i.e., when the stimuli are applied with frequencies higher than 0.1Hz (less than 10s interval) a depression in H-reflex amplitude is observed supposedly due to a reduced release of neurotransmitter in the Ia terminal [37, 38]. The HD is also exemplified in the upper panel of Figure 13b (green curve) that shows an averaged reflex response evoked at every 1s (1Hz stimulus frequency).

It is interesting to note a further decrease in H-reflex amplitude when both presynaptic mechanisms are present (PSI+HD; see the blue trace in Figure 13b). This result might be related to the increased frequency used for the conditioning stimulus (1Hz as compared to 0.1Hz used to obtain the trace in green) delivered 100ms before the test stimulus (also delivered at 1Hz to induce HD). Indeed, it was recently shown that an increased conditioning stimulus frequency enhances PSI of both H- [39] and T-reflexes [36].

4.2. The T-reflex

In section 4.1 we presented a technique for the assessment of stretch reflex excitability based on transcutaneous electrical stimulation (the H-reflex). Here we are going to discuss another way to investigate the same pathway by using a mechanical stimulus applied to the tendon in opposition to the electrical current applied to a peripheral mixed nerve. The target again will be the SO muscle. This technique has been used by clinicians to assess the integrity of the spinal cord after injury or in neuropathologies [40]. Perhaps, the main concern about the use of this technique in scientific research is to maintain the mechanical stimulus consistent throughout the experiment. Several investigators have used an instrumented hammer [41, 42] designed to apply a somewhat controlled mechanical percussion to the tendon. An alternative approach is to use a powerful electromechanical shaker to achieve tendon mechanical stimulation [43]. The tip of the shaker is lightly pressed against the Achilles tendon to ensure reasonable stimulus reproducibility. The shaker can be controlled via software that provides the desired input waveform shape, amplitude and duration (e.g., a sinusoidal cycle with 10ms duration and excursion of ~3mm). An inbuilt accelerometer is a reliable alternative to provide a feedback from the shaker tip excursion and monitoring stimulus consistency [3, 43].

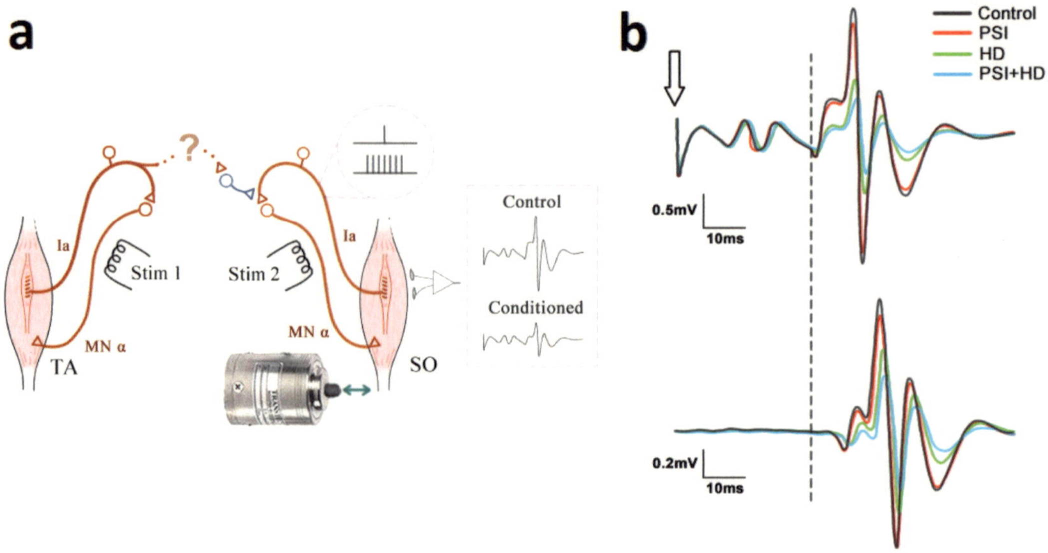

Figure 13. a) Schematic of the experimental setup for testing the presynaptic inhibition pathway. The test stimulus was either electrical (Stim2) or mechanical (indicated by the shaker in contact with the SO tendon). The interval between conditioning (Stim 1) and test stimuli (CT interval) was 100ms. SO afferent activation is shown in the dashed circle. For the H-reflex a single action potential is generated per Ia fiber, whereas the tendon stimulus evokes a burst of firing in Ia afferents. This difference might be responsible for the lesser sensitivity of the T-reflex to PSI as compared to the H-reflex (see text for details). **b)** Upper panel: Averaged H-reflex waveforms obtained in the SO muscle under different conditionings as compared to the control or no-conditioning case (in dark gray). The trace in red shows an H-reflex conditioned by a 1ms stimulus to the CPN to induce PSI on the afferent terminals of the SO muscle. The green trace represents the H-reflex under homosynaptic depression, HD (stimulus applied to the PTN at 1Hz). When the test and conditioned responses were obtained with interval of 1s (conditioned and test stimuli applied at 1Hz) an additional inhibition was observed (blue trace; HD+PSI). The vertical arrow shows the instant of stimulus delivery. Lower panel: the same as for upper panel showing the T-reflex. Note the longer delay as compared to the H-reflex (indicated by a horizontal dashed line). Results similar to those observed in H-reflex were attained for condition PSI+HD. Data based on [36], but figures are unpublished.

The main difference between both techniques (H and T reflexes) is that in the case of the H-reflex the stimulus bypasses the muscle spindles (it is applied directly to the nerve, see Figure 6). To generate the T-reflex the stimulus is applied distally, on the tendon of the muscle of interest. The mechanical percussion induces a brief muscle stretch leading to the activation of spindle afferents. As a consequence, the mechanical stimulus generates a burst of firing in each afferent axon (mainly in Ia afferents). In contrast, the electrical stimulation produces only one spike per axon and at a more fixed latency (less sparse spikes arriving to the MN pool) than the burst due to the tendon tap [20] (see dashed circle in Figure 13). Therefore, the effect of asynchronous afferent bursts on the Ia-MN synapses will be different from a less dispersed volley of single action potentials. The MN depolarization (sum of EPSPs) generated by a more asynchronous afferent volley would produce a long rising time course in the membrane of the MN, giving time to other inputs (e.g., Ib afferents; see also Figure 6) mediated by oligosynaptic pathways to exert influence on the membrane of the postsynaptic cell [20]. Therefore, conditioning effects on T-reflex might be different from effects observed on H-reflex. For instance, T-reflex has been shown to be less responsive to a conditioning that induces PSI compared to the H-reflex [44] (see Figure 13). Despite the relatively lower sensitivity to PSI, the T-reflex also showed a stronger inhibitory effect when the conditioning stimulus was applied at higher frequency (1Hz), as for the H-reflex (see previous section) [36]. However, postsynaptic effects (e.g., mediated by RI) may have similar strength for both reflexes (see section 5.2.1; [44, 45]) regardless of the stimulus frequency.

Another important difference is related to the sensitivity of reflex responses to the fusimotor system excitability. T-reflexes are differentially susceptible to γ-MN activity (that regulates the muscle spindle sensitivity) as compared to H-reflexes [46]. All these aspects need to be taken into account in the interpretation of results and/or comparisons between both types of reflex responses.

4.3. The F-wave

F-waves are recorded routinely in clinical neurophysiological practice [47]. The F wave is a late response that occurs in a muscle following stimulation of its motor nerve, evoked by antidromic activation ("backfiring") of a fraction of the MNs. Typically, F-waves are evoked in response to a strong electrical stimulus (supramaximal stimulation) applied to a peripheral nerve. Action potentials traveling orthodromically reach the muscle fiber, thereby eliciting a strong M-response (M_{MAX}). The action potentials traveling antidromically (see arrows in Figure 6) reach the cell bodies of the MNs making a small fraction of them to fire. This causes orthodromic action potentials to travel back towards the muscle, generating a relatively small amplitude CMAP called F-wave. Several measurements can be done on the F responses, including peak-to-peak amplitude, duration, latency (period between stimulation and F-wave response), and persistency (number of F-waves obtained per number of stimulations). Most electrophysiologists agree that F-wave latency constitutes a valuable parameter that reflects conduction properties of motor axons, being even more reliable than distal motor conduction measurements used to detect mild or early generalized abnormalities [48]. Although the use of F waves for assessing MN excitability is controversial [49], they are sensitive to changes in MN excitability [48] and have been used to assess it in a variety of protocols [50, 51]. In contrast to the H-reflex, which is influenced by presynaptic effects (PSI and HD), the F response is not a reflex (is not elicited by Ia volley), hence its generation is related solely to the MN membrane potential, which depends on the EPSPs and IPSPs the MN is receiving. Figure 14 shows F-wave recordings from the SO muscle (in response to supramaximal stimulation to the PTN) obtained in a subject at rest.

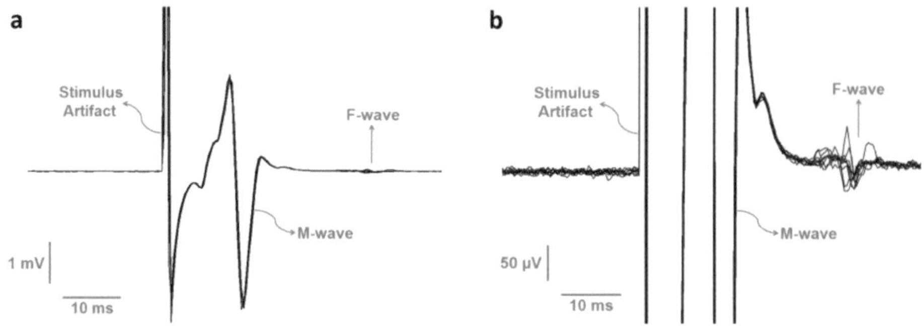

Figure 14. Nine superimposed EMG signals from the SO muscle showing stimulus artifacts, M-waves (M_{MAX}) and F-waves obtained in response to supramaximal stimulation (rectangular pulses with 0.2ms duration) delivered to the PTN of a resting subject (unpublished data). Surface stimulating electrodes were positioned with the cathode ($2cm^2$) on the popliteal fossa and the anode ($8cm^2$) on the patella. The stimulus intensity used to elicit F-waves was above that necessary to elicit M_{MAX}. The same recordings are shown in **a** and **b**, with different amplitude gains (note the calibration bars).

4.4. The V-wave

As described in section 4.1, when a supramaximal stimulus is delivered to the nerve of a relaxed muscle, an M-wave is observed in the EMG with short latency and no H-reflex is observed due to the collision (see Figure 8) between antidromic and orthodromic spikes (there could be F-waves, but they are not our focus here). However, if the subject maintains a steady voluntary contraction, and the same supramaximal stimulus is delivered to the peripheral nerve, a reflex response appears at a latency equal to the H-reflex. This reflex response, frequently referred to as a V-wave (associated with a voluntary drive), is an electrophysiological variant of the H-reflex and is used to measure the level of efferent drive [52-54].

The rationale behind the genesis of this response is that the descending drive activates a subset of MNs in the spinal cord making their axons conduct action potentials orthodromically. These action potentials collide with the antidromic volley generated at the electrical stimulation site by the supramaximal stimulus applied to the peripheral mixed nerve. Thus, this subset of MNs (recruited by the descending command) will be susceptible to be activated by the reflex afferent volley generated by the supramaximal electrical stimulus. Hence, the V-wave amplitude roughly reflects the number of spinal MNs being activated by the volitional drive, as well as the excitability associated with the stretch reflex pathway (previously discussed in section 4.1).

This electrophysiological measure has been used in several human neurophysiology studies, for instance: (1) neuronal plasticity associated with resistance training in healthy subjects [52]; (2) short-term effects of neuromuscular electrical stimulation [55]; (3) multiple sclerosis [56].

In the next section, we will present simulation results regarding the mechanisms behind the genesis of the V-wave.

5. Results from simulations

5.1. General description of the simulator

In this section, we will present simulation results that are valuable to better understand some mechanisms underlying the conditioning of muscle activity discussed previously in this chapter. The simulations were carried out in a multi-scale web-based neuromuscular simulator (dubbed ReMoto) that is freely accessible at http://remoto.leb.usp.br. A complete description of the simulator may be found elsewhere [4, 5]. Briefly, the simulator provides a detailed modeling of four spinal motor nuclei that command leg muscles responsible for ankle extension (SO; medial gastrocnemius - MG; lateral gastrocnemius - LG) and ankle flexion (TA). Each nucleus encompasses a MN pool and spinal INs mediating recurrent inhibition (by means of Renshaw cells), RI (by means of inhibitory Ia INs that receive inputs from antagonist muscles), and Ib inhibition. Individual spinal neurons are modeled following biophysical data from both cat MNs and INs, including active ionic channels responsible for the genesis of action potentials (sodium and fast potassium) and afterhyperpolarization (slow potassium). MN dendrites have an L-type calcium channel yielding a persistent inward current that is activated by the presence of neuromodulators in the spinal cord [57]. Ia and Ib afferents are present in ReMoto so as to allow studies on spinal reflexes (e.g., H-reflex) generated by electrical stimulation applied to a nerve (PTN for SO, LG and MG; CPN for TA). Model parameter values (e.g., axon conduction velocity, ionic channel time constants, maximum synaptic conductances) and default numbers of elements (i.e. spinal neurons and afferents) are based on experimental data from cats or humans. Some of the parameter values were adjusted so that the dynamic behavior of an individual model matches those experimentally observed in cats or humans, for example, MN frequency-current (*f-I*) curves, post-synaptic potentials time course, and IN discharge patterns.

The MN pool drives muscle units, which generate both electrical (MUAPs) and mechanical activity (force twitches). For each muscle, one output is the EMG, expressed as the sum of all MUAPs, and the other output is force, being the sum of the twitches of all muscle units. Muscle twitches are modeled as the impulse responses of second-order critically-damped systems [58]. MUAPs occurring at the muscle surface are modeled by first- and second-order Hermite-Rodriguez functions [59], which are randomly attributed to each MU. MUAP amplitude and durations are chosen to match intramuscular MUAPs recorded from humans. To model the MUAP recorded by bipolar surface electrodes at the muscle's surface, each intramuscular signal is re-scaled depending on the MU positioning within the muscle cross-section [60], thus representing the spatio-temporal filtering due to the volume conductor (see section 2.2). A white Gaussian noise is added to the resultant surface EMG and this signal is band-pass filtered to mimic a real EMG signal recorded in experiments.

Volitional muscle control is represented by the generation of random trains of action potentials in the DTs, which are modeled by independent nonhomogeneous renewal point processes with Gamma-distributed ISIs. The instantaneous firing rate or the ISI of these point processes can be modulated by mathematical functions (e.g., sinusoid and ramp) in order to generate dynamic motor behaviors, such as rhythmic muscle activity.

Recently, a detailed muscle spindle model was added to the simulator's structure, so that stretch reflex responses can be studied with the simulator [61]. This model (fully described in [62]) represents the nonlinear dynamics of three intrafusal muscle fibers (bag 1, bag 2 and chain). The combination of the fibers' tensions yields the instantaneous activity of the Ia and II afferents. Each intrafusal fiber has an active element, which represents the static and dynamic fusimotor activity coming from gamma MNs. A single muscle spindle model lies in parallel with each muscle model so that muscle stretch and stretch velocity modulate intrafusal fiber tension and consequently the afferent activity. Primary (Ia) and secondary (II) afferent activities are translated into spike trains that are transmitted to the spinal cord through an ensemble of peripheral nerve axons with an associated distribution of conduction velocities (type II afferents are at the moment available only in a downloadable version at the website). In order to represent the ISI variability observed in afferent axons [63], each spike train is represented by a non-homogeneous renewal point process with Gamma-distributed ISIs, whose intensity is modulated by the correspondent muscle spindle output (i.e., Ia or II). In addition, a linear recruitment of afferents is adopted so that during low afferent activity only a small fraction of afferents are discharging and the increase in afferent activity (from muscle spindle model) results in the recruitment of additional afferent axons.

5.1.1. Simulated H and T reflexes

H and T reflexes can be studied in ReMoto by activating (electrically or mechanically) the monosynaptic pathway encompassing Ia afferents, MN pool, and muscle (including the spindle). Oligosynaptic pathways [23] that may contribute to the H and T reflexes are not yet available in the simulator. Due to its multi-scale structure one may evaluate neurophysiological mechanisms and test hypotheses that are unfeasible with human experiments. Recent results [64] of conditioning effects on H and T reflexes are presented below, with emphasis on RI, which is an important inhibitory pathway associated with the control of movements [65, 66].

The friendly interface of ReMoto allows the easy set up of H- and T-reflex simulations using the structure depicted in Figure 15. The SO motor nucleus encompasses 900 type-specified MNs (800 S-type, 50 FR-type, and 50 FF-type), which receives synaptic contacts from Ia afferents (400 with 90% connectivity) of the PTN. In order to generate test H-reflexes, electrical stimuli (1ms rectangular pulses) are delivered at the nerve in a point equivalent to the popliteal fossa (0.66m from the spinal cord and 0.14m to the muscle end-plate). Figure 16a shows the M-wave and H-reflex generated by a 13mA stimulus without conditioning, as well as the discharge times of Ia afferents and MUs that were recruited directly by the electrical stimulus (early recruited MUs) and reflexively by Ia-to-MN excitation, respectively.

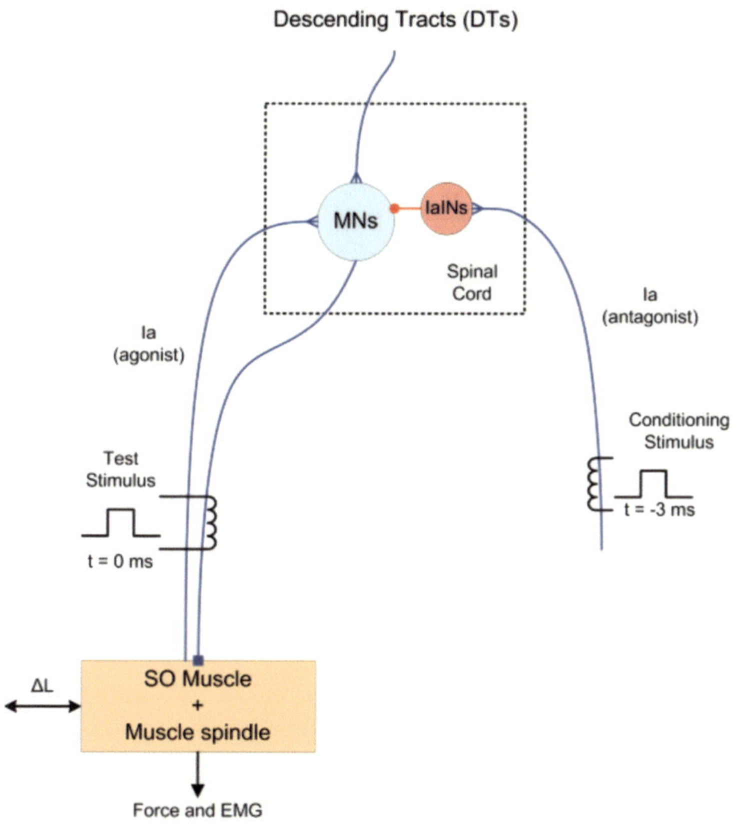

Figure 15. Schematic diagram of the neuromuscular system used to simulate H-reflex, T-reflex and V-wave of the SO muscle. An electrical pulse with appropriate amplitude delivered to the PTN elicits a direct M-wave and a test reflex (H-reflex), which can be observed in the simulated EMG. Similarly, the V-wave can be generated after a supramaximal stimulus delivered to the PTN during a sustained voluntary contraction evoked by the activity of DTs. Test T reflexes can be observed in the EMG after the application of an idealized SO muscle stretch (ΔL) that evokes a phasic response of muscle spindles and a burst of firing in Ia afferents. To simulate a conditioned H- or T-reflex due to RI, the antagonist CPN was stimulated with a CT interval equal to -3ms. For the T-reflex, an additional 7ms interval was added to account for the difference in reflex latencies.

Test T-reflexes can be simulated by applying an idealized stretch (10ms triangular-shaped stretch) to muscle fibers (see the schematic in Figure 15 and the time course in the lower panel of Figure 16b) in order to evoke a response in the muscle spindle model, which reflexively activates the spinal MNs by means of Ia afferents. The upper panel in Figure 16b shows the T-reflex generated with amplitude similar to the H-reflex described in the paragraph above (~25%M_{MAX}). It is worth noting that in these simulations a similar number of spinal MNs were recruited by the afferent volley evoked by the electrical (H-reflex) and mechanical stimulus (T-reflex), suggesting that despite the asynchronous discharge in Ia fibers during the T-reflex (see Ia afferent discharges in Figure 16b; [20]), the excitatory post-synaptic effect is similar between the electrically- and mechanically-evoked reflexes. A remarkable difference between these reflexes is the latency in which each wave is observed in the simulated EMG. The T-reflex is shifted by approximately 7ms with respect to latency of the H-reflex, which represents the conduction time between the point of mechanical (muscle tendon) and electrical (popliteal fossa) stimulations [44, 45] (see also the vertical line in Figure 13b for experimental data).

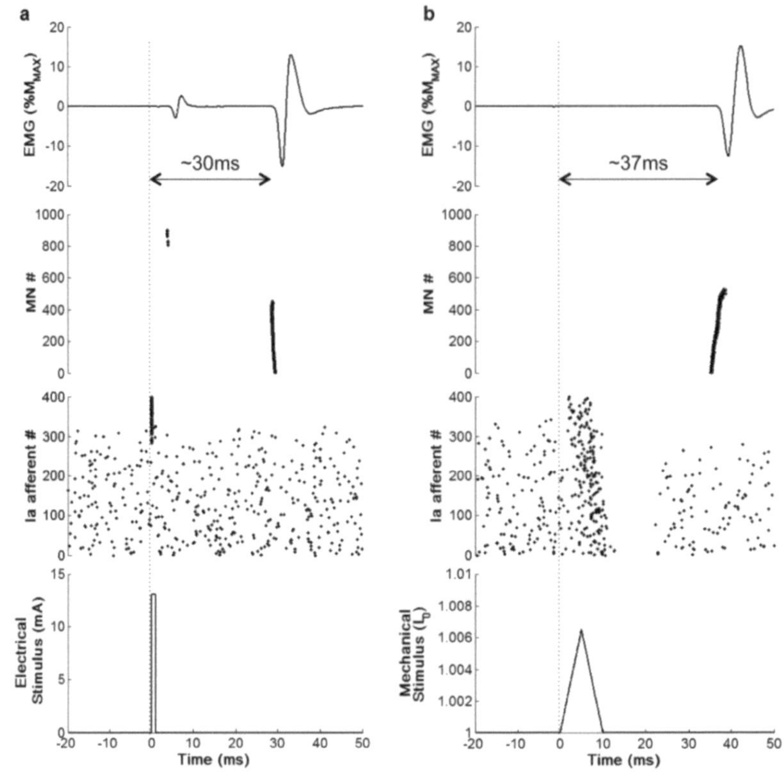

Figure 16. Simulated H and T reflexes (data based on [64], but figures are unpublished). **a)** From top to bottom: SO EMG showing the M-wave and the test H-reflex; raster plots of MU discharges at the muscle end-plate; raster plots of Ia afferent discharges at the popliteal fossa; and electrical stimulus delivered to the PTN at the popliteal fossa. **b)** From top to bottom: SO EMG showing the test T-reflex; raster plots of MU discharges at the muscle end-plate; raster plots of Ia afferent discharges at the popliteal fossa; and idealized mechanical stimulus (normalized to the optimal muscle length, L_0) delivered directly to the muscle spindle model. In both simulations, Ia afferents had a random low-frequency background discharge, which is compatible with the experimental data recorded from humans [63, 67]. Differences in latencies between the H- and T-reflex are due to the different places of stimulus application.

5.1.2. Conditioning effects from the activation of the reciprocal inhibition pathway

In this set of simulations, we have evaluated the conditioning effects of the RI pathway on the amplitude of H and T reflexes. Test reflexes were evoked as described in the preceding section; nevertheless, a conditioning stimulus was applied to the CPN, which innervates the antagonist muscle (see schematic in Figure 15), in order to elicit an afferent volley to the inhibitory Ia INs (IaINs) that make inhibitory synapses on the SO MN pool. The stimulus amplitude (1ms duration) delivered to the CPN was 1.1MT (i.e. 10% above the MT). In addition, the connectivity between Ia afferents and IaINs was set at 100%, while a 20% connectivity was adopted in the IaINs-to-MNs pathway. Similarly to experimental studies, a CT interval equal to -3ms was adopted for the H-reflex simulations (i.e. the conditioning stimulus was delivered 3ms before the test stimulus). To account for the difference in reflex latencies, 7ms was added to the CT interval in T-reflex simulations [44, 45].

Top panels in Figure 17 (a and b) show the EMGs of the SO muscle for a control condition (red curves) and when a conditioning stimulus was applied to the CPN (black curves). RI reduced the H-reflex amplitude by ~40% of its control value (Figure 17a), whereas the amount of inhibition observed in T-reflex was ~53% of its control value (Figure 17b). This difference was not statistically significant (t-Student test; $p > 0.05$; $n = 5$), supporting the hypothesis that the post-synaptic effect is similar in both H and T reflexes [45].

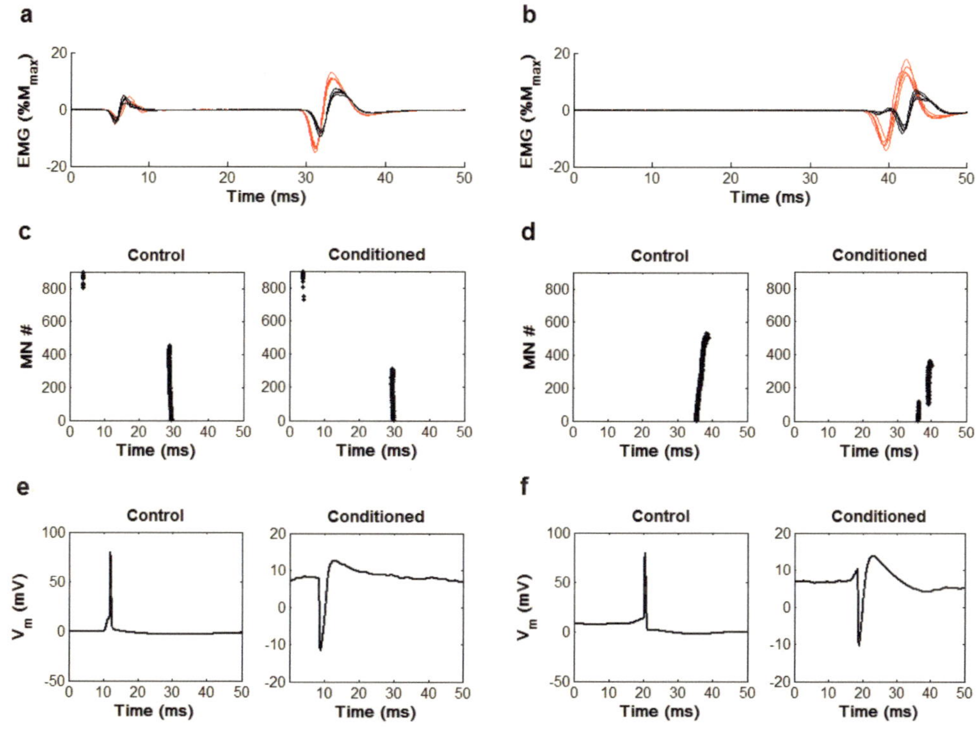

Figure 17. Conditioning effects of the reciprocal inhibition (RI) on H and T reflexes. Data based on [64], but figures are unpublished. **a)** Simulated SO EMGs showing M waves and the H reflexes evoked with (black curves) and without (red curves) a conditioning stimulus delivered to the CPN (five repetitions for each condition). **b)** The same as **a** but for T reflexes. **c)** Raster plots of MU discharges at the muscle end-plate for a single simulation of H-reflex in a control condition (left-side graph) and with a conditioning stimulus delivered to the CPN (right-side graph). **d)** The same as **c** but for a single simulation of T-reflex. **e)** Membrane potential time course of a single MN during a H-reflex simulation. The left-side graph shows an action potential generated in a control condition, whereas the right-side graph shows the post-synaptic potentials observed when a conditioning stimulus is delivered to the CPN. **f)** The same as **e** but for a single MN during a T-reflex simulation. The zero in all displayed abscissas indicates the moment when the stimulus (either electrical or mechanical) was delivered.

Approximately the same number of spinal MNs was de-recruited by the RI in both reflexes (see Figure 17c and d), with a more pronounced effect on high-threshold neurons. This finding (which is readily accessible in the simulator, but not in human experiments) can be explained by the higher input conductance of these cells, which yield smaller compound excitatory post-synaptic potentials (EPSP). Hence, these cells will be operating near their firing thresholds, which means that they will be more easily de-recruited by the arrival of small IPSPs (see right-side graphs in Figure 17e and f). Another result that is unique to the simulations is the recording of intracellular membrane potentials. In the lower panels of Figure 17 (e and f), the membrane potential of a single MN is shown. In a control condition (i.e. without conditioning), this MN is recruited by both electrically- and mechanically-evoked synaptic volleys (left-side graphs). Similarly, the arrival of an IPSP is effective in de-recruiting this MN in both reflexes (right-side graphs), suggesting that RI has a similar effect on these responses. In addition, the compound EPSP observed in the MN soma has a similar time course for both reflexes, reinforcing the hypothesis that post-synaptic effects are similar between H- and T-reflexes [45].

5.2. Simulated V-wave

As described in section 4.4, the V-wave is believed to reflect the level of the efferent drive maintained by a voluntary command. To test this hypothesis, we have used the neuromuscular simulator described above to generate V waves in the SO muscle [68]. The structure depicted in Figure 15 (with exception of the conditioning stimulus) was also used in this simulation, with the MN pool encompassing 900 type-identified MNs and 100 independent axons representing the DTs. The spike train associated to each DT axon was modeled as Poisson point processes with a given mean intensity and the connectivity between DTs and the MN pool was fixed at 30%. At time 1s, a supramaximal electrical stimulus was delivered to the PTN evoking an M_{MAX} and subsequently a V-wave. Changes in V-wave amplitude (normalized with respect to the M_{MAX}) were evaluated by changes in the mean ISI of DTs, mimicking the neuronal plasticity that is supposed to occur after training [52, 55, 56].

Figure 18 shows the simulated SO EMG (upper panels) for two different intensities of the descending drive (mean ISI equal to 3.8ms in Figure 18a and 3ms in Figure 18b), which were chosen to match the ratio V/M_{MAX} observed in the literature [52]. The increase in the ratio reflects the increase in the number of active MNs (from 233 to 426; see lower panels in Figure 18), which roughly corresponded to the number of MNs discharging before the electrical stimulation. This information cannot be accessed in human experiments, emphasizing, therefore, the relevance of mathematical modeling and computer simulations.

The reader can notice that the background EMG activity before the stimulus delivery is slightly different between the two simulated conditions. However, the interference pattern is more susceptible to nonlinear summation and cancellation of MUAPs. Therefore, the V-wave may be a more reproducible and reliable measure of the efferent drive, which can increase or decrease due to different factors, e.g, neuronal plasticity following training and hyper-excitability of spinal MNs following neurological diseases, such as stroke and amyotrophic lateral sclerosis [54, 56].

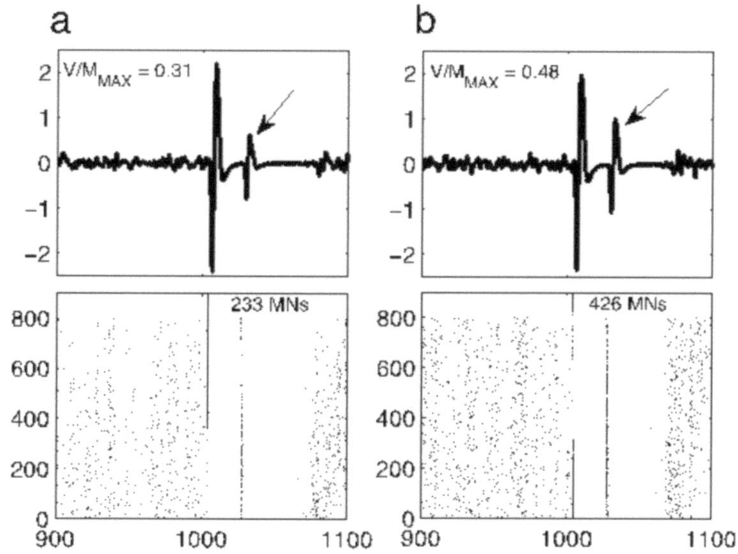

Figure 18. V-waves (arrows) preceded by M-waves in ReMoto simulation of SO EMG (upper panels). Raster plots of MN spikes (lower panels). **a)** Lower-intensity descending drive. **b)** Higher intensity descending drive. Data based on [68].

6. Conclusion

In this chapter we have discussed several aspects regarding the use of surface EMG in a variety of human neurophysiology protocols. Different conditioning effects on the interference pattern and phasic responses, which can be used to infer spinal cord mechanisms, were presented and discussed. Finally, in order to refine the understanding of some underlying mechanisms involved in motor control, as well as to facilitate the interpretation of EMG data, we have introduced a comprehensive web-based simulator of the neuromuscular system with open-access and a friendly interface. The simulation results can be used to test hypothesis raised from the analysis of experimental data and to propose new questions to be addressed in different experimental protocols. The techniques and models presented here might be useful for researchers/clinicians who intend to conduct experiments on both healthy subjects and patients with neuromuscular disorders.

Acknowledgements

The authors are grateful to CNPq (Brazilian Science Foundation), FAPESP (São Paulo Research Foundation) and Canadian Bureau for International Education (PDRF Program) for their financial support.

Author details

Rinaldo André Mezzarane, Leonardo Abdala Elias, Fernando Henrique Magalhães, Vitor Martins Chaud and André Fabio Kohn

Biomedical Engineering Laboratory, University of São Paulo, São Paulo, Brazil

References

[1] Pierrot-Deseilligny E, Burke D. The circuitry of the human spinal cord: Spinal and corticospinal mechanisms of movement. Cambridge: Cambridge University Press; 2012.

[2] Hultborn H, Meunier S, Morin C, Pierrot-Deseilligny E. Assessing changes in presynaptic inhibition of Ia fibres: a study in man and the cat. Journal of Physiology. 1987;389:729-56.

[3] Mezzarane RA, Kohn AF, Couto-Roldan E, Martinez L, Flores A, Manjarrez E. Absence of effects of contralateral group I muscle afferents on presynaptic inhibition of Ia terminals in humans and cats. Journal of Neurophysiology. 2012;108:1176-85.

[4] Cisi RRL, Kohn AF. Simulation system of spinal cord motor nuclei and associated nerves and muscles, in a Web-based architecture. Journal of Computational Neuroscience. 2008;25(3):520-42.

[5] Elias LA, Chaud VM, Kohn AF. Models of passive and active dendrite motoneuron pools and their differences in muscle force control. Journal of Computational Neuroscience. 2012;33(3):515-31.

[6] Merletti R, Parker PA. Electromyography: physiology, engineering, and noninvasive applications. Hoboken: Wiley; 2004.

[7] De Luca CJ. Electromyography. In: Webster JG, editor. Encyclopedia of medical devices and instrumentation. New York: John Wiley & Sons; 2006. p. 98-109.

[8] Kandel ER, Schwartz JH, Jessell TM, Siegelbaum SA, Hudspeth AJ. Principles of neural science. 5 ed. New York: McGraw-Hill; 2013.

[9] De Luca CJ, Adam A, Wotiz R, Gilmore LD, Nawab SH. Decomposition of surface EMG signals. Journal of Neurophysiology. 2006;96(3):1646-57.

[10] Mezzarane RA, Klimstra M, Lewis A, Hundza SR, Zehr EP. Interlimb coupling from the arms to legs is differentially specified for populations of motor units comprising the compound H-reflex during "reduced" human locomotion. Experimental Brain Research. 2011;208:157-68.

[11] DeLuca CJ. The use of surface electromyography in biomechanics. Journal of Applied Biomechanics. 1997;13(2):135-63.

[12] Dumitru, D. Electrodiagnostic Medicine. Philadelphia: Hanley & Belfus; 1995

[13] Merletti R, Knaflitz M, DeLuca CJ. Electrically evoked myoelectric signals. Critical Reviews in Biomedical Engineering. 1992;19(4):293-340.

[14] Mezzarane RA, Kohn AF. A method to estimate EMG crosstalk between two muscles based on the silent period following an H-reflex. Medical Engineering & Physics. 2009;31(10):1331-6.

[15] Capaday C, Cody FW, Stein RB. Reciprocal inhibition of soleus motor output in humans during walking and voluntary tonic activity. Journal of Neurophysiology. 1990;64:607-16.

[16] Petersen N, Morita H, Nielsen J. Evaluation of reciprocal inhibition of the soleus H-reflex during tonic plantar flexion in man. Journal of Neuroscience Methods. 1998;84:1-8.

[17] Magladery JW, McDougal DB, Jr. Electrophysiological studies of nerve and reflex activity in normal man. I. Identification of certain reflexes in the electromyogram and the conduction velocity of peripheral nerve fibres. Johns Hopkins Medicine Journal. 1950;86:265-90.

[18] Burke D, Gandevia SC, McKeon B. Monosynaptic and oligosynaptic contributions to human ankle jerk and H-reflex. Journal of Neurophysiology. 1984;52(3):435-48.

[19] Knikou M. The H-reflex as a probe: pathways and pitfalls. Journal of Neuroscience Methods. 2008;171(1):1-12.

[20] Burke D, Gandevia SC, McKeon B. The afferent volleys responsible for spinal proprioceptive reflexes in man. Journal of Physiology. 1983;339:535-52.

[21] Schieppati M. The Hoffmann reflex: a means of assessing spinal reflex excitability and its descending control in man. Progress in Neurobiology. 1987;28:345-76.

[22] Henneman E, Mendell LM. Functional organization of motoneuron pool and its inputs. Handbook of Physiology The nervous System. Bethesda (MD): American Physiological Society; 1982. p. 423-507.

[23] Misiaszek JE. The H-reflex as a tool in neurophysiology: its limitations and uses in understanding nervous system function. Muscle & Nerve. 2003;28(2):144-60.

[24] Klimstra M, Zehr EP. A sigmoid function is the best fit for the ascending limb of the Hoffmann reflex recruitment curve. Experimental Brain Research. 2008;186(1):93-105.

[25] Crone C, Hultborn H, Mazieres L, Morin C, Nielsen J, Pierrot-Deseilligny E. Sensitivity of monosynaptic test reflexes to facilitation and inhibition as a function of the test reflex size: a study in man and the cat. Experimental Brain Research. 1990;81:35-45.

[26] Stein RB, Capaday C. The modulation of human reflex during functional motor tasks. Trends in Neurosciences. 1988;11:328-32.

[27] Ashby P. Some Spinal Mechanisms of Negative Motor Phenomena in Humans. Negative Motor Phenomena. 1995;67:305-20.

[28] Mcnamara DC, Crane PF, Mccall WD, Ash MM. Duration of Electromyographic Silent Period Following Jaw-Jerk Reflex in Human Subjects. Journal of Dental Research. 1977;56(6):660-4.

[29] Nozaki D, Kawashima N, Aramaki Y, Akai M, Nakazawa K, Nakajima Y, et al. Sustained muscle contractions maintained by autonomous neuronal activity within the human spinal cord. Journal of Neurophysiology. 2003;90(4):2090-7.

[30] Rudomin P, Schmidt RF. Presynaptic inhibition in the vertebrate spinal cord revisited. Experimental Brain Research. 1999;129(1):1-37.

[31] Frigon A, Collins DF, Zehr EP. Effect of rhythmic arm movement on reflexes in the legs: Modulation of soleus H-reflexes and somatosensory conditioning. Journal of Neurophysiology. 2004;91(4):1516-23.

[32] Mezzarane RA, Zehr EP. Locomotor-related descending regulation and voluntary motor output interact to modulate H-reflex variability in leg muscles. 39th Annual Meeting of the Society for Neuroscience; 2009; Chicago.

[33] Faist M, Dietz V, PierrotDeseilligny E. Modulation, probably presynaptic in origin, of monosynaptic Ia excitation during human gait. Experimental Brain Research. 1996;109(3):441-9.

[34] Mezzarane RA, Kohn AF. Control of upright stance over inclined surfaces. Experimental Brain Research. 2007;180(2):377-88.

[35] Iles JF. Evidence for cutaneous and corticospinal modulations of presynaptic inhibition of Ia afferents from the human lower limb. Journal of Physiology. 1996;491:197-207.

[36] Mezzarane RA, Magalhães FH, Chaud VM, Elias LA, Kohn AF. Responsiveness of H- and T-reflexes of soleus muscle to presynaptic inhibition induced by a low frequency train of stimuli. 42nd Annual Meeting of the Society for Neuroscience; 2012; New Orleans.

[37] Hultborn H, Illert M, Nielsen J, Paul A, Ballegaard M, Wiese H. On the mechanism of the post-activation depression of the H-reflex in human subjects. Experimental Brain Research. 1996;108(3):450-62.

[38] Kohn AF, Floeter MK, Hallett M. Presynaptic inhibition compared with homosynaptic depression as an explanation for soleus H-reflex depression in humans. Experimental Brain Research. 1997;116(2):375-80.

[39] Roche N, Achache V, Lackmy A, Pradat-Diehl P, Lamy JC, Katz R. Effects of afferent stimulation rate on inhibitory spinal pathways in hemiplegic spastic patients. Clinical Neurophysiology. 2012;123(7):1391-402.

[40] Mezzarane RA, Nakajima T, Zehr EP. Modulation of soleus stretch reflex amplitude during rhythmic arm cycling movement after stroke. 41st Annual Meeting of the Society for Neuroscience; 2011; Washington.

[41] Archambeault M, de Bruin H, McComas A, Fu W. Tendon reflexes elicited using a computer controlled linear motor tendon hammer. 2006 28th Annual International Conference of the IEEE Engineering in Medicine and Biology Society, Vols 1-15. 2006:2342-5.

[42] Chung SG, Van Rey E, Bai ZQ, Rymer WZ, Roth EJ, Zhang LQ. Separate quantification of reflex and nonreflex components of spastic hypertonia in chronic hemiparesis. Archives of Physical Medicine and Rehabilitation. 2008;89(4):700-10.

[43] Fornari MCD, Kohn AF. High frequency tendon reflexes in the human soleus muscle. Neuroscience Letters. 2008;440(2):193-6.

[44] Morita H, Petersen N, Christensen LO, Sinkjaer T, Nielsen J. Sensitivity of H-reflexes and stretch reflexes to presynaptic inhibition in humans. Journal of Neurophysiology. 1998;80(2):610-20.

[45] Enriquez-Denton M, Morita H, Christensen LO, Petersen N, Sinkjaer T, Nielsen JB. Interaction between peripheral afferent activity and presynaptic inhibition of ia afferents in the cat. Journal of Neurophysiology. 2002;88(4):1664-74.

[46] Rossi-Durand C. The influence of increased muscle spindle sensitivity on Achilles tendon jerk and H-reflex in relaxed human subjects. Somatosensory and Motor Research. 2002;19(4):286-95.

[47] Daube JR, Rubin DI. Clinical Neurophysiology. 3rd ed. Oxford: Oxford University Press; 2009.

[48] Panayiotopoulos CP, Chroni E. F-waves in clinical neurophysiology: a review, methodological issues and overall value in peripheral neuropathies. Electroencephalography and Clinical Neurophysiology. 1996;101(5):365-74.

[49] Espiritu MG, Lin CS, Burke D. Motoneuron excitability and the F wave. Muscle & Nerve. 2003;27(6):720-7.

[50] Magalhaes FH, Kohn AF. Vibration-induced extra torque during electrically-evoked contractions of the human calf muscles. Journal of NeuroEngineering and Rehabilitation. 2010;7:26.

[51] Salih F, Steinheimer S, Grosse P. Excitability and recruitment patterns of spinal motoneurons in human sleep as assessed by F-wave recordings. Experimental Brain Research. 2011;213(1):1-8.

[52] Aagaard P, Simonsen EB, Andersen JL, Magnusson P, Dyhre-Poulsen P. Neural adaptation to resistance training: changes in evoked V-wave and H-reflex responses. Journal of Applied Physiology. 2002;92(6):2309-18.

[53] Pensini M, Martin A. Effect of voluntary contraction intensity on the H-reflex and V-wave responses. Neuroscience Letters. 2004;367(3):369-74.

[54] Solstad GM, Fimland MS, Helgerud J, Iversen VM, Hoff J. Test-retest reliability of v-wave responses in the soleus and gastrocnemius medialis. Journal of Clinical Neurophysiology. 2011;28(2):217-21.

[55] Gondin J, Duclay J, Martin A. Soleus- and gastrocnemii-evoked V-wave responses increase after neuromuscular electrical stimulation training. Journal of Neurophysiology. 2006;95(6):3328-35.

[56] Fimland MS, Helgerud J, Gruber M, Leivseth G, Hoff J. Enhanced neural drive after maximal strength training in multiple sclerosis patients. European Journal of Applied Physiology. 2010;110(2):435-43.

[57] Elias LA, Kohn AF. Individual and collective properties of computationally efficient motoneuron models of types S and F with active dendrites. Neurocomputing. 2013;99:521-33.

[58] Milner-Brown HS, Stein RB, Yemm R. The contractile properties of human motor units during voluntary isometric contractions. Journal of Physiology. 1973;228(2): 285-306.

[59] Lo Conte LR, Merletti R, Sandri GV. Hermite expansions of compact support waveforms: applications to myoelectric signals. Ieee Transactions on Biomedical Engineering. 1994;41(12):1147-59.

[60] Fuglevand AJ, Winter DA, Patla AE, Stashuk D. Detection of motor unit action-potentials with surface electrodes - Influence of electrode size and spacing. Biological Cybernetics. 1992;67(2):143-53.

[61] Chaud VM, Elias LA, Watanabe RN, Kohn AF. A simulation study of the effects of activation-dependent muscle stiffness on proprioceptive feedback and short-latency reflex. 4th IEEE RAS/EMBS International Conference on Biomedical Robotics and Biomechatronics; Rome: IEEE; 2012. p. 133-8.

[62] Mileusnic MP, Brown IE, Lan N, Loeb GE. Mathematical models of proprioceptors. I. Control and transduction in the muscle spindle. Journal of Neurophysiology. 2006;96(4):1772-88.

[63] Matthews PB, Stein RB. Regularity of primary and secondary muscle spindle afferent discharges. Journal of Physiology. 1969;202(1):59-82.

[64] Elias LA, Chaud VM, Magalhaes FH, Mezzarane RA, Kohn AF. H and T reflexes evaluated by a biologically-realistic neuromuscular model. 42nd Annual Meeting of the Society for Neuroscience; 2012; New Orleans.

[65] Hyngstrom AS, Johnson MD, Miller JF, Heckman CJ. Intrinsic electrical properties of spinal motoneurons vary with joint angle. Nature Neuroscience. 2007;10(3):363-9.

[66] Di Giulio I, Maganaris CN, Baltzopoulos V, Loram ID. The proprioceptive and agonist roles of gastrocnemius, soleus and tibialis anterior muscles in maintaining human upright posture. The Journal of Physiology. 2009;587(Pt 10):2399-416.

[67] Aniss AM, Diener HC, Hore J, Gandevia SC, Burke D. Behavior of human muscle receptors when reliant on proprioceptive feedback during standing. Journal of Neurophysiology. 1990;64(2):661-70.

[68] Elias LA, Chaud VM, Watanabe RN, Kohn AF. Application of a web-based simulator to a study of neuromuscular training in humans. BMES 2011 Annual Meeting; 2011; Hartford.

Chapter 5

Clinical Quantitative Electromyography

Tameem Adel and Dan Stashuk

Additional information is available at the end of the chapter

http://dx.doi.org/10.5772/56033

1. Introduction

Human muscles are composed of motor units and each motor (MU) unit is composed of a specific α-motor neuron and the muscle fibres it innervates. A motor neuron innervates the muscle fibres of a MU via the neuromuscular junction (NMJ) formed at the terminal end of each branch of its axon. Voluntary muscle contractions are initiated when the central nervous system recruits MUs by activating their motor neurons, which in turn, via their NMJs, activate their muscle fibres. At each NMJ, a region of transmembrane current is produced across the sarcolemma membrane of its corresponding fibre when the motor neuron is activated (i.e. discharges an action potential). This transmembrane current creates a change in transmembrane potential (or action potential) which propagates along the fibre and initiates/co-ordinates its contraction [1]. The currents creating the action potentials of the activated fibres of recruited MUs summate to create dynamic electric fields in the volume conductor in and around muscles. Electrodes placed in these electric fields detect time changing voltage signals which are the electromyographic (EMG) signals discussed in this chapter. When a muscle is affected by a neuromuscular disorder, characteristics of its action potentials, and as a result of the EMG signals they create, change depending on whether the muscle is affected by a myopathic or neurogenic disorder and the extent to which the muscle is affected. Therefore, quantitative EMG signal analysis can be used to support the diagnosis of neuromuscular disorders. Clinical quantitative electromyography (QEMG) attempts to use the information contained in an EMG signal to characterize the muscle from which it was detected to support clinical decisions related to the diagnosis, treatment or management of neuromuscular disorders.

The main objective of this chapter is to provide an overview of different clinical EMG (detection, measurement and analysis) techniques and the information available in an EMG signal depending on how it was detected (i.e. what type of electrode was used and during what type of muscle activation protocol). How to extract and utilize information from EMG signals to clinically characterize the corresponding MUs and subsequently the whole muscle will also be covered. Descriptions of muscle electrophysiology, EMG detection electrodes and information extraction techniques for surface and intramuscular electrodes are provided. A review and comparison of applications of EMG techniques for clinical decision support concludes the chapter.

2. Muscle morphology, physiology and electrophysiology

2.1. Morphological and physiological description of a muscle

2.1.1. MU structure and layout

Each muscle consists of muscle fibres. The muscle fibres of a muscle are grouped according to their innervating α-motor neuron. A MU refers to a single α-motor neuron and the muscle fibres it innervates [5]. A voluntary muscle contraction is initiated by the activation of motor neurons whose axons propagate action potentials to their terminal ends where they join with a muscle fibre via a NMJ as shown in Fig.1. More specifically, a NMJ is the area where the axon terminal of a motor neuron axon innervates a muscle fibre. In a normal muscle, when a motor neuron is activated (i.e. discharges an action potential) each of its innervated muscle fibres are also activated via their respective NMJ. At each NMJ, following the arrival of the action potential at its axon nerve terminal, a region of transmembrane current is produced across the sarcolemma membrane of its corresponding fibre which creates a change in muscle fibre transmembrane potential (or a muscle fibre action potential) which propagates along the fibre and initiates/co-ordinates its contraction. Therefore, in normal muscle, activation of a motor neuron causes all of its innervated muscle fibres to contract and contribute to the force generated by the muscle.

For each muscle, there is a pool (or group) of motor neurons which are activated during a voluntary muscle contraction. The number of muscle fibres in a certain motor unit and the diameter of these fibres determine the size of the motor unit or the magnitude of its contribution to the muscle force created. The number of muscle fibres within a motor unit is not constant. Most muscles have large numbers of smaller MUs and smaller numbers of larger MUs. The distribution of the MU sizes of a muscle determines how precisely its force can be controlled; the smaller the motor unit, the more precise its force and function.

A MU territory is the cross-sectional area of a muscle in which the fibres of a MU are randomly located. For a normal MU, its MU fibres are randomly positioned throughout its territory. MU territories can be conceived to be circular, with diameters taking values between 10 and 15 mm depending on the size of the MU. In addition, the MU territories of the MUs of a muscle are greatly overlapped. Therefore, in a normal muscle, adjacent muscle fibres rarely belong to the same MU. Instead, the muscle fibres of a MU are interdigitated with muscle fibres of many other motor units. The interdigitation and spatial distribution of the fibres of the MUs of a muscle, help evenly distribute the contributions of MUs to muscle force.

http://dx.doi.org/10.5772/56033

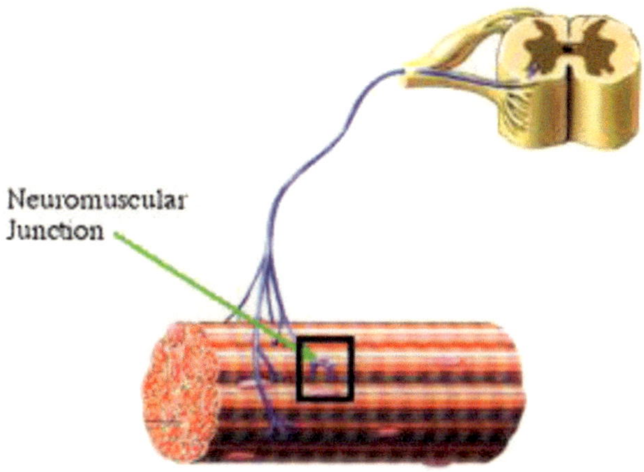

Figure 1. A motor unit [30]

2.1.2. MU activation (recruitment and rate coding)

When a MU is recruited, its motor neuron discharges a train of action potentials that propagate along its axon and, as described above, cause the muscle fibres of the MU to contract. The recruitment of only one MU leads to a weak muscle contraction. The recruitment of additional MUs leads to the activation of more muscle fibres and, as a result, muscle contraction becomes gradually stronger. Changing the rate at which a MU fires (i.e. the rate at which its motor neuron discharges an action potential) can also change the average force produced by a muscle. Therefore, muscle force is modulated by concurrent changes in the number of MUs recruited and their rates of firing.

Motor unit recruitment or derecruitment refers to the activation or deactivation of a MU or population of MUs and thus the subsequent addition or subtraction of the forces produced by its or their muscle fibres, respectively, to the overall muscle force. Motor unit recruitment strategies vary depending on the inherent properties of the specific motor neuron pools of a muscle. Smaller muscles with smaller pools or numbers of MUs tend to recruit all of their MUs earlier during an increasing force contraction and often have all of their MUs recruited at 30% of maximal voluntary contraction. Larger muscles with large numbers of MUs recruit MUs throughout the entire range of force generation.

In general, the firing times of a healthy MU can be modeled as a Gaussian renewal point process and the firing times of different MUs are usually independent of one another. Intervals between the firing times of a particular MU are referred to as inter-discharge intervals (IDIs) and the rate at which a MU fires is simply called its firing rate and often measured in pulses per second (pps)... MU rate coding refers to changing the firing rate of a MU (i.e. the inter-discharge intervals between motor neuron discharges). MUs are initially recruited with firing rates of about 8 – 10 pps and can increase their firing rates up to 25 to 50 pps. In general, as the intended force of a contraction exceeds the recruitment threshold of a MU, its firing rate will increase.

In general, MUs are recruited in order of their size. When the muscle is initially activated, small MUs are recruited first. As the strength of a muscle contraction increases, MUs of progressively larger size are recruited [25]. The result of this process of adding sequentially larger MUs is a smooth increase in the created muscle force [32]. This orderly recruitment of sequentially larger MUs is referred to as the "Henneman size principle" or simply the "size principle" [32], [34], [35]. Henneman et al. noted that motor axon diameter, conduction velocity and, by further investigation, motor neuron size all increase with functional threshold [32]. There are exceptions to the size-ordered activation of MUs. For example, MU recruitment patterns can vary for different movement tasks, depending on muscle function, sensory feedback, and central control [34]. The force produced by a single MU is partly determined by the number and sizes of the muscle fibres in the motor unit (i.e. the MU size). Another important determinant of force is the frequency with which the muscle fibres are activated. Due to the Henneman size principle mentioned above, force increments due to recruitment are small, whereas during higher force contractions, force increments become much larger.

2.2. Muscle electrophysiology

An innervated muscle fibre is activated when the currents created by the activity of its NMJ create a transmembrane action potential that then propagates in both directions along the muscle fibre away from the NMJ initiating and coordinating contraction of the fibre. In other words, action potentials propagate along the axon of a motor neuron to activate the muscle fibres of a MU. The currents creating the action potentials of the activated muscle fibres linearly contribute to a spatially and temporally dynamic electric field created in the volume conductor in and around a muscle. The strength and spatial and temporal complexity of the created electric field is determined by the number of MUs active and their size and spatial extent. Electrodes placed in this electric field can be used to detect a time changing voltage signal (i.e. an EMG signal).

3. EMG signals

3.1. Volume conduction and detection of EMG signals

"Volume conduction is the spread of current from a potential source through a conducting medium, such as body tissues" [6]. Simulation models have been devised so that the effects of having different kinds of volume conductors and arrangements of detection electrodes on an EMG signal can be studied [67].

The voltage signal detected when measuring the dynamic electric field created in the volume conductor surrounding a muscle fibre by the currents that flow to create and propagate a muscle fibre action potential, is called a muscle fibre potential (MFP). In turn, the detected voltage signal associated with the firing of a MU is called a motor unit potential (MUP). A

MUP is actually the sum of the MFPs of it muscle fibres. The train of detected MUPs created by the repeated firing of the same MU is referred to as a motor unit potential train (MUPT). Thus, a MU can be represented by its MUPT or by a MUP template; which is an estimate of its typical or expected MUP shape. The detected MUPTs created by all of the active MUs during a muscle contraction summate to comprise a detected EMG signal. Thus, a detected EMG signal contains contributions from all of the muscle fibres active during a muscle contraction. The term "interference pattern" is also used to refer to the EMG signal detected during a muscle contraction.

Due to different distances between a detection electrode surface and the individual muscle fibres of a MU, the size and frequency content of the MFP contributions of the various fibres to the MUPs generated by a MU vary among the different fibres of the MU. There is an inverse relationship between both the amplitude and high frequency content of MFPs, and the distance between the contributing muscle fibre and the electrode detection surface such that muscle fibres that are closer to the detection surface [6] contribute larger and higher frequency content MFPs. In addition, the peaks of individual MFP contributions occur at different times, indicating that their associated muscle fibre action potentials are not synchronously propagating past or "arriving" at the electrode detection surface [6]. The difference in their arrival times is referred to as their temporal dispersion. Temporal dispersion is caused by the different conduction distances between the NMJs of the fibres of a MU and the electrode detection surface and the different muscle fibre action potential conduction velocities of the fibres of a MU. The number of muscle fibres contributing significant MFPs to a MUP and their respective temporal dispersions will determine the size and complexity of a detected MUP. The stability of the MUPs of a MU refers to how similar its detected MUPs are across multiple motor neuron discharges. MUP stability is primarily dependent on the consistency of the times required by the NMJs of a MU to initiate a muscle fibre action potential on their respective muscle fibre and the consistency of the propagation velocities of the initiated muscle fibre action potentials.

In addition to the concepts of MFPs, MUPs and MUPTs, there are additional extrinsic and intrinsic factors that impact the characteristics of a detected EMG signal. The extrinsic factors depend on the structure and placement of the electrode detection surface. Extrinsic factors include: the area, shape and distance between electrode detection surfaces; the location of the electrode detection surface with respect to the NMJs of the muscle; the location of the electrode detection surface with respect to the lateral edge of the muscle; and the orientation of the electrode detection surface with respect to the direction of muscle fibre action potential propagation [45]. Specific electrode configurations and their applications are described below. Intrinsic factors are related to inherent characteristics within the muscle itself. Intrinsic factors include: the number of active MUs, the fibre type composition of the muscle, the amount of blood capable of flowing through the muscle during the contraction, the diameters, depths and locations of the active fibres, and, for surface EMG signals, the amount of tissue between the surface of the muscle and the electrode detection surface [45].

3.2. Specific electrode configurations for detecting EMG signals

One way of envisaging an EMG electrode is to compare it to a receiving antenna. For telecommunications, dynamic electromagnetic signals propagate throughout air and an antenna detects these signals. Air in this case is analogous to the volume conductor throughout which currents spread. An EMG electrode acts as an antenna detecting, in this case, dynamic voltage signals generated by the activity of muscle fibres from which currents propagate throughout the volume conductor surrounding the muscle fibres and muscles [24].

Electrodes used to detect EMG signals are actually transducers that allow the electric fields created in the volume conductor surrounding muscle fibres by the ionic currents associated with muscle contraction to be detected and amplified using standard instrumentation amplifiers which are dependent on electronic currents. EMG signals can be detected using a bipolar electrode configuration; measuring the voltage difference using two, or more, active electrodes, or a monopolar electrode configuration; with one reference (passive) electrode and one active electrode. In general, an EMG signal can be detected using a surface or intramuscular electrode configuration. Accordingly, there are two classes or types of EMG signals, surface and intramuscular EMG signals, respectively.

3.2.1. Surface electrodes

Surface EMG electrodes are placed on the skin overlying a muscle. It is typical for surface EMG signals to be detected using a bipolar electrode configuration consisting of two electrodes with surface areas approximately equivalent to that of a 1 cm by 3 cm rectangle and with approximately 1 cm spacing. However, surface electrode arrays with more than 2 electrodes, smaller detection surfaces and electrode spacing have been developed. Huppertz et al. used two columns of electrodes [7] to detect surface EMG. In [13], a 2-dimensional array of electrodes, which consisted of 128 electrodes in total, was used.

3.2.2. Intramuscular electrodes

Intramuscular (or needle) electrode configurations are inserted through the skin and into a muscle. Intramuscular EMG signals can be detected using various needle electrode configurations. Below are some characteristics of clinically used needle electrodes. (Concentric and monopolar needle electrodes are the most commonly used needle electrodes.)

3.2.2.1. Needle electrodes

1. Concentric needle electrodes

A concentric needle electrode consists of a needle cannula in which an insulated core conductor is positioned. The cannula and core conductor are cut at a 15° angle to expose the active detection surface. A concentric needle electrode usually has an elliptical active detection surface area of 0.07 to 0.08 mm^2 provided by its core conductor while its cannula serves as the reference electrode [6].

http://dx.doi.org/10.5772/56033

2. Monopolar needle electrodes

A monopolar needle electrode consists of a solid stainless steel needle coated with insulation except for its distal tip, which serves as the active detection surface. The reference detection surface consists of either another monopolar needle electrode or a surface electrode. Compared to a concentric needle electrode, a monopolar needle electrode has a larger active detection surface area of about 0.2 mm^2. [6].

3. Single fibre needle electrodes

A single-fibre EMG (SFEMG) needle electrode consists of a hollow cannula, which contains an insulated core exposed through a side port 7.5 mm from the tip of the cannula. The circular active detection surface has a diameter of 25 μm [6]. The surface of the cannula serves as the reference electrode.

3.3. Potential Information content

The electrode configuration and muscle activation protocol used to detected EMG signals depends on the objectives of the investigation being completed

3.3.1. Surface EMG signals

Because surface electrodes are placed on the skin overlying a muscle, whose muscle activation related electric fields they are detecting, the various distances between specific MUs and the muscle fibres of those MUs to the electrode detection surface(s) are large and relatively equal. As such, the MUPs of different MUs are composed of primarily of low frequency components (50 to 200Hz) and quite similar in shape and it is difficult to discriminate between the activities of different MUs. As the detection surface area increases more MUs become essentially equidistant from the electrode. This increases the number of MUs able to make significant contributions to a detected signal (or the uptake volume of the electrode) lowers there frequency content and reduces the ability to discriminate individual MU contributions. Reducing the inter-electrode spacing for bipolar electrode configurations can only somewhat counter the effects of increased detection surface area. Alternatively, as the detection surface area decreases, the uptake volume of the electrode reduces, the MUPs are composed of relatively higher frequency content components, and it is easier to discriminate individual MU contributions. Therefore, depending on the amount of detection surface area and the inter-electrode spacing, surface electrodes generally sample from a large number of MUs over a large portion of a muscle. Therefore, surface EMG signals primarily contain information regarding the overall activity of a muscle and are primarily used to assess muscle activation patterns and muscle fatigue [4].

Stalberg [19] was the first to introduce the idea of spike triggered averaging a macro detected EMG signal (i.e. an EMG signal detected using an electrode with a large detection surface) using individual motor unit firing times as triggers [18]. He used a macro electrode that had a cannula of length 15 mm centered on a single fibre needle (SFN) detection surface to acquire the signal triggering potentials. For each MUPT, the motor unit firing times are used as triggers for locating 100 ms epochs in the macro detected signal. Each located interval is ensemble averaged to extract the macro MUP for the MU [18]. The size parameters of the macro MUPs, such as peak-to-peak voltage or area are related to the overall size of the contributing MU [15], [16]. When used with spike-triggered-averaging techniques surface EMG can be used to extract surface motor unit potentials (SMUPs) which are useful for assessing MU sizes [45] and can be used for estimating the number of motor units in a muscle [45].

An exception to conventional surface EMG signals are multi-channel signals simultaneously detected using arrays of surface electrodes with small detection surface areas and small inter-electrode spacing. These signals can be used for surface EMG signal decomposition [13] applications. Detecting surface EMG signals using multi-electrode arrays provides information about the spatial distributions of MU fibres under the electrode array, which in turn enhances the ability to discriminate individual MU activity relative to standard surface EMG electrode configurations.

One other application multi-channel surface EMG was to use a multi-channel electrode with four detection surfaces linearly positioned along the direction of the muscle fibres and with each detection surface aligned perpendicular to this direction [22]. Using a linear array of detection electrodes increases the possibility of interpreting EMG signal features compared to single-channel surface signals. Using a linear array of detection surfaces makes it possible to investigate in detail the processes of the generation, propagation, and extinction of muscle fibre action potentials.

3.3.2. Intramuscular EMG signals

Intramuscular or needle EMG electrodes are inserted through the skin and into the muscle and can be positioned at specific locations within a contracting muscle. As such, the various distances between specific MUs and the muscle fibres of those MUs to the electrode detection surface(s) can be significantly different. Therefore, intramuscular EMG electrodes can be positioned to preferentially detect the activity of MUs whose muscle fibres are closest to the detection surface(s) of the intramuscular electrode. This can result in the MUPs of different MUs being quite different in shape making it easier to discriminate between the activities of different MUs.

Intramuscular EMG signals can be acquired using selective electrodes with a small detection surface (e.g. concentric or monopolar needle electrodes) or using an electrode with a large detection surface (e.g. macro electrodes [19]) [17]. Generally, MUPTs detected using intramuscular electrodes provide local information about their respective MUs. The MUPs comprising intramuscular EMG signals can provide information related to MU size, MU muscle fibre distribution and the stability of time it takes for NMJs to depolarize their connected muscle fibre. In addition, MUPTs can provide information about MU recruitment and firing rates.

4. Neuromuscular disorders

Neuromuscular disorders change both the morphology and activation patterns of the MUs of the muscles affected. Therefore, the shapes of MUPs detected in muscles affected by neuromuscular disorders will differ from those detected in healthy or normal muscles. In addition, for a given level of muscle activation the number of MUPTs contributing to a detected signal, which reflects the level of MU recruitment, and the rates at which MUPs occur in detected MUPTs, which reflect MU firing rates, will differ.

A normal muscle at rest will have no electrophysiological activity (i.e. there will be no electric field created in its surrounding volume conductor). Muscles affected by a neuromuscular disorder can have spontaneous muscle fibre activity called fibrillations and/or spontaneous MU activity called fasiculations.

Myopathic disorders cause muscle fibre atrophy, splitting, hypertrophy and necrosis. Examples of atrophic and hypertrophic muscle fibres are diagrammed in Fig 2. Atrophic and split muscle fibres have smaller diameters and slower muscle fibre action potential propagation velocities. They therefore produce in general smaller and wider MFPs with later occurring peak vales. Hypertrophic muscle fibres have larger diameters and faster muscle fibre action potential propagation velocities. They therefore produce in general large and narrower MFPs with earlier occurring peak values. Necrotic fibres are not active and do not contribute to detected MUPs or muscle force. As such, myopathic MUPs, in general, are composed of fewer MFP contributions of varying size and with larger temporal dispersion than in MUPs detected in normal muscles. Myopathic MUPs are therefore generally smaller in size and more complex than normal MUPs. The variation in muscle fibre action potential propagation velocity in a muscle fibre affected by a myopathic process can be greater than normal. This in turn can increase the instability of myopathic MUPs across the MUPs of a MUPT.

Because the MUs of a myopathic muscle are generally smaller during equivalent muscle activations more of them must be recruited and they need to be activated at higher firing rates compared to a normal muscle [6]. Therefore, at equivalent levels of muscle activation, EMG signals detected in a myopathic muscle can become more complex than EMG signals detected in a normal muscle (see Fig 3).

In contrast, neurogenic disorders cause the loss of MUs and muscle fibre denervation. Subsequent to reinnervation of the denervated muscle fibres the surviving MUs have increased numbers of fibres with greater and clustered spatial fibre densities relative to normal muscle as seen in Fig.2. The increased number of MU fibres result in MUPs comprised of larger numbers of MFP contributions. The greater and clustered spatial fibre densities result in grouped MFP contributions. Consequently neurogenic MUPs tend to be larger and more complex than normal MUPs sometimes with distinct components or phases (e.g. satellite potentials). During the acute phase of reinnervation newly formed NMJs have larger variations in the time taken to initiate a muscle fibre action potential in their respective muscle fibres. This results in increased instability of neurogenic MUPs across the MUPs of a MUPT.

Because the MUs of a neurogenic muscle are generally larger and because they are fewer in number during equivalent muscle activations, fewer of them must be recruited but they need to be activated at higher firing rates compared to a normal muscle [6]. Therefore, at equivalent levels of muscle activation, EMG signals detected in a myopathic muscle can become more complex than EMG signals detected in a normal muscle. Therefore, at equivalent levels of muscle activation, EMG signals detected in a neurogenic muscle are generally less complex than (or sparse compared to) EMG signals detected in a normal muscle (See Fig 3).

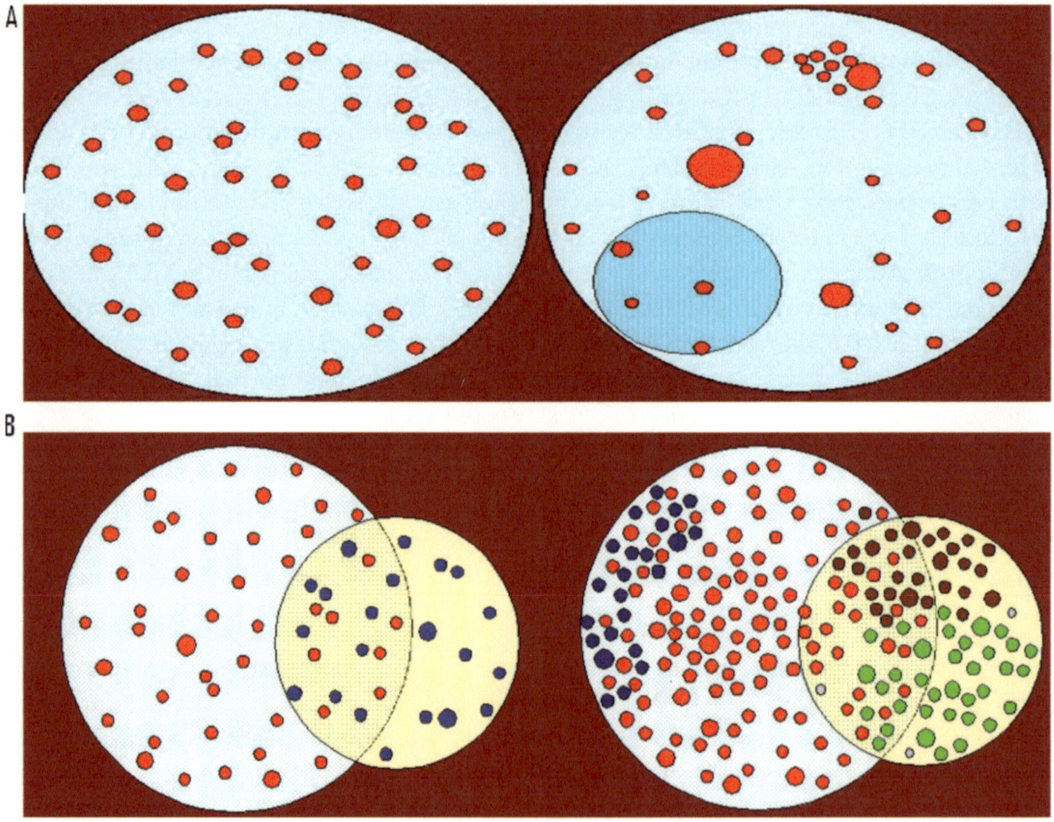

Figure 2. A. Normal MU vs. myopathic MU; B. Normal MU vs. neurogenic MU [43]

http://dx.doi.org/10.5772/56033

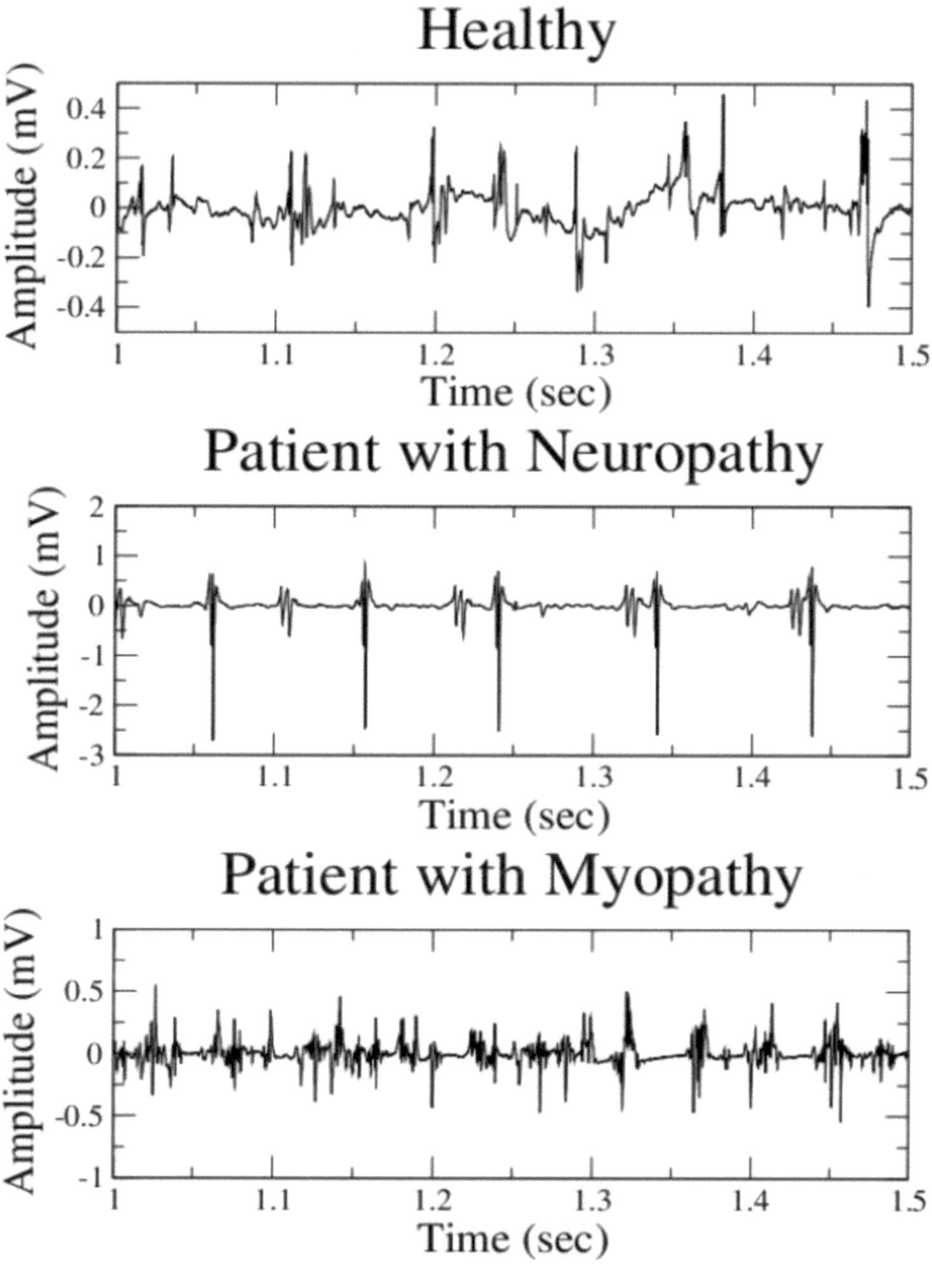

Figure 3. Examples of healthy, neurogenic and myopathic EMG signals [38]

5. How to extract clinically important information

Suitably detected EMG signals can contain information that can be used to assist with the diagnosis of neuromuscular disorders. Specific characteristics of a detected EMG signal can be related to the type of neuromuscular disorder present (i.e. myopathic or neurogenic) as well as the degree to which the muscle may be affected by a disorder. As described above, the changes in MU morphology and activation created by a disease process lead to expected changes in MUP shapes and stability as well as the level of EMG signal complexity. However, in order to use EMG signals to support clinical decisions, the EMG signals must be acquired from a contracting muscle during specific activation protocols and using specific detection electrode configurations. The activation protocol and detection electrode configuration used should provide EMG signals in which the effect of the changes in MU morphology and activation created by a disease process are emphasized. Specific aspects of the detected EMG signals can then be analyzed to determine if they were most likely detected in a myopathic, normal or neurogenic muscle. It this last step qualitative or quantitative analysis can be applied.

5.1. Qualitative electromyography

The current status quo for assessing the clinical state of a muscle is to qualitatively analyze EMG signals detected using needle electrodes following abrupt movement of the electrode, while the muscle is at rest and during low levels of muscle activation. Characteristics of the detected signals are subjectively compared to those expected to be detected in normal muscle. The signals detected following abrupt needle movement and while the muscle is at rest are grouped into what is classified as spontaneous activity. Following abrupt needle movement, if the muscle remains active (i.e. significant signals are detected) for a prolonged period of time this is a sign of abnormality. Likewise, if while the muscle is at rest, potentials related to muscle fibre fibrillation or MU fasciculation are detected the muscle is considered abnormal. The degree of spontaneous muscle activity is often subjectively graded using a discrete 4 or 5 level scale. MUPs contained in EMG signals detected during low levels of muscle activation are visually and aurally analyzed to assess their shape, size and stability either as they are presented in a free running or triggered raster display.

The firing rates of MUs and the number of recruited MUs are also estimated.

The advantage of analyzing an IP detected during minimal muscle activation is that individual MUPs can be recognized. Therefore information about their recruitment information and their firing rates can be obtained [21]. In order to estimate MU firing rates, a 500 ms epoch is displayed [6]. This technique depends on visual inspection to identify individual MUP discharges. The number of discharges of an MU in this 500 ms epoch is multiplied by 2 to get the firing rate [6]; to obtain the number of discharges in one second.

This is a semi-quantitative approach to implement IPA where an IP is detected during maximal force of contraction [14]. The IP is considered full when the signal baseline is completely obscured by MUP spikes [6]. If the baseline can be seen between MUP discharges, the IP is considered incomplete, while if individual MUPs can be recognized, the IP is considered discrete [6]. One border of the EMG envelope is defined by connecting the negative peaks while the other is defined by connecting the positive peaks. The voltage difference between these lines (borders) is the envelope amplitude [6]. The criteria are as follows [14]: if the IP is full and the envelope amplitude is small, this is a myopathic pattern, and if the IP is discrete and the envelope amplitude is larger than its normal value, this is a neurogenic pattern.

The objectives of this qualitative analysis and characterization of the needle-detected EMG signals is to extract information regarding the morphology of a representative sample of MUs of the muscle being examined. Experienced and skilled clinicians can use these qualitative analyses to assist with the diagnosis of an examined muscle with respect to which, if any, specific disease processes may be present and if present, to what extent.

One of the main disadvantages of qualitative EMG analysis is inter and intra-rater variability. Specific assessments made and the consistency with which they are made depend on the training, experience and skill of the examiner. In addition, no more than a few MUPs can be qualitatively analyzed at a time [4]. Therefore, qualitative analysis is restricted to low levels of muscle activation where only a few MUs are recruited and consequently the EMG signals detected are the aggregation of only a few MUPTs.

5.2. Clinical Quantitative EMG (QEMG)

Quantitative electromyography (QEMG) is an objective assessment of several aspects of detected EMG signals to assist with the diagnosis of a muscle under examination and also to assess the severity of an existing disorder if one is detected. QEMG is also sometimes used to assess the status of a detected disorder (active or not) and its time course (chronic or acute) [6]. Quantitative analysis is an automated process, unlike qualitative analysis, which typically requires comparing measured feature values of an EMG signal detected in a muscle under examination to standard or training set values from EMG signals detected in muscles of know clinical state (i.e. myopathic, normal or neurogenic). As a result, standardization or the collection of training data needs to be completed properly; for instance, data should be grouped based on age, gender, and specific muscle. In addition, the EMG signals need to be acquired using a standardized and consistent technique regarding the electrode used, the detection protocol, etc [4]. QEMG aims at increasing diagnostic sensitivity and specificity. Unlike qualitative analysis, quantitative analysis is not limited to studying just the first few recruited MUs and EMG signals detected at higher levels of muscle activation can be analyzed.

Accuracy and transparency are two important factors that must be taken into consideration when selecting or designing a QEMG technique for clinical use. Accuracy is a major issue for any supervised learning problem as the ultimate purpose is to correctly categorize, a muscle being examined so that its condition can be correctly weighted in determining the overall patient diagnosis. Transparency is essential here as well because a clinician should be able to clearly understand the rationale behind the characterization process. A clinician is expected to have moderate knowledge of statistics and if the complexity of a certain technique is beyond that, it is considered as a non-transparent characterization technique. Rule-based classifiers usually provide this required transparency when they are used in QEMG but their accuracy levels are not as high as support vector machines or neural networks.

To perform QEMG, the complete EMG signal, or interference pattern, can be analyzed or individual MUP activity can be isolated from an EMG signal using level or window triggering or EMG signal decomposition methods. If EMG signal decomposition methods are used, individual MUPT can be analyzed which allow information about typical MUP shape, MUP shape stability and MU activation patterns to be used. The next sections discuss QEMG methods based on interference pattern and individual MUPT analysis, respectively.

5.2.1. Interference Pattern (IP) analysis

As mentioned earlier, the term "interference pattern" is used to refer to the complete EMG signal detected from a contracting muscle. The term "interference pattern" is sometimes used to describe the EMG signal detected during a maximal contraction only but the former definition is more common. The characteristics of an interference pattern (IP) depend on the level of muscle activation maintained during its detection and the type of electrode used. The level of activation determines the number of recruited MUs and their firing rates. The type of electrode used determines the shape characteristics of the MUPs (duration, area, amplitude, etc.) that are created by the active MUs and which in turn comprise the IP.

The term "interference pattern analysis" (IPA) refers to those techniques that analyze an IP. IPA is used when a global analysis of an EMG signal is desired. IPA is a quantitative analysis which can be completed using either a frequency or time domain representation of the IP [6]. Following are brief descriptions of common IPA techniques.

5.2.1.1. Frequency domain analysis

Any signal of time can be represented by a summation of sinusoidal functions of several frequency values, phase shifts and magnitudes. Therefore, a frequency domain representation of an IP can be obtained if these frequency values, phase shifts and magnitudes of the signal are identified. A frequency domain representation reveals information about MUP amplitudes, and durations as well MU firing patterns. For instance, high frequency components are representative of MUPs with short durations and short rise times, while low frequency components are representative of to MUPs with long durations and long rise times [8].

5.2.1.2. Time domain analysis

Time domain analysis basically depends on detecting the main characteristics of the time domain representation of an IP. Detecting changes in the sign and slope of an IP was how it was initially performed [8]. Later, more specific characteristics of the time domain signals were found to be important. For instance, the number of turns and their amplitude are important features for discriminating between IPs detected in myopathic, normal and neurogenic muscles. A peak is identified to be a turn if the change in amplitude between this peak and the previous peak exceeds a prespecified threshold, while the amplitude is the difference in voltage values between successive peaks of opposite polarity [8].

5.2.1.3. Clouds analysis

Clouds analysis uses the number of turns and the mean turn amplitude features of IPs detected during several contractions maintained at different levels of muscle activation ranging from slight effort to maximal. The number of turns and the mean turn amplitude for each IP define points in a two dimensional plot in which is overlaid a cloud or region [8]. The cloud defines the area in which 90% of data from IPs detected in normal muscle are expected to be. Accordingly, a muscle is considered diseased if more than 10% of its IPs provides data points which are outside of the cloud.

One of the limitations of IPA is that because of superpositions of MUPTs it is difficult to detect marginal levels of disorders. Small numbers of abnormal MUPTs may be lost in IPs generated by a majority of normal MUPTs.

5.2.2. MUP template / MUPT characterization

A MUPT is composed of the MUPs created by a single MU. The typical MUP shape of a MUPT is represented by its MUP template. The stability of the MUPs with in a MUPT can be estimated as can the firing behavior of the MU that created the MUPT. MUPT characterization refers to performing supervised learning to determine if a MUPT was created by a normal or abnormal (disordered) MU, if just two categories are considered or by a myopathic, normal or neurogenic MU if three categories are considered. This characterization is based on a training stage that is performed using training data suitably representing each category. MUPT features used for MUPT characterization often consist of MUP template morphological features; features extracted from the time domain representation of the MUP template [4] as well as spectral features; those extracted from its frequency domain representation [4]. MU firing pattern features have not yet be effectively used. Typically, a feature selection step is performed to select the best feature subset. As is the case with any supervised learning problem, feature selection can be filter-based (quality metric of the feature subset depends on information content like interclass distance or correlation) or wrapper-based (quality metric of the feature subset depends on the accuracy of the characterization process using such feature set). However, wrapper-based feature selection techniques are used more frequently [56].

In addition to the intrinsic MUP template features, like turns, duration, amplitude, etc, combinations of features can be used if they improve the characterization results. For instance, MUP template thickness (area/amplitude) can be added to the features used for characterization to improve classification performance as the discriminative power of the feature set would be higher.

5.2.2.1. Signal detection and preprocessing

1. Level and/or window triggering

Individual MUPTs can be extracted for quantitative analysis using level or window triggering methods. These methods allow the MUPs created by a single MU to be extracted, but only if their amplitudes are unique with respect to the amplitudes of MUPs created by other MUs.

These methods can be used with careful positioning of the needle and during low level of muscle activation. Only one MUPT can be extracted from the EMG signal detected during muscle contraction. Therefore, for each MUPT to be extracted a separate contraction must be performed.

2. EMG signal decomposition

EMG signals are the linear summation of the MUPTs created by the MUs active in a muscle. EMG signal decomposition extracts individual MUPTs from an EMG signal. Unlike level or window triggering, EMG signal decomposition allows several MUPTs created by MUs concurrently active during a single muscle contraction to be analyzed. The accuracy of the MUPTs extracted by an EMG signal decomposition algorithm determines the type of analyses that can be successfully applied to the extracted MUPTs. The MUPTs extracted during EMG signal decomposition can be further analyzed to assist in diagnosing neuromuscular disorders.

EMG signal decomposition involves three main steps, described in the following paragraphs.

The first step is to detect the MUPTs comprising an EMG signal. Some EMG signal decomposition algorithms attempt to detect all the MUPTs that existed in the EMG signal while others attempt to extract only MUPTs that had a major contribution to the EMG signal. The following step is to determine the shapes of the different MUPs. This can be done by categorizing the MUPs in the signal based on their shapes and sizes. This categorization, if implemented properly, reveals clusters of MUPs with similar shapes and sizes. As a result, MUPs with different shapes and sizes should belong to different clusters. MUPs with similar shapes and sizes were most probably created by different discharges of the same MU, while MUPs with unique shapes and sizes (i.e. not belonging to cluster or to a cluster with very few members) are most probably superpositions. The main outcome of this step is to identify the number of MUs that contributed significant MUPs to the EMG signal (i.e. to estimate the number of MUPTs with significant MUPs) and to estimate the MUP template of each discovered MUPT.

The second step is to determine the class of every template. Superpositions of MUPs are harder to deal with in the first step as well as in this step. If the overlap is only slight, the constituents might still be recognizable. But if the overlap is complete it might be necessary to try different alignments of the templates to see which gives the closest fit. The motor unit discharge patterns can also be used to help determine which MUs are involved in a superimposed MUP [36]. As discharge rates are assumed to be rather orderly (i.e. IDIs can be assumed to follow a Gaussian distribution), the time at which a particular discharge took place can be estimated from the time at which the preceding or following discharge took place.

The final step in decomposition is to validate the results to ensure they are consistent with the expected physiological behavior of MUs. If there are unexpected short IDI in any of the discharge patterns, or if there are detected MUPs that have not been assigned to a MUPT, then the decomposition is probably not correct or incomplete. On the other hand, if all the activity in the signal (i.e. the detected MUPs) has been adequately accounted for by the set of extracted MUPTs which in turn represent MUs with physiologically realistic discharge patterns, then there is a good chance that the decomposition is substantially complete and accurate [36].

5.2.2.2. Non-transparent classification techniques

MUPT characterization can be performed using probabilistic techniques. Probabilistic techniques provide a MUP characterization in terms of conditional probabilities that sum to 1 across all of the categories considered. For instance, a probabilistic technique can suggest that considering the features of a MUPT there is a 10% probability it was detected in a myopathic muscle, a 70% probability it was detected in a normal muscle and a 20% probability it was detected in a neurogenic muscle neurogenic if three categories are considered.

Various methods have been used in the literature to perform MUP template characterization, ranging from conventional to advanced classifiers. For example, linear discriminant analysis (LDA), decision trees and a standard Naive Bayes (NB) classifier were implemented and compared in [9]. LDA attempts to find a linear combination of features that maximizes the between class variance and minimizes the within class variance and it relies on this as a basis for optimal classification. Using these trivial classifiers has the advantage of being rather more transparent than using more advanced pattern recognition techniques like neural networks and support vector machines.

Artificial neural networks were first used for MUP template characterization in [10] and [11]. More progress in this direction was achieved in [12] as artificial neural networks were used along with radial basis functions and probabilistic neural networks in a two-phase classifier, which increased MUPT characterization accuracy. In the second phase of the classification, a C4.5 decision tree was used to determine whether the disorder was myopathic or neurogenic, if any. Another example of using neural networks in MUP analysis can be found in [63].

In [53] autoregressive (AR) modeling and cepstral analysis were applied to characterize MUP templates and the training dataset was built on normal MUP templates as well as MUP templates taken from myopathic muscles. It was concluded in [53] that using AR modeling and cepstral analysis along with time domain features (in particular duration) led to categorizations with high accuracy in the assessment of myopathic MUP templates (in this work two categories were used; normal and myopathic). In [54], MUP templates were classified into three categories; normal, myopathic and neurogenic using support vector machines (SVM).

Using artificial neural networks in classification could lead to over-fitting; a classifier that has difficulty in producing the same accuracy with new or more generalized data. As mentioned earlier, using a SVM and artificial neural networks does not provide enough transparency and renders it more difficult for clinicians to understand how a certain classification decision was made.

5.2.2.3. Transparent rule-based MUPT classification techniques

An example of a transparent rule-based classification technique is the two-stage classifier developed in [55]. This two-stage classifier is based on utilizing radial basis function artificial neural networks and decision trees. The combined use of an artificial neural network and a decision tree reduces the number of tuned parameters required and allows an interpretation of the classification decisions to be provided [55].

Techniques based on pattern discovery (PD) represent another example of transparent rule-based techniques used for MUPT characterization. Pattern discovery is an information theory based technique established to detect significant patterns in data and then to use these patterns for classification [5]. PD was first introduced by Wong and Wang [57]-[60]. PD is applied on discrete data and, as a result, a quantization step is required for each feature that has continuous values, which is the case with most MUPT features. The number of discretization bins can be identified according to the nature of the problem at hand and the dataset used. For instance, if the number of bins is three; low, medium and high for each feature, there might be some loss of accuracy resulting from placing "very high" and "slightly high" values in the same bin. On the other hand, using five bins; very low, low, medium, high and very high can solve such a problem but more training examples are needed to keep the same number of expected occurrences per bin. In the PD classification algorithm, the first step is to discover the "significant" patterns; patterns that are repeated more often than expected assuming a random occurrence [56]. Rules are composed of patterns that include a muscle category. The order of a rule is equal to the number of MUPT features plus the muscle category. For example, high amplitude values in neurogenic MUPTs are a 2nd order rule [5]. Each rule has an associated weight of evidence (WOE) that denotes how much evidence the rule holds in support of a certain category [9]. For rule selection during testing, the highest order rule for each category is selected first. WOEs of selected rules are added to be normalized and this process continues until there are no more rules or all features have already been included in the previously selected rules [56]. In addition to the well-known pros and cons of discretization, characterizations performed by PD are transparent as the technique is rule-based which makes it feasible to explain to a clinician the rationale behind the classification decisions. However, when PD is used, there is a decrease in accuracy due to the discretization performed on the continuous MUPT feature values.

In [61], a fuzzy inference system was introduced. This system is based on using PD in combination with fuzzy logic theory to yield a hybrid system. The idea was to reduce quantization error via assigning memberships for every MUPT feature value based on their position within their assigned bin. The fuzzy membership values allow the same MUPT feature value to be considered in more than one rule simultaneously. Using this technique for establishing rules is similar to the method by which humans manually interpret certain data values and then attempt to classify these values, which makes it very useful, at least in terms of transparency, in a clinical decision support system.

5.2.3. Muscle categorization

The ultimate purpose of characterizing MUPTs is to characterize the muscle from which they were detected. The statistical method for muscle characterization can be performed by calculating mean values for sampled MUPT features and comparing them to expected normative mean values (Note: comparisons should be standardized with respect to age, gender, muscle, EMG detection technique, etc.). Using the expected normative mean and outlier threshold values the overall category of a muscle is then determined based on the mean values of the sampled MUPT feature values with respect to these thresholds. For instance,

Stalberg identified the outlier range to be outside of the mean ± 2 × standard deviations range. This way, a categorization of the muscle being examined can be obtained. As an example for standard feature values, MUP template values documented in [62] are still considered standard values for MUP template duration, amplitude and shape.

The above muscle categorization techniques do not provide any measure of confidence. Probabilistic muscle categorization, on the other hand, addresses this weakness as it provides probabilities describing MUPT characterizations as well as the overall muscle characterization. More formally, a probabilistic MUPT characterization technique assigns a likelihood measure to each MUPT category under consideration. For each MUPT characterization, a set of n likelihood measures is obtained, where n is number of muscle categories under consideration (2 or 3) [4]. For each MUPT, this set of likelihood measures should sum to 1.

5.2.3.1. Aggregation of MUPT characterizations

Characterizations of MUPTs must be aggregated to obtain the overall muscle characterization of the muscle from which these MUPTs were detected. As with MUPTs, a set of n muscle likelihood measures is obtained, where n is the number of muscle categories and the muscle is considered to belong to the category that has the highest category likelihood value. Muscle likelihood values can be considered confidence measures in a particular characterization. In [64], [65], the idea of implementing probabilistic characterization and aggregating MUP template characterizations using Bayes' rule was first introduced. MUP template characterization was performed using Fisher's LDA. Other techniques used Bayes' rule to aggregate MUP template likelihood measures obtained from multiple classifiers like decision trees, LDA and Naive Bayes [56].

5.2.3.2. Measures of confidence and involvement

A muscle characterization likelihood value (measure) indicates the probability that the muscle, from which the characterized MUPTs were detected, actually belongs to the given category, conditioned on the evidence provided by the set of MUPT characterizations. Thus, a muscle characterization likelihood measure can be considered a measure of confidence in making a particular categorization based on the available evidence. For instance, a muscle confidence score of 75% for a given category means that, out of all the muscles that are assigned that score, 75% of such muscles actually belong to that category.

Another relevant concept in the context of muscle categorization is that of the level of involvement (LOI). When the values of the arithmetic mean of MUPT features are used to aggregate MUPT probabilities, the conditional probabilities resulting from a muscle characterization technique correlate well with the level of involvement (LOI) of a disease [66].

It is not easy to predict LOI due to the fact that confidence in making a correct muscle categorization decision at lower levels of disease involvement is low, which results in greater variability and lower accuracy in the LOI measurement [4].

6. Summary

An overview of the basis of EMG signals and the types of information they may contain depending on how they are detected was provided in addition to descriptions of various clinical QEMG techniques. The main objective was to emphasize the specific information targeted for extraction by clinical QEMG techniques and how this information can be extracted so that the sampled MUs, that created the MUPs comprising an EMG signal, can be accurately characterized and subsequently used to characterize and then categorize an examined muscle. Different clinical QEMG techniques were described. The bulk of the ongoing research in clinical QEMG is centered around improving muscle categorization accuracy using transparent clinical QEMG techniques so that characterization results can be explained to clinicians.

Author details

Tameem Adel* and Dan Stashuk

Department of Systems Design Engineering, University of Waterloo, Waterloo, Canada

References

[1] Campbell Biology, 6th edition

[2] Windhorst U, Johansson H. Modern techniques in neuroscience research. Springer; 1999

[3] H. Parsaei, D. W. Stashuk, S. Rasheed, C. Farkas, and A. Hamilton-Wright, "Intramuscular EMG Signal Decomposition," Crit Rev Biomed Eng, vol. 38, no. 5, pp. 435–465, 2010

[4] C. Farkas, A. Hamilton-Wright, H. Parsaei, and D. W. Stashuk, "A review of clinical quantitative electromyography," Crit Rev Biomed Eng, vol. 38, no. 5, pp. 467–485, 2010

[5] T. Adel, D. Stashuk, Muscle categorization using PDF estimation and Naïve Bayes classification," embc, 2012

[6] D. Dimitru, A. Amato, M. Zwarts, Electrodiagnostic Medicine, second edition.

[7] H. J. Huppertz et al., Muscle Nerve 20, 1360, 1997.

[8] William F. Brown, Charles F. Bolton, Michael J. Aminoff, Neuromuscular Function and Disease, Basic, Clinical, and Electrodiagnostic Aspects

[9] Pino L, Stashuk D, Boe S, Doherty T. Motor unit potential characterization using "pattern discovery". Medical Engineering & Physics. 2008 Jun;30(5):563-573.

[10] Christodoulou C, Pattichis C. Unsupervised pattern recognition for the classification of EMG signals. IEEE Trans. Biomed. Eng. 1999 Feb;46(2):169-178.

[11] Schizas CN, Middleton LT, Pattichis CS. Neural network models in EMG diagnosis. IEEE Transactions on Biomedical Engineering. 1995;42(5):486-496.

[12] Katsis CD, Exarchos TP, Papaloukas C, Goletsis Y, Fotiadis DI, Sarmas I. A two-stage method for MUAP classification based on EMG decomposition. Comput. Biol. Med. 2007;37(9):1232-1240.

[13] J. Blok, J. Van Dijk, G. Drost, M. Zwarts and D. Stegeman, A high-density multichannel surface electromyography system for the characterization of single motor units, Rev. Sci. Instrum. 73, 1887 (2002).

[14] Buchthal F, Kamieniecka Z, The diagnostic yield of quantified electromyography and quantified muscle biopsy in neuromuscular disorders. Muscle Nerve;2:265-280, 1982.

[15] Roeleveld K, Stegman DF, Falck B, Stalberg E. Motor unit size estimation: confrontation of surface EMG with macro EMG. EEG Clin Neurophysiol;105:181–8, 1997.

[16] Doherty TJ, Age-related changes in the numbers and physiological properties of human motor units. PhD Thesis, University of Western Ontario, 1993.

[17] Stashuk D. Decomposition and quantitative analysis of clinical electromyographic signals. Med Eng Phys; 21:389–404, 1999.

[18] Dan Stashuk, EMG signal decomposition: how can it be accomplished and used?, Journal of Electromyography and Kinesiology 11, 151–173, 2001.

[19] Stalberg EV. Macro EMG, a new recording technique. J Neurol Neurosurg Psychiat; 43:475–82, 1980.

[20] J.V. Basmajian, W. J. Forrest, G. Shine, A simple connector for fine-wire EMG electrodes. J Appl Physiol 21:1680, 1966.

[21] Petajan JH, AAEM Minimonograph # 3: Motor Unit Recruitment. Muscle Nerve; 14:489-502, 1991.

[22] Roberto Merletti, Dario Farina, Marco Gazzoni, The linear electrode array: a useful tool with many applications Journal of Electromyography and Kinesiology 13, 37–47, 2003.

[23] G. E. Loeb and C. Gans. Electromyography for Experimentalists, chapter 6, pages 60-70. The University of Chicago Press, Chicago, 1986

[24] Saksit, PhD Thesis, chapter 2: physiology of EMG

[25] American Association of Electrodiagnostic Medicine. Glossary of terms in electrodiagnostic medicine. Muscle Nerve. 2001;Suppl 10:S1-50.

[26] Ounjian, M., R.R. Roy, E. Eldred, A Garfinkel, J.R. Payne, A. Armstrong, A. Toga, and V.R. Edgerton Physiological and Developmental Implications of Motor Unit Anatomy. J. Neurobiol. 22:547-559, 1991. Motor unit territory.

[27] Bodine-Fowler, S., Garfinkel, A., Roy, Roland R., and Edgerton, V. Reggie. Spatial distribution of muscle fibres within the territory of a motor unit. Muscle and Nerve 13:1133-1145, 1990.

[28] Garnett, R. & Stephens, JA. The reflex responses of single motor units in human first dorsal interosseous muscle following cutaneous afferent stimulation. J. Physiol. Land. 303: 351-364, 1980.

[29] Kanda, K., Burke, R. E., & Walmsley, B. Differential control of fast and slow twitch motor units in the decerebrate cat. Exp. Brain Res. 29:57-74, 1977.

[30] Jennifer Hill, Exercise Physiology Student, Spring 2010 [http://www.unm.edu/~lkravitz/Exercise%20Phys/motorunitrecruit.html]

[31] Carlo DeLuca. Control Properties of Motor Units. J. exp. Biol. 115, 125-136, 1985

[32] Henneman, E., Somjen, G. & Carpenter, D. O. (1965). Functional significance of cell size in spinal motoneurons. J. Neurophysiol. 28, 560-580.

[33] Adrian ED & Zotterman Y. (1926). "The impulses produced by sensory nerve endings: Part II: The response of a single end organ.". J Physiol (Lond.) 61: 151–171.

[34] Hodson-Tole EF, Wakeling JM. Motor unit recruitment for dynamic tasks: current understanding and future directions. J Comp Physiol B. Jan 2009;179(1):57-66

[35] Gordon T, Thomas CK, Munson JB, Stein RB. The resilience of the size principle in the organization of motor unit properties in normal and reinnervated adult skeletal muscles. Can J Physiol Pharmacol. Aug-Sep 2004;82(8-9):645-61

[36] Miki Nikolic, PhD Thesis, Univ. of Copenhagen, 2001.

[37] Yamada R, Ushiba J, Tomita Y, Masakado Y. Decomposition of Electromyographic Signal by Principal Component Analysis of Wavelet Coefficient. IEEE EMBS Asian-Pacific Conference on Biomedical Engineering; Keihanna, Japan. pp. 118-119, 2003

[38] Zennaro D, Welling P, Koch VM, Moschytz GS, Laubli T. A Software Package for the Decomposition of Long-Term Multichannel EMG Signal Using Wavelet Coefficients. IEEE Trans Biomed Eng, 50(1):58–69. doi: 10.1109/TBME.2002.807321, 2003

[39] K. Roeleveld, J. H. Blok, D. F. Stegeman, A. van Oosterom, Volume Conduction Models for Surface EMG; Confrontation with Measurements

[40] Plonsey R: Bioelectric Phenomena. McGraw Hill, New York, 1969.

[41] Stegeman DF, Dumitru D, King JC, Roeleveld K: Near and far-fields: source characteristics and the conducting medium in neurophysiology. J Clin Neurophysiol (In press).

[42] Fang J, Agarwal GC, Shahani BT, Decomposition of EMG signals by wavelet spectrum matching. Procedures of the 19th Annual International Conference of the IEEE Engineering in Medicine and Biology Society; Chicago, IL, USA. pp. 1253-1256, 1997.

[43] Barkhaus PE, Nandedkar SD: Recording characteristics of the surface EMG electrodes. Muscle Nerve 17:1317–1323, 1994.

[44] Walter, C.B. Temporal quantification of electromyography with reference to motor control research. Human Movement Science 3: 155-162, 1984.

[45] M. Raez, M. Hussain, F. Mohd-Yasin, Techniques of EMG signal analysis: detection, processing, classification and applications

[46] Stashuk DW, Kassam A, Doherty TJ, Brown WF. Motor Unit Estimates Based on the Automated Analysis of F-Waves. Proceedings of the Annual International Conference on Engineering in Medicine and Biology Society. 1992;14:1452–1453.

[47] Micera S, Vannozzi G, Sabatini AM, Dario P. Improving detection of muscle activation intervals. IEEE Engineering in Medicine and Biology Magazine. 2001;20(6):38–46.

[48] Thexton AJ. A randomization method for discriminating between signal and noise in recordings of rhythmic electromyographic activity. J Neurosci Meth. 1996;66:93–98.

[49] Bornato P, de Alessio T, Knaflitz M. A statistical method for the measurement of the muscle activation intervals from surface myoelectric signal gait. IEEE Trans Biomed Eng. 1998;45:287–299. doi: 10.1109/10.661154.

[50] Determination of an optimal threshold value for muscle activity detection in EMG analysis Kerem Tuncay Ozgunen, Umut Celik and Sanli Sadi Kurdak, Journal of Sports Science and Medicine (2010) 9, 620-628

[51] Di Fabio, R.P, Reliability of computerized surface electromyography for determining the onset of muscle activity. Physical Theraphy 67(1), 43-48, 1987.

[52] Gary Kamen, David A. Gabriel, Essentials of Electromyography

[53] Pattichis CS, Elia AG. Autoregressive and cepstral analyses of motor unit action potentials. Med Eng Phys. 1999 Sep; 21(6-7):405-419.

[54] Katsis C, Goletsis Y, Likas A, Fotiadis D, Sarmas I. A novel method for automated EMG decomposition and MUAP classification. Artificial Intelligence in Medicine. 2006 May;37(1):55-64.

[55] Katsis CD, Exarchos TP, Papaloukas C, Goletsis Y, Fotiadis DI, Sarmas I. A two-stage method for MUAP classification based on EMG decomposition. Comput. Biol. Med. 2007;37(9):1232-1240.

[56] Pino L. Neuromuscular clinical decision support using motor unit potentials characterized by 'pattern discovery'. Ph.D. dissertation, Dept. Syst. Des. Eng., Univ. Waterloo, Waterloo, ON, Canada, 2009.

[57] A. Wong, and Y. Wang, "Pattern discovery: a data driven approach to decision support," IEEE Trans Syst Man Cybern Part C: Appl Rev, vol. 33, pp. 114–124, 2003.

[58] A. Wong and Y. Wang, "High-order pattern discovery from discrete valued data," IEEE Trans Knowled Data Eng vol. 9, pp. 877–893, 1997.

[59] A. Wong and Y. Wang "Discovery of high order patterns," IEEE Trans Syst Man Cybern, vol. 2, pp. 1142–1147, 1995.

[60] Y. Wang, "High-order pattern discovery and analysis of discrete valued data sets," Ph.D. Thesis, Univ. of Waterloo, Waterloo, 1997.

[61] Hamilton-Wright A, Stashuk DW. Clinical characterization of electromyographic data using computational tools. (2006). 2006 IEEE Symposium on Computational Intelligence and Bioinformatics and Computational Biology, 1-7, 2006.

[62] Buchthal F, Pinell P, Rosenfalck P. Action potential parameters in normal human muscle and their physiological determinants. Acta Physiol. Scand. 32(2-3):219-229, 1954.

[63] Xie H, Huang H, Wang Z. Multiple Feature Domains Information Fusion for Computer-Aided Clinical Electromyography, Computer Analysis of Images and Patterns, 304-312, 2005.

[64] Pfeiffer G, Kunze K. Discriminant classification of motor unit potentials (MUPs) successfully separates neurogenic and myopathic conditions. A comparison of multi- and univariate diagnostical algorithms for MUP analysis. Electroencephalography and Clinical Neurophysiology/Electromyography and Motor Control, 97(5):191-207, 1995.

[65] Pfeiffer G. The diagnostic power of motor unit potential analysis: An objective Bayesian approach. Muscle & Nerve, 22(5):584-591, 1999.

[66] Pino LJ, Stashuk DW. Using motor unit potential characterizations to estimate neuromuscular disorder level of involvement. In: 2008 30th Annual International Conference of the IEEE Engineering in Medicine and Biology Society. Vancouver, BC: 4138-4141, 2008.

[67] J. Malmivuo, R. Plonsey, Bioelectromagnetism, 1995.

Chapter 6

Age-Related Neuromuscular Adjustments Assessed by EMG

Adalgiso Coscrato Cardozo, Mauro Gonçalves,
Camilla Zamfolini Hallal and Nise Ribeiro Marques

Additional information is available at the end of the chapter

http://dx.doi.org/10.5772/55053

1. Introduction

Aging is characterized by changes in the neuromuscular system that decrease muscle strength, balance, proprioception and reaction time (Bassey, 1997). Aging may be accompanied by adjustments in muscle activation such as a decrease in voluntary activation and alterations in the rate of agonist/antagonist coactivation (Häkkinen et al., 1998). This progressive decline in physical capacities reduces the ability of older adults to perform complex motor tasks and is associated with impaired mobility and a reduction in the ability to live independently (Meuleman et al., 2000).

Assessment of muscle activation by electromyography (EMG) provides important information about age-related neuromuscular adjustments (Schmitz, et. al., 2009). EMG contributes to the identification of factors that generate impairments to the performance of daily activities and an increase in the risk of falls for older adults. Additionally, identifying age-related abnormal muscle activation may be helpful in preventing mobility impairments.

The aim of this chapter is to provide a global understanding of the EMG parameters used to identify age-related neuromuscular fatigability alterations. Towards this end, issues that affect EMG results in older adults will be presented, such as weakness and muscle activation abnormalities, muscle activation and fatigability, performance in daily activities, postural control changes, and the effects of physical activity on the neuromuscular system.

2. Weakness and muscles activation abnormalities

It is well described that age-related muscle strength loss causes a reduction in maximal voluntary joint torque and power production, resulting in clinical implications for older adults, particularly when this strength loss involves weakness in the lower limbs (Bento et al., 2010, LaRoche et al., 2010). It is also clear that this age-related weakness is not fully explained by muscle mass loss (Clark & Fielding, 2012). Recent studies have demonstrated that the decline of muscle mass only explains 6-10% of strength impairments and that muscle mass gains in older adults do not prevent this age-related weakness (Clark et al., 2006a, Clark et al., 2006b, Delmonico et al., 2009). Explanations of these phenomena have proposed that age-related loss of muscle strength is associated with impaired intrinsic force generation capacity and abnormalities in muscle fiber contractile and metabolic properties, excitation-contraction coupling and patterns of muscle activation (Clark & Fielding, 2012, Manini & Clark, 2012).

EMG is widely used to assess muscle activation and is used to highlight the relationship between muscle recruitment and age-related weakness (Clark et al., 2010, Ling et al., 2009, Watanabe et al., 2012, Wheeler et al., 2011). Muscle activation is a result of the excitation of motor neurons leading to force production in muscle fibers (Clark et al., 2010). Additionally, the quantity of motor units and the firing rates of these motor neurons play important roles in determining the intrinsic muscular force (Clark et al., 2010). Along these lines, age-related losses may be related to a suppressed ability of the central nervous system to maximize motor unit recruitment, resulting in a lower activation of agonist muscles (Clark et al., 2010). Other studies have proposed that age-related weakness is also associated with increased antagonist activation (Macaluso et al., 2002).

Recent studies showed that muscle strength is a good predictor of mobility and disability in older adults (Clark & Field, 2012). Clark et al. (2010) assessed the isometric strength of knee extensors (3 maximal trials of 3-5 seconds at 60º of knee flexion), the isokinetic strength of knee extensors (5 consecutive contractions at 60, 90, 180 and 240°.s^{-1}) and the EMG activation of knee extensors (Vastus Medialis, Vastus Lateralis and Rectus Femoris) and knee flexors (Biceps Femoris and Semimembranosus) in older adults with normal and impaired mobility. These authors identified that older adults with impaired mobility had lower activation of knee extensor muscles in all maximal isokinetic voluntary contractions. Additionally, the lower activation of knee extensor muscles was associated with lower torque and power in all isokinetic trials. Thus, the most novel result of this study is the demonstration that agonist muscle activation deficits may contribute to reduced lower limb strength. However, the findings of this study did not support the hypothesis that increases in antagonist coactivation leads in strength deficits during fast contractions (Clark et al., 2010).

Higher antagonist coactivation may not limit strength in older adults with different levels of mobility (Clark et al., 2010). However, age-related weakness may be influenced by increased antagonist coactivation (Macaluso et al., 2002). Macaluso et al. (2002) assessed vastus lateralis and biceps femoris activation during isometric contractions of knee extensors and knee flexors in young and older women. This study demonstrated that older women were on average 45% weaker than young women in knee flexor and extensor maximal torque. However, only in the

http://dx.doi.org/10.5772/55053

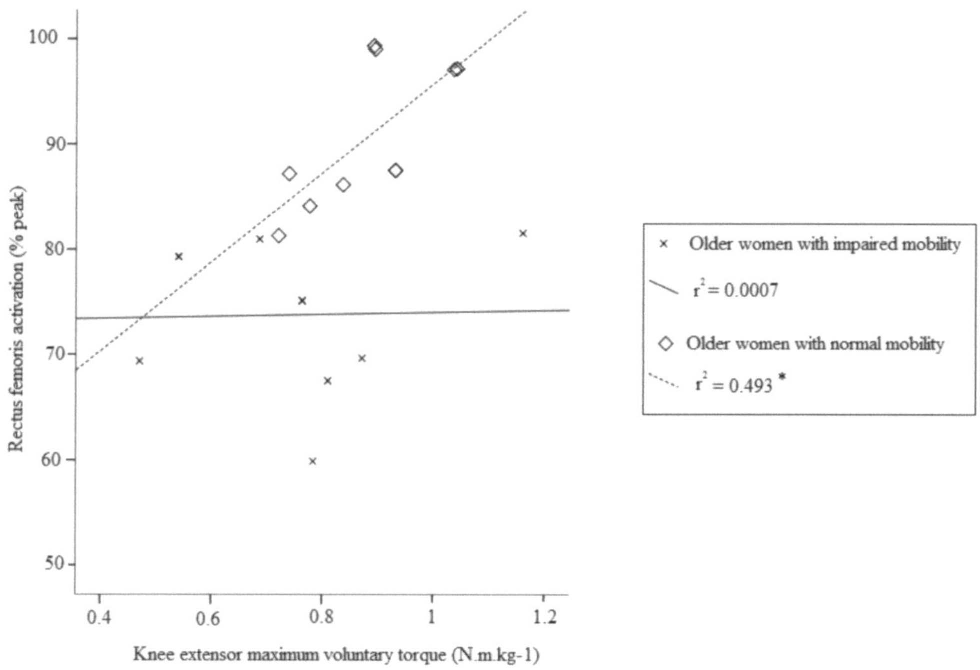

Figure 1. The relationship between knee extensor maximum voluntary torque and rectus femoris activation during a knee extensor isokinetic concentric movement in older women with impaired or normal mobility. * $p < 0.05$ (Cardozo et al., unpublished data).

contraction of knee extensors was a significantly higher antagonist coactivation found in older women. Thus, antagonist coactivation may contribute to decreased strength in older adults and, in agreement with Clark et al (2010), Macaluso et al. (2002) also proposed that decreased neural activation of the agonist muscles is another potential explanation for age-related weakness.

Ling et al. (2009) compared the surface-represented motor unit size and firing rate of the vastus medialis (VM) during knee extension at 10, 20, 30 and 50% of maximal voluntary contraction in young and old adults. These authors used EMG positioned at the VM motor point and discharged supramaximal stimulation on the femoral nerve. This study demonstrated that aging causes neuromuscular compensations that counteract Henneman's size principle (Henneman & Olson, 1965; Ling et al, 2009). According to this principle, the recruitment of larger motor units and the increase in their firing rates are progressive and consistent with increases in force level (Henneman & Olson, 1965, Ling et al., 2009). However, Ling et al. (2009) demonstrated that in contrast to young adults, old adults recruit larger motor units and have higher firing rates at low loads.

Figure 1 presents the relationship between knee extensor maximum voluntary torque and rectus femoris activation during a knee extensor isokinetic concentric movement in older women with impaired or normal mobility.

Thus, we can see that age-related muscle strength loss decreases maximal joint torque and power production, yet the muscle activation mechanisms that promote this behavior are still not well described.

3. Muscles activation and fatigability

Despite is expected a reduced fatigability in older adults, the findings of several studies is controversial (Allman & Rice, 2002, Avin & Frey Law, 2011).

During muscular fatigue, there are changes in the amplitude and frequency of the EMG signal (Cardozo & Gonçalves, 2003, Cardozo et al., 2011), which is dependent on the number of active motor units, their firing rates and the conduction velocity (Oliveira & Gonçalves, 2009). These changes are described in figure 2. Along these lines, EMG is widely used to highlight the muscular fatigue phenomenon in several populations, including people who suffer from back pain, athletes and, recently, older adults (Croscato et al., 2011, Fraga et al., 2011, Hunter et al., 2004, Lindström et al., 2006).

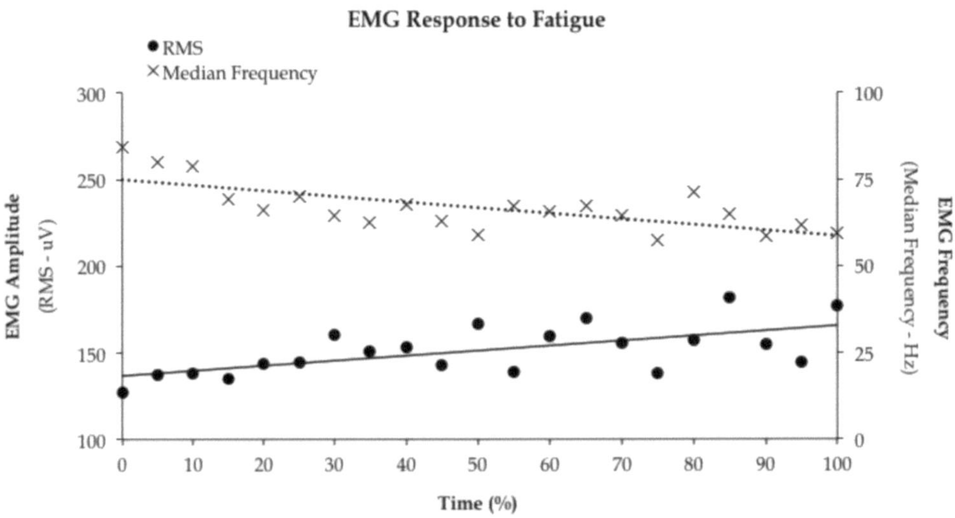

Figure 2. Amplitude (root mean square-RMS) and frequency (median frequency) behavior due to an isometric fatiguing protocol (Cardozo et al., unpublished data).

Hunter et al. (2004) compared the time to task failure, physiological responses (mean arterial pressure, heart rate, and rating of perceived exertion) and EMG responses at a sustained submaximal isometric contraction (20% of MVC) for elbow flexion in young and old men and women. The main finding of this study was that the time to task failure was longer with older adults, regardless of gender, and longer with young women than with young men. However, older adults had a reduced rate of increase in physiological parameters (mean arterial pressure, heart rate and rating of perceived exertion) and in EMG burst relative to younger adults. The authors speculated that changes in the EMG pattern were related to torque fluctuations. The authors concluded that motor unit activity increased most slowly during fatiguing submaximal efforts in older adults, possibly leading to increases in the time of task failure (Hunter et al., 2004).

Lindstrom et al. (2006) assessed the EMG activation of the vastus lateralis and rectus femoris during 100 repeated maximum knee extension contractions at $90^{\circ}.s^{-1}$ in young and old men and women. The authors found that older male adults were most fatigable according to the peak torque and EMG parameters (with a higher area based fatigue index and lower root mean square for the vastus lateralis in older men), but this group did not see the greatest fatigue according to the Borg scale. The authors suggested that the EMG amplitude revealed that fatigue is a combination of age-related changes in muscle and central activation failure (Lindstrom et al., 2006).

Aging leads to selective atrophy of type II fibers and increases the contribution of type I fibers to the generation of torque (Avin et al., 2011). However, even in low intensity activities (e.g., rising from a sitting position and walking) when torque is generated by the recruitment of type I fibers, older adults have a higher metabolic cost and higher fatigability than young subjects (Hortobágyi et al., 2011, Wert et al., 2010). This phenomenon is related to a declining VO2max (which occurs at a rate of approximately 8% per decade) and leads to older adults performing their daily activities at higher relative intensities (as measured by percentage of VO2max) than young people (Wilson and Tanaka, 2000). Additionally, recent studies have shown that the rate of consumption of VO_2 during walking is also related to the EMG activation pattern (Peterson & Martin, 2010, Hortobágyi et al., 2011).

Peterson and Martin (2010) and Hotobágyi et al. (2011) found a moderate association between higher Cw and increased antagonist coactivation of the thigh and calf muscles in older adults (Peter & Martin, 2010, Hortobágyi et al., 2011). According to Hortobágyi et al. (2011), older adults had an 18.4% higher Cw than young adults and this higher Cw was associated with increased antagonist coactivation (Vastus Lateralis x Biceps Femoris and Tibialis Anterior x Gastrocnemius Lateralis). Peterson and Martin (2010) determined that antagonist coactivation of the thigh (vastus medialis, biceps femoris and semitendinosus) had a higher contribution to the increase in Cw than the contribution from the shank (tibialis anterior, lateral soleus and medial gastrocnemius). Both studies suggested that age-related neuromuscular adaptations in the lower limbs decrease the joint instability and that a higher antagonist coactivation is required to maintain dynamic stability during a normal gait, which increases the Cw.

4. Performance in daily activities

Everyday tasks are motor acts performed during a day that contribute to physical independence, such as rising from a seated position, ascending or descending stairs, walking and taking a shower. Challenges encountered during daily activities, which are easily overcome by young adults, may represent a potential risk for falls among the elderly. Functional motor activities are especially difficult for older adults due to sensorimotor deficits related to age, exposing these older adults to fatal accidents and serious injuries (Korteling, 1994, Roeneker et al., 2003).

An age-related decline in the ability to perform physical tasks associated with daily living as well as in strength and muscle size may occur regardless of physical fitness or amount of training (Klitgaard et al., 1990, Schulz & Curnow, 1998). The decline in force and task performance may be related to alterations in the activation of motor units, decreases in muscle mass and increases in fat mass (Lexell, 1995).

Performance in daily tasks may be investigated by EMG in young and old persons. A study performed by Landers et al. (2001) analyzed integrated electromyography (IEMG) in two tasks of daily living: while the subjects sat down on a chair and while they carried a small load. The muscles analyzed were rectus femoris and biceps brachii. The raw EMG signal was recorded over six seconds for each collection point at a sample rate of 100 Hz. Subjects were given three practice trials, followed by three maximum isometric contractions at each test angle. The results showed that higher normalized integrated EMG values indicate greater muscular effort and, when combined with other tests, that biomechanical measures can provide information about muscle function in older adults.

The ability to walk efficiently and safely is important to maintain independence (Callisaya et al., 2010). However, the energy cost of gait in the elderly is higher than in young people, which can cause early fatigue (Hortobagyi et al., 2009). However, little is known about what makes the elderly more prone to fatigue during the gait, but existing hypotheses are that this fatigue is related to neuromuscular mechanisms, such as increased muscle coactivation (Burnett et. al., 2000, Hortobagyi et al., 2009, Macaluso et al., 2002). Increased coactivation might be used to optimize power generation and compensate for aging-related decline of neuromotor functioning, as manifested by reduced strength and power of muscles, reduced proportions of fast twitch muscle fibers and increased response times (Ishida et al., 2008).

Older adults also require greater effort relative to their available maximal capacity to execute daily motor tasks when compared with younger adults (Hortobagyi et al., 2003). This is due to a change in muscle fiber type with aging and a higher percentage of peak oxygen uptake required to perform daily tasks (Astrand et al., 1973, Waters et al., 1983). Higher physiological relative effort in elderly people may be the cause of premature fatigue associated with decline of motor function and, consequently, falls. Hortobagyi et al. (2003) tested the hypothesis that the relative effort to execute daily activities is higher in old adults compared with young adults. They assessed the vastus lateralis and biceps femoris muscles by EMG during the ascent and descent of stairs, the rise from a chair and the performance of maximal-effort isometric supine leg presses. The EMG signals were sampled at 1000 Hz, and the dependent variables included the average root mean square (RMS) EMG and EMG coactivity, expressed as a ratio of biceps femoris root mean square EMG with vastus lateralis RMS EMG activity. The results show that the relative vastus lateralis EMG activity is higher in old adults than young adults during some daily activities, and an association exists between the increased relative effort at the knee joint and increased muscle activation.

Stair descent and ascent are also important functional abilities (Holsgaard et al., 2011). Studies indicate that the elderly operated at a higher proportion of their maximal capacity than did young adults when performing tasks such as the safe descent of stairs (Reeves et al., 2008). Hinman et al. (2005) used EMG to record muscle activity during stair descent. They determined the effects of age on the onset of vastus medialis obliquus activity relative to that of vastus lateralis and the onset of quadriceps activity in the terminal swing relative to heel-strike during stair descent. Muscle onset was identified from individual EMG traces with a computer algorithm and was validated visually. The results show that older adults activated their quadriceps significantly earlier than the younger group during stair descent. Thus, quadricep activation may compensate for strength and balance impairments in older people during challenging activities.

Dexterous manipulations, such as eating and writing, may deteriorate due to aging (Keogh et al., 2007). Reduced hand function is related to the loss of finger-pinch force control (Keogh et al., 2006, Lazarus & Haynes, 1997, Ranganathan et al., 2001). Keogh et al. (2007) determined the effect of unilateral upper-limb strength training on the finger-pinch force control of older men by EMG. The EMG activity of the flexor pollicis brevis and flexor digitorum superficialis muscles was recorded using a sample rate of 1000 Hz, and the EMG data were subsequently filtered with a second-order Butterworth low-pass filter with the cutoff frequency set at 400 Hz. The amplitude of the electromyographic signals was obtained by using the RMS procedure with a bin size of 100 ms. The results show that a nonspecific upper-limb strength-training program may improve the finger-pinch force control of older men. However, additional studies are required to create strategies for the improvement of hand-held movements in older adults.

5. Changes in postural control

The capacity to maintain the body in an upright position in a stable state is critical to prevent falls in old people. This capacity requires the integration of visual feedback, the vestibular system, proprioception, reaction times and muscular responses. However, these mechanisms are negatively affected by aging, and therefore, the adaptive reflexes that respond to disturbances of balance are damaged (Abreu & Caldas, 2008). As a result of these changes, the elderly become more prone to falls (Tinetti, 2003).

EMG can evaluate the response of muscles during postural control in different situations requiring the integrity of the neuromuscular system. Figure 3 presents the time delay between a perturbation (accelerometer signal) and the muscle activation (EMG onset) response obtained by EMG analyses of the tibialis anterior muscle. This time delay is negatively affected by the aging process, promoting slower responses in old adults. This behavior may increase the risk of falls in this population when the muscle activation may not be fast enough to maintain stability after a perturbation.

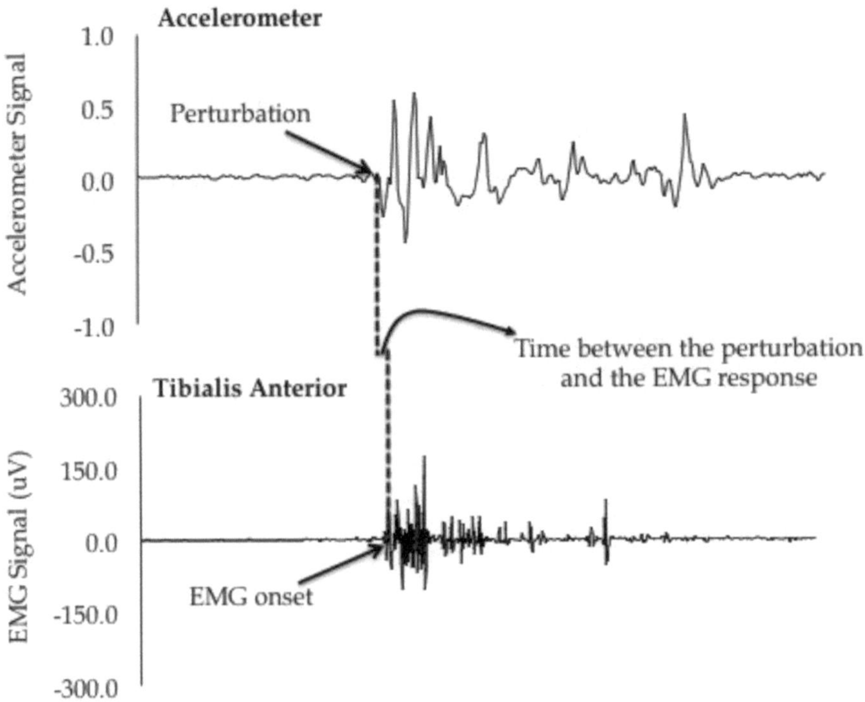

Figure 3. EMG response due to perturbation (Cardozo et al., unpublished data).

Older people have different strategies to maintain posture in balance situations: the ankle strategy responds to slow disturbances; the hip strategy is used on larger and faster displacements of the center of pressure (COP); and the step strategy is used when the others are not able to return the COP to the support base, using quick jumps or steps (Vanicek et al., 2009).

Another strategy used by older adults is an increase in antagonistic muscle activation during balance recovery (Mixco et al., 2012). This coactivation can be a necessary change to compensate for the decline in postural control associated with aging (Nagai et al., 2011). Additionally, Freitas et al. (2009) have shown that older adults activated their muscles and were able to reach the peak of activation. However, they retained a higher level of activation longer than younger adults.

As a result of the aging process, reaction time tends to increase due to the atrophy of fast twitch fibers with aging. This atrophy contributes to a lower power output, slower sensory feedback and slower muscle onset, resulting in ineffectiveness of equilibrium recovery after disturbances (Pijnappels et al., 2008).

Due to physiological changes resulting from the aging process, recovery strategies are slower and therefore less effective in old adults (Mian et al., 2007). Thus, to minimize these changes, physical activity is highly recommended and widely used as an intervention to prevent falls.

6. Effects of physical activity on the neuromuscular system

Decreases in maximal isometric, concentric, and eccentric forces, force development rate and muscle power are all age-related effects (Granacher et al., 2010, Petrella et al., 2005, Skelton et al., 1994). Regular physical exercise for the elderly population has been identified as an important intervention in the treatment and recovery of some diseases (Bassey, 1997). As the functional benefit of exercise may be greatest in older adults, in recent years, there have been several studies about the effects of physical activity on the neuromuscular system of this population.

Traditional strength training protocols can still be recommended to improve muscle strength and voluntary neural activity in older adults (Fung & Hughey, 2005, Runge et. al., 1998). However, other types of training have been shown to develop strength, power and balance in this population. Resistance training with power training and ballistic strength training may be effective for improving explosive force production and functional performance in old age (Granacher et al., 2011). Orr et al. (2006) show that power training at low intensities can improve balance, power, strength and endurance in the lower limb muscles of older adults. Recent studies have also shown that whole body vibration and resistance exercises combined with vascular occlusion may improve muscle strength (Granacher et al., 2012, Rabert et al., 2011, Takarada et al., 2000). Figure 4 shows the influence of an active lifestyle on increasing healthy life expectancy.

The assessment of lower limb muscle activity provides important information about neuromuscular behavior before and after physical activities (Schmitz et al., 2009). EMG can identify changes in the motor skills of older adults and help create prevention strategies for age-associated changes in neuromuscular factors that can impair daily activities and increase the rate of falls among this population.

A recent study investigated the effects of strength and endurance exercises over the course of 12 weeks in older adults. The maximal neuromuscular activity of agonist muscles was evaluated using EMG (RMS) in the vastus lateralis and rectus femoris and antagonist co-activation in the biceps femoris long head. The sampling frequency was 2000 Hz, and the data were filtered using a Butterworth band-pass filter of the fourth order with a cutoff frequency between 20 and 500 Hz. The RMS values of the antagonist biceps femoris muscle were normalized by the maximum RMS values of this muscle. After determination of the maximal neuromuscular activity, the submaximal neuromuscular activity was evaluated to determine the isometric neuromuscular economy. The results show that training in older adults resulted in greater changes in neuromuscular economy as assessed by EMG (Cardore et al., 2012). Similarly, Cardore et al. (2011) investigated the effects of concurrent training on endurance capacity and dynamic neuromuscular economy in elderly men. During the maximal test, muscle activation was measured at each intensity by means of electromyographic signals from the vastus lateralis, rectus femoris, biceps femoris long head, and gastrocnemius lateralis to determine the dynamic neuromuscular economy. Changes in the myoelectric activity of the Rectus Femoris and Vastus Lateralis muscles were observed as an adaptative response after strength and endurance training.

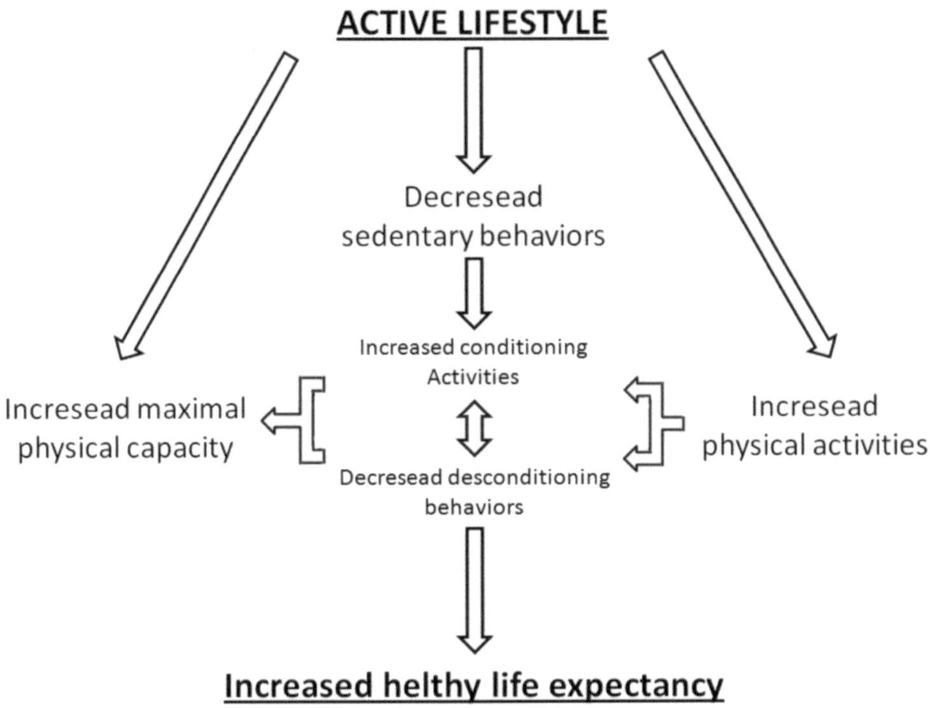

Figure 4. An active lifestyle enhances physical activity and decreases sedentary behaviors (Cardozo et al., unpublished data).

Valkeinen et al. (2006) examined the EMG activity after a 21 week strength training period in elderly woman with fibromyalgia. The EMG activity of the right vastus lateralis and vastus medialis muscles was recorded during maximal isometric leg extensions, and the results were expressed as the mean integrated EMG activity. There was a large increase in the maximal force and EMG activity of the muscles, indicating that strength training for elderly people can increase neuromuscular functional performance. Hakkinen et al. (2001) examined neuromuscular adaptations in middle-aged and older men and women during a resistance training period of 6 months. The EMG activity during the unilateral extension actions of the knee muscles was recorded from the agonist muscles vastus lateralis and vastus medialis and from the biceps femoris. The EMG signal was collected at 1000Hz, full wave rectified and integrated. The results show that there were increases in the EMG integrated magnitude of the agonist muscle during isometric and concentric leg extensions at maximal voluntary contraction in older women after training. This finding may be related to changes in the muscle activation pattern providing a recruitment pattern (Hakkinen et al., 1998, Hakkinen et al., 2001, Ling et al., 2009). Additionally, the EMG changes can also be related to reduced antagonist muscle coactivation (Hakkinen et al., 2001). This phenomenon may enhance the agonists' force production, which is important in older adults during multijoint actions (Hakkinen et al., 1998).

Furthermore, the maintenance of balance during daily activities may represent a challenge for older adults (Bugnariu & Fung, 2007). Aging is also associated with a decrease in the ability to control the body's position, requiring input from the afferent receptor systems to generate an appropriate motor response in dynamic and static activities (Alexander, 1994, Granacher et al., 2012, Woollacott & Shumway-Cook, 2002). Due to age-related decline in the integrity of many postural regulating systems, rehabilitation is needed to promote the re-acquisition of motor skills (Maki & Mcllroy, 1996). Along these lines, physical exercise is the most common intervention to prevent the consequences of balance perturbations, such as falls, fractures and death (Alfieri et al., 2012, Morey et al., 2008).

To improve balance, physical activity protocols include progressively difficult postures that reduce the base of support as well as dynamic movements that perturb the center of gravity, stress postural muscle groups and reduce sensory input (Granacher et al., 2012). In addition, multisensory exercises that stimulate all three afferent systems can be a good strategy for intervention (Alfieri et al., 2010, Bruin & Murer, 2007, Nitz & Choy, 2004, Orr et al., 2008;). Bugnariu & Fung (2007) investigated the effects of aging and adaptation on the capability of the central nervous system to select pertinent sensory information and resolve sensory conflicts. EMG activity was collected from the tibialis anterior, gastrocnemius medialis, vastus lateralis, semitendinosus, tensor fascia lata, erector spinae, neck extensor and neck flexor sternocleidomastoideus. Functional balance and mobility were assessed before and after virtual environment exposure and perturbation trials. The group found that after exposure to sensory conflicts, the central nervous system can adapt to the changes and improve balance capability in the elderly.

7. Conclusion

This chapter presents a global understanding of age-related neuromuscular alterations, such as weakness and fatigue, and the use of EMG parameters in their identification. Neuromuscular adaptations due to aging influence the ability of the elderly to maintain the capacity to perform daily activities and to modulate their postural control. Additionally, physical activity can improve neuromuscular functional ability in older people.

Acknowledgements

The authors would like to thank the Biomechanics Laboratory of the Department of Physical Education (Instituto de Biociências de Rio Claro, UNESP – Univ Estadual Paulista) and the Fundação de Amparo à Pesquisa do Estado de São Paulo (FAPESP).

Author details

Adalgiso Coscrato Cardozo, Mauro Gonçalves, Camilla Zamfolini Hallal and Nise Ribeiro Marques

UNESP – Univ Estadual Paulista, Brazil

References

[1] Abreu SSE & Caldas CP. Velocidade de marcha, equilíbrio e idade: um estudo correlacional entre idosas praticantes e idosas não praticantes de um programa de exercícios terapêuticos. *Rev Bra. Fisioter* 2008; 12(4): 324-330.

[2] Alexander NB. Postural control in older adults. *J Gerontol A Biol Sci Med Sci.* 1994; 42: 93-108.

[3] Alfieri FM, Guirro RRJ & Teodori RM. Postural stability of elderly submitted to multisensorial physical therapy intervention. *Electromyogr Clin Neurophysiol* 2010; 50: 113–119.

[4] Alfieri FM, Riberto M, Gatz LS, Ribeiro CPC, Lopes JAF & Battistella LR. Comparison of multisensory and strenght training for a postural control in the elderly. *Clin Interv in Aging* 2012; 7: 119-125.

[5] Allman BL & Rice CL. Neuromuscular fatigue and aging: central and peripheral factors. *Muscle and Nerve* 2002: 25: 785-796.

[6] Astrand I, Astrand PO, Hallback I & Kilbom A. Reduction in maximal oxygen uptake with age. *J Appl Physiol* 1983; 35: 649–654.

[7] Avin KG & Frey Law LA. Age-related differences in muscle fatigue vary by contraction type: a meta-analysis. *Physic Ther J* 2011; 91: 1153-1165.

[8] Bassey EJ. Physical capabilities, exercise and aging. *Rev Clin Geront* 1997; 7: 289-297.

[9] Bento PCB, Pereira G, Ugrinowitsch C & Rodacki ALF. Peak torque and rate of torque development in elderly with and without fall history. *Clin Biomech* 2010; 25: 450–454.

[10] Bruin ED & Murer K. Effect of additional functional exercises on balance in elderly people. *Clin Rehabil* 2007; 21: 112–121.

[11] Bugnariu N & Fung J. Aging and selective sensoriomotor strategies in the regulation of upright balance. *J NeuroEng Rehab* 2007; 4: 1-7.

[12] Burnett RA et al. Coactivation of the antagonist muscle does not covary with steadiness in old adults. *J Appl Physiol* 2000; 89: 61-71.

[13] Callisaya ML et al. Ageing and gait variability - a population - based study on older people. *Age and Ageing* 2010; 39: 191-197.

[14] Cardore EL et al. Effects of strength, endurance, and concurrent training on aerobic power and dynamic neuromuscular economy in elderly men. *J Strenght Cond Res* 2011; 25(3):758-766.

[15] Cardore, EL et al. Neuromuscular adaptations to concurrent training in the elderly: effects of intrasession exercise sequence. *Age* 2012 (Epub ahead of print).

[16] Cardozo AC & Gonçalves M. Eletromyographic fatigue threshold of erector spinae muscle induced by a muscular endurance test in health men. *Electromyogr Clin Neurophysiol* 2003; 43: 377-380.

[17] Cardozo AC, Gonçalves M & Dolan P. Back extensor muscle fatigue at submaximal workloads assessed using frequency banding of the electromyographic signal. *Clin Biomech* 2011; 26: 971-976.

[18] Charansonney OL. Physical activities and aging: A life-long story. *Discov Med* 2011; 12: 177-185.

[19] Clark BC, Fernhall B & Ploutz-Snyder LL. Adaptations in human neuromuscular function following prolonged unweighting: I. Skeletal muscle contractile properties and applied ischemia efficacy. *J Appl Physiol* 2006a; 101: 256–263.

[20] Clark BC, Manini TM, Bolanowski SJ & Ploutz-Snyder LL. Adaptaptions in human neuromuscular function following prolonged un-weighting: II. Neurological properties and motor imagery efficacy. *J Appl Physiol* 2006b; 101: 264–272.

[21] Clark DJ & Fielding RA. Neuromuscular contributions to age-related weakness. *J Gerontol A Biol Sci Med Sci* 2012; 67A: 41-47.

[22] Clark DJ, Patten C, Reid KF, Carabello RJ, Phillips EM & Fielding RA. Impaired voluntary neuromuscular activation limits muscle power in mobility-limited older adults. *J Gerontol A Biol Sci Med Sci* 2010; 65: 495-502.

[23] de Freitas PB, Knight CA & Barela JA. (2009). Postural reactions following forward platform perturbation in young, middle-age, and old adults. *Conf Proc IEEE Eng Med Biol Soc* 2009; 6271-6275.

[24] Delmonico MJ, Harris TB, Visser M, Park SW, Conroy MB, Velasquez-Mieyer P et al. Longitudinal study of muscle strength, quality, and adipose tissue infiltration. *Am J Clin Nutri* 2009; 90: 1579–1585.

[25] Geel SE & Robergs RA. The effect of graded resistance exercise on fibromyalgia symptoms and muscle bioenergetics: a pilot study. *Arthritis Rheum* 2002; 47: 82–86.

[26] Granacher U, Gruber M & Gollhofer A. Force production capacity and functional reflex activity in young and elderly men. *Aging Clin Exp Res* 2010; 22: 374–382.

[27] Granacher U, Muehlbauer T & Gruber M. A Qualitative review of balance and strength performance in healthy older adults: impact for testing and training. J Aging Res 2012 (Epub ahead of print).

[28] Granacher U, Muehlbauer T, Zahner L, Gollhofer A & Kressig RW. Comparison of traditional and recent approaches in the promotion of balance and strength in older adults. *Sports Medicine* 2011; 41: 377–400.

[29] Hakkinen A, Hakkinen K, Hannonen P & Alen M. Strenght training induced adaptations in neuromuscular function of premenopausal women with fibromyalgia: comparison with healthy women. *Ann Rheum Dis* 2001; 60: 21-26.

[30] Hakkinen K, Hakkinen A, Kraemer WJ, Hakkinen A, Valkeinen H & Alen M. Selective muscle hypertrophy, changes in EMG and force, and serum hormones during strength training in older women. *J Appl Physiol* 2001; 91: 569-580.

[31] Hakkinen K, Kallinen M, Izquierdo M, Jokelainen K, Lassila H, Malkia E, Kraemer WJ, Newton RU & Alen M. Changes in agonist-antagonist EMG, muscle CSA and force during strength training in middle-aged and older people. *J Appl Physiol* 1998; 84: 1341–1349.

[32] Hakkinen K, Kraemer WJ, Newton RU. Changes in electromyographic activity, muscle fiber and force production characteristics during heavy resistance/power strength training in middle-aged and older men and women. *Acta Physiol Scand* 2001; 171: 51–62.

[33] Henneman E & Olson CB. Relationship between structure and function in the design of skeletal muscles. *J Neurophysiol* 1965; 28: 581-590.

[34] Hinman RS et al. Age-related changes in electromyographic quadriceps activity during stair descent. *J Orthop Res* 2005; 23(2): 322-326.

[35] Holsgaard LA et al. Stair-ascent performance in elderly women: effect of explosive strength training. *J aging Phys Act* 2011; 19(2): 117-136.

[36] Hortobagyi T, Mizelle C, Beam S & DeVita P. Old adults perform activities of daily living near their maximal capabilities. *J Gerontol A Biol Sci Med Sci* 2003; 58(5): 453–460.

[37] Hortobágyi T et al. Interaction between age and gait velocity in the amplitude and timing of antagonist muscle coactivation. *Gait & Posture* 2009; 29: 558-564.

[38] Hortobágyi T, Finch A, Solnik S et al. Association between muscle activation and metabolic cost of walking in young and old adults. *J Gerontol A Biol Sci Med Sci* 2011; 66A: 541-547.

[39] Hunter SK, Critchlow A & Enoka RM. Influence of aging and sex differences in muscle fatigability. *J Appl Physiol* 2006; 97: 1723-1732.

[40] Ishida A et al. Stability of the human upright stance depending on the frequency of external disturbances. *Med Biol Eng Comput*. 2008; 46: 213-221.

[41] Keogh J. W, Morrison S, Barrett R. (2006). Age-related differences in interdigit coupling during finger pinching. Eur J Appl Physiol, Vol. 97, pp. 76-88.

[42] Keogh J. W, Morrison S, Barrett R. (2007).Strength Training Improves the Tri-Digit Finger-Pinch Force Control of Older Adults. Arch Phys Med Rehabil, Vol. 88, pp. 1055-1063.

[43] Klitgaard H, Mantoni M, Schiaffino S. (1990). Function, morphology and protein expression of ageing skeletal muscle: a cross-sectional study of elderly men with different training backgrounds. Acta Physiol Scand, Vol. 140, pp. 41–54.

[44] Korteling, J. (1994). Effects of aging, skill modification and demand alternation on multiple-task performance. *Hum Factors*, Vol. 32, No.5, pp. 597-608.

[45] Landers K. A., Hunter G. R., Wetzstein C. J., Bamman M. M., Weinsier R. L. (2001). The interrelationship among muscle mass, strength, and the ability to perform physical tasks of daily living in younger and older women. Journal of Gerontology, Vol. 56 (10), pp. 443-448.

[46] Laroche, D. P., Cremin, K. A., Greenleaf, B., Croce, R. V. (2010). Rapid torque development in older female fallers and nonfallers: A comparison across lower-extremity muscles. *Journal of Electromyography and Kinesiology*, Vol.20, pp. 482-488.

[47] Lazarus J. C, Haynes J. M. (1997). Isometric pinch force control and learning in older adults. Exp Aging Res, Vol. 23, pp. 179-199.

[48] Lexell J. (1995). Human aging, muscle mass, and fiber type composition. J Gerontol Biol Sci Med Sci, Vol. 50, pp. 11–16.

[49] Lindström, B., Karlsson J. S., Lexell J. (2006). Isokinetic torque and surface electromyography during fatiguing muscle contraction in young and older men and women. *Isokinetic and Exercise Exercise*, Vol.14, pp. 225-234.

[50] Ling SM, Conwit RA, Ferrucci L, Metter EJ. (2009). Age-associated changes in motor unit physiology: observations from the Baltimore Longitudinal Study of Aging. *Archive of Physical Medicine and Rehabilitation*, Vol.90, pp. 1237-1240.

[51] Macaluso, A. et. al. (2002). Contractile muscle volume and agonist-antagonist coactivation account for differences in torque between young and older women. Muscle Nerve, Vol. 25, pp. 858-863.

[52] Macaluso, A., Nimmo, M.A., Foster, J.E., Cockburn, M., McMillan, F.R.C.P., DeVito, G. (2002). Contractile muscle volume and agonist-antagonist coactivation account for differences in torque between young and older women. *Muscle & Nerve*, Vol.25, pp. 858-863.

[53] Maki B. E, McIlroy W. E (1996). Postural control in the older adult. Clin Geriatr Med, Vol. 12, pp. 635-658.

[54] Manini, T. M., Clark, B. C. (2012). Dynapenia and Aging: an Update. *The Journal of Gerontology Series A: Biological Science and Medicine Science*, Vol.67A, pp. 28-40.

[55] Meuleman, J. R. et. al. (2000). Exercise training in the debilitates aged: strength and functional outcomes. *Arch. Phys. Rehabil*, Vol.81, pp. 312-318.

[56] Mixco A., Reynolds M., Tracy B., Reiser R. F. (2012). Aging-related cocontraction effects during ankle strategy balance recovery following tether release in women. *J Electromyogr Kinesiol*, Vol. 22(1), pp. 31-36.

[57] Morey M. C, Sloane R, Pieper C. F. (2008). Effect of physical activity guidelines on physical function in older adults. J Am Geriatr Soc, Vol. 4, pp. 1873-1878.

[58] Nagai K., Yamada M., Uemura K., Yamada Y., Ichihashi N., Tsuboyama T. (2011). Differences in muscle coactivation during postural control between healthy older and young adults. *Age*, Vol. 33(3), pp. 393-407.

[59] Nitz J. C, Choy N. L. (2004). The efficacy of a specific balance-strategy training program for preventing falls among older people: a pilot randomized controlled trial. Age Agein, Vol. 33, pp. 52–58.

[60] Orr R, Raymond J, Sigh M. F. (2008). Efficacy of progressive resistance training on balance performance in older adults. Sports Med, Vol. 38, pp. 317–343.

[61] Orr R, Vos N. J, Singh N. A, Ross D. A, Stavrinos T. M, Fiatarone-Singh M. A. (2006). Power training improves balance in healthy older adults. The Journals of Gerontology, Vol. 61, pp. 78–85.

[62] Peterson, D. S., Martin, P. E. (2011). Effects of age and walking speed on coactivation and cost of walking in healthy adults. *Gait and Posture*, Vol.31, pp. 355-359.

[63] Petrella J. K, Kim J. S, Tuggle S. C, Hall S. R, Bamman M. M. (2005). Age differences in knee extension power, contractile velocity, and fatigability. Journal of Applied Physiology, Vol. 98, pp. 211–220.

[64] Pijnappels M, Reeves ND, Maganaris CN, Van Dieen JH. (2008). Tripping without falling; lower limb strength, a limitation for balance recovery and a target for training in the elderly. J. Electromyogr. Kinesiol. Vol. 18(12), p. 188-196.

[65] Rabert M. S, Zapata M. J. M, Vanmeerhaeghe A. F, Abella F. R, Rodríguez D. R, Bonfill X. (2011). Whole body vibration for older persons: an open randomized, multicentre, parallel, clinical trial. BMC Geriatrics, Vol. 11, pp. 1-6.

[66] Ranganathan V. K, Siemionow V, Saghal V, Yue G. (2001). Effects of aging on hand function. J Am Geriatr Soc 2001;49:1478-84. 3. Carmeli E, Patish H, Coleman R. The aging hand. J Gerontol A Biol Sci Med Sci, Vol. 58, pp. 146-152.

[67] Reeves, N. D. et. al. (2008). The demands of stair descent relative to maximum capacities in elderly and young adults. *J Electromyogr Kinesiol*, Vol. 12, No. 2, pp. 218-227.

[68] Roeneker D. et al. (2003). Speedof-processing and driving simulator training result in improved driving performance. *Hum Factors*, Vol. 45, No.2, pp. 218-234.

[69] Russ, D.W., Kent-Braun, J.A. (2003). Sex difference in human skeletal muscle fatigue are eliminate under ischemic condition. *Journal of Applied Physiology*, Vol.94, pp. 2412-2422.

[70] Schmitz, A. et. al. (2009). Differences in lower-extremity muscular activation during walking between healthy older and young adults. Journal of Electromyography and Kinesiology, Vol. 19, pp. 1085-1091.

[71] Schulz R, Curnow C. (1998). Peak performance and age among superathletes: track and field, swimming, baseball, tennis, and golf. J Gerontol, Vol. 43, pp. 113–120.

[72] Skelton D. A, Greig C. A, Davies J. M., Young A. (1994). Strength, power and related functional ability of healthy people aged 65–89 years. Age & Ageing, Vol. 23, pp. 371–377.

[73] Takarada Y, Takazawa H, Sato Y, Takebayashi S, Tanaka Y, Ishii N. (2000). Effects of resistance exercise combined with moderate vascular occlusion on muscular function in humans. J Appl Physiol, Vol. 88, PP. 2097–2106.

[74] Tinetti M. (2003) Preventing falls in elderly persons. N. Eng. J. Med. Vol. 348(1), pp. 42-49.

[75] Valkeinen H, Alen M, Hannonen P, Hakkinen A, Airaksinen O, Hakkinen K. (2004). Changes in knee extension and flexion force, EMG and functional capacity during strength training in older females with fibromyalgia and healthy controls. Rheumatology (Oxford), Vol. 43, pp. 225–228.

[76] Valkeinen H, Hakkinen A, Hannonen P, Hakkinen K, Alen M (2006). Acute heavy-resistance exercise induced pain and neuromuscular fatigue in elderly women with fibromyalgia and healthy controls: effects of strength training. Arthritis & Rheumatism, Vol. 54, pp. 1334-1339.

[77] Vanicek N, Strike S, McNaughton L, Polman R. (2009). Postural responses to dynamic perturbations in amputee fallers versus nonfallers: a comparative study with able-bodied subjects. Arch. Phys. Med. Rehabil. Vol. 90(6), pp. 1018-1025.

[78] Watanabe, K., Kouzaki, M., Merletti, R., Fujibayashi, M., Moritani, T. (2012). Spatial EMG potential distribution pattern of vastus lateralis muscle during isometric knee extension in young and elderly men. *Journal of Electromyography and Kinesiology*, Vol.22, pp. 74-79.

[79] Waters R. L., Hislop H. J., Perry J, Thomas L, Campbell J. (1983). Comparative cost of walking in young and old adults. J Orthop Res, Vol. 1, pp. 73–76.

[80] Wheeler, K. A., Kumar, D. K., Shimada, H., Arjunan, S. P., Kalra, C. (2011). Surface EMG model of the bicep during aging: a preliminary study. *Conference Procedures of IEEE Engenering in Medicine and Biological Society*. 2011;2011:7127-30.

[81] Woollacott M, Shumway-Cook A. (2002). Attention and the control of posture and gait: a review of an emerging area of research. *Gait Posture*, Vol. 16, pp. 1-14.

[82] Mian, OS, Baltzopoulos V, Minetti AE, Narici MV. The impact of physical training on locomotor function in older people. Sports Med.2007; 37(8):683-701.

Chapter 7

SYNERGOS: A Multiple Muscle Activation Index

Amir Pourmoghaddam, Daniel P O'Connor,
William H Paloski and Charles S Layne

Additional information is available at the end of the chapter

http://dx.doi.org/10.5772/56168

1. Introduction

An important movement control strategy used by the central nervous system (CNS) is the activation of multiple muscles acting in concert with each other to achieve a specific movement [1-6]. The specific temporal pattern of motor unit firing, the number of recruited motor units, and the intensity of the firing units result in a state of Multiple Muscle Activation (MMA) during each movement. We hypothesized that quantifying the MMA would provide information about certain states of muscle activation used by the CNS at any moment of a given movement activity. As neuromuscular disorders disrupt the firing characteristics of the motor units by which the CNS controls human movement, quantifying the degree of MMA might be useful as an assessment tool for these disorders. Additionally, monitoring changes in MMA over time might provide valuable information about the progression of a disease state or conversely, a recovery profile. Currently, no easily implemented screening technique for use in clinical settings exists that allow the changes in the MMA to be measured and tracked over time. Therefore, developing a single value that quantifies the degree of activation among multiple muscles that accounts for temporal and magnitude changes in muscle activity in a combinatorial fashion may be of value to clinicians and researchers interested in evaluating alterations in muscle activation due to different physiological and environmental constraints. In this chapter, a new index, "SYNERGOS" (from the Greek word for "working together") is introduced to quantify the level of MMA. At its core, SYNERGOS systematically identifies the changes in muscle activity depicted by electromyography (EMG) signals obtained from multiple muscles and summarizes the coactivity among these muscles into a single scalar quantifying the MMA over a predefined period (i.e. in this report, the gait cycle) during a variety of movements.

Surface EMG is commonly used to investigate neuromuscular activation during human movements. EMG can provide insight into the relationship between the underlying activity of the CNS and the resulting muscle contractions that produce the observable movement. Such insight sheds light on the different neuromuscular activation patterns in both healthy movements and disease states [7, 8]. However, several studies identified the inherent stochastic characteristics of EMG signals and recommended applying nonlinear data analysis to investigate the underlying nonlinear features (i.e. determinism) of the signal [9-16]. Recurrence Quantification Analysis (RQA) has shown promising results to detect subtle changes in EMG signals which can be missed by the application of linear data analysis. RQA quantifies several parameters such as percentage of recurrence (% REC) and percentage of determinism (% DET) to detect such subtle changes in dynamical state of EMG signal [13, 15-18]. % DET is an indication of the underlying deterministic patterns in a dynamical system that is associated with the degree that an EMG signal "recurs," or is predictable [15, 16, 18] as a result of increasing firing rate in recruited motor units [9, 10, 16, 18]. % DET has shown significant sensitivity to the change in the amount of loading and duration of a movement during both static and dynamic movements [13-18]. In this study, the % DET obtained from the RQA for each recorded muscle during predefined duration (i.e. gait cycles within each gait speed) is a single value used as an input for calculation of SYNERGOS index for each gait cycle.

Previous authors have proposed techniques that have demonstrated that individual muscles are not independently controlled by the CNS during movement [2, 4, 6, 19]. These methods of quantifying multiple muscle activities provide several time-variant and time-invariant parameters [2, 4] or several modes [6, 20, 21] demonstrating the level of activation of each muscle during a movement. These techniques share some features in common with SYNERGOS, namely the application of EMG to detect the multi-muscle actions during various activities and the use of sophisticated techniques to explore the underlying dynamics associated with the muscle activation controlling limb motion. While having these features in common with SYNERGOS, these techniques are designed to investigate and parameterize the underlying synergies by quantifying different modes of multiple muscle actions during body movements so that relative time-invariant contributions of different muscles can be identified. Conversely, SYNERGOS is not designed to identify multiple modes of activation synergies but rather SYNERGOS is unique in that a single index value accounting for the simultaneous activity of all muscles during a given movement, or over time in the case of cyclical movements (e.g., one index for each gait cycle), can be conveniently assessed.

In this report, we assess the potential of the SYNERGOS technique to evaluate changes in MMA between walking and running conditions that use different muscle activation strategies due to differences in the complexity of these movements [22]. We hypothesized that the SYNERGOS method can detect significant differences in quantified MMA during walking vs. running due to higher level of coactivities resulted from more frequent and intense simultaneous neuromuscular activities depicted by EMG signals. Additionally we hypothesized that the SYNERGOS method was significantly sensitive to identify the changes in MMA associated with small but incrementally increasing gait speed beginning with a slow walk and concluding with running. These hypotheses were based on previous studies indicating an elevated muscle coactivation associated with higher gait speed (modeled by faster knee extension/flexion) [23, 24]. In this study, the cyclic movement of walking and running was chosen, which by their nature, maintain their general kinematic form as speed increases but the underlying MMA is modulated in concordance with increasing speed. We believe that if SYNERGOS can detect minute changes in MMA associated with slight increases in locomotion speed it may have functional utility to evaluate MMA during a variety of movements.

2. Method

2.1. Subjects

Ten, healthy University of Houston students participated in the study at the Laboratory of Integrated Physiology (5 male and 5 female; age range: 20-25 years, Mean 22, SD 2.3 years, weight: 55-80Kg Mean 67.45, SD 12.90 Kg.). The exercise readiness of each subject was monitored by using a physical activity questionnaire (modified International Physical Activity Questionnaire) in which several wellness aspects such as cardiovascular fitness, discomfort during exercise, history of dizziness, joint problems, pregnancy, diabetes, breathing problems, and history of major surgery were questioned [25]. In addition, the subjects were required to report any history of neuromuscular disorder and lower extremity injury. No subject reported any of the aforementioned exercise readiness risks. These selection criteria were chosen to minimize the known effects of neuromuscular disorders and aging on changes in neuromuscular activation. [26, 27]. All procedures were reviewed and approved by the University of Houston Committee for the Protection of Human Subjects. The subjects were fully informed about the test protocol and provided signed consent prior to participating.

2.2. Experimental protocol

Each experiment was conducted in a single laboratory session. To alter the gait pattern from walking to running, the participants were instructed to walk at a comfortable initial speed (different between subjects) on a treadmill whose speed increased by 0.045 m/s every five strides up to a maximum duration of 180 seconds. Subjects were encouraged to stop the trial if at any point they became uncomfortable. All subjects successfully completed this protocol by transitioning their gait from walking to running. The transition speed (speed in which gait pattern was changed from walk to run) was recorded for each subject by observation to be used during analyses (see Statistical Analysis below). In addition, to verify the transition between walk and run, the vertical hip velocity and the stride time variability were evaluated. Both of these measures are sensitive to the sudden changes in gait pattern (i.e. walk to run transition). This approach confirmed the observed transitional strides [28]. The mean initial speed across all participants was a slow walk at 1.12 ± 0.13 m/s with final speed at a run of 3.30 ± 0.11 m/s.

2.3. Material and data collection

2.3.1. EMG activity

EMG signals were collected using six preamplifier bipolar active electrodes (EMG preamplifier, Type No: SX230, Biometrics Ltd., Gwent, UK) with a fixed electrode distance of 20 mm from rectus femoris (RF), tibialis anterior (TA), lateral gastrocnemius (GA), soleus (SO), vastus medialis (VM), and biceps femoris (BF) of the right lower limb using double sided tape. The electrodes were connected to a DataLINK base-unit DLK900 of the EMG acquisition system which was connected to a PC using USB cable. To achieve acceptable impedance level the skin over the location of each electrode was shaved and cleaned with alcohol swabs. EMG data were collected at 1000 Hz and passed through an amplifier with the gain set at 1000. The amplification bandwidth was 20–460 Hz (input impedance =100 MV, common mode rejection ratio >96 dB (~110dB) at 60 Hz). A zeroing reference electrode was placed above the right lateral malleolus bone and was secured by elastic wrap and tapes. There was no excessive filtration of the EMG data during collection but a digital filter was applied during data processing (see below). During the collection session, the electrodes were not removed from the subjects until data collection was completed.

2.3.2. Apparatus

Kinematic data were also collected at 200Hz using VICON motion capture device (Oxford Metrics, Oxford, UK) to identify the gait cycles by detecting each heel strike (i.e. right heel strike to heel strike). The kinematic markers were located on the hip, knee, ankle, heel, and toe. An electronic trigger was used to synchronize the EMG and kinematic data and to determine the events in which the treadmill speed increased (one trigger per gait speed increase).

2.4. Data processing

The data were processed by using a customized Matlab script (Mathworks, USA R2007a). The detailed specifications of each are provided below.

2.4.1. Recurrence Quantification Analysis (RQA)

The first step was to calculate the % DET by using RQA (RQASP program [29]; also see details in Appendix-RQA formulation). The EMG signals were band-pass filtered from 10-500 Hz [30, 31] however, no other smoothing techniques were used for the remaining signals to maximize the exposure of the raw signals to the nonlinear analysis method [16, 32]. To minimize the potential effect of any noise in the raw EMG signal on the outcome of RQA, the initial parameters (i.e. time delay and embedding dimension) were selected by following the recommended settings (i.e. embedding dimension, time lag, and radius) [29].

For each walking speed and each muscle, the EMG signal was clustered into five data bins that were defined as the epochs of recorded data between each right foot heel strike (i.e. each gait cycle). For each subject, the percentage of recurrence (% REC) and % DET of the clustered EMG signals was calculated for all muscles within each speed condition (% REC is required for the control during the selection of radius, see Appendix-RQA formulation for more details). As the RQA processes the time-delayed reconstructed space phase of the EMG signal, several parameters were defined prior to performing the analysis. The data were analyzed using an embedding dimension of m=6 based on the False Nearest Neighbor technique [33] and time delay of 5 (τ = 0.005 second) based on the Mutual Information (MI) technique [34]. In the MI technique, the first local minimum of the average mutual information is used to detect the time delay. The proximity radius (see Appendix-RQA formulation) was selected as 2 to 10 units of the rescaled "Maximum" unit of the Distance Matrix to keep the percentage of the recurring points in the recurrence plot (RP) of the signal less than 2% , as has been recommended [18].

2.4.2. *Shuffled surrogates tests*

While many studies have indicated a nonlinear dynamical pattern for EMG signals [10, 14, 15, 17, 18, 35] the nonlinearity of such signals was tested to justify the application of RQA in SYNERGOS [15, 17, 35-38]. A common practice to test the assumption of nonlinearity in a signal (i.e. EMG) is using surrogate data testing [15, 35-37, 39]. During this test the original EMG data are randomly shuffled using different algorithms namely time shuffling to generate random signals. It is expected that the randomization of the signal has significant effects on the nonlinear characteristics of the signal while keeping the linear characteristics of the signal unchanged which verifies the nonlinear behavior of the signal (i.e. EMG). In this study, 20 series of surrogate data using three algorithms were generated for each set of muscles per gait cycle [15, 35-38]. The approximate entropy (ApEn) and % DET of the original data were used to monitor the changes in the underlying dynamics of the EMG data after shuffling [40-42]. It was hypothesized that the value of % DET would significantly decrease while the value of ApEn would significantly increase for the shuffled data (see Appendix-Shuffled Surrogate Tests of EMG). By rejecting the null hypotheses of this testing procedure the existence of underlying nonlinear dynamics of the EMG signal could be assumed and therefore the application of RQA was justified.

2.4.3. *SYNERGOS*

We developed the SYNERGOS method to assess the level of MMA based on the activation of each muscle with all possible sets of the other muscles. SYNERGOS employs a two-step method for quantifying MMA. The first step is using RQA to analyze the EMG signals of each recorded muscle separately. The calculated % DET of the EMG signal obtained from each muscle serves as an input variable for the second step of SYNERGOS in which the inputs are combined by using a novel method that quantifies the level of MMA. SYNERGOS accounts for the concomitant activation of all measured muscles rather than only pairs of muscles. This measure results in a single scalar value indicating the overall activity among the set of multiple muscles representing the overall activation of these muscles during the course of the movement. Fig. 1 shows the schematic of the algorithm.

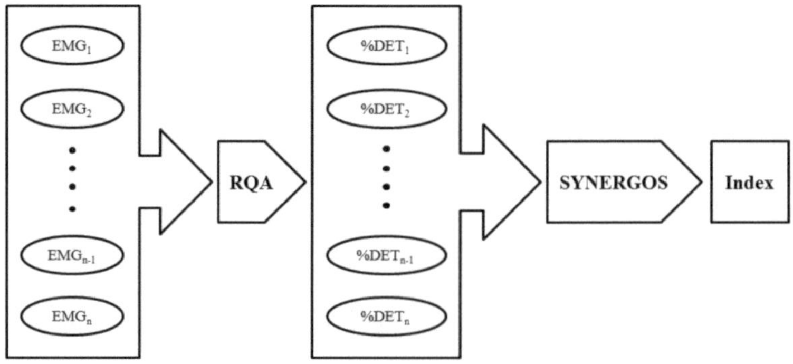

Figure 1. The schematic view of the SYNERGOS algorithm. EMG signals are analyzed using the RQA and the output, % DET for each muscle is imported into the SYNERGOS algorithm which eventually provides a single scalar index representing the state of MMA.

In this method, the average of several components is calculated. Each component is an average of the mth roots of the products (m= 2, 3, …, n while n= number of recorded muscles) of % DET of EMG signals for sets of m different muscles (i.e., pairs, triplets, quartets, etc.), where the final component is the nth root of the products of % DET of all n muscles being analyzed (i.e. the geometric mean). The SYNERGOS index was calculated based on the equation (1) by using the % DET derived for each muscle.

$$SYNERGOS = \frac{1}{n-1}\left[SYN_{bi} + SYN_{tri} + SYN_{quad} + \ldots + SYN_{n-muscle}\right] \tag{1}$$

SYN_{bi} represents the paired-muscle coactivities with $\binom{n}{2}$ possible elements (see equation 2). While SYN_{tri} depicts the contribution of simultaneous coactivity among three-muscle sets to SYNERGOS index with $\binom{n}{3}$ possible combinations. The same strategy is used to calculate the higher order muscular coactivity among other multiple-muscle sets. SYNERGOS index is elaborated in equation (2) as:

$$SYNERGOS = \frac{1}{n-1}\left[\begin{array}{l} \frac{1}{\binom{n}{2}} \sum_{i=1}^{n}\sum_{j=i}^{n} \sqrt{\left(1-\delta_{ij}\right) DET_i DET_j} + \\ \frac{1}{\binom{n}{3}} \sum_{i=1}^{n}\sum_{j=i}^{n}\sum_{k=j}^{n} \sqrt[3]{\left(1-\aleph_{ijk}\right) DET_i DET_j DET_k} + \\ \frac{1}{\binom{n}{4}} \sum_{i=1}^{n}\sum_{j=i}^{n}\sum_{k=j}^{n}\sum_{l=k}^{n} \sqrt[4]{\left(1-\aleph_{ijkl}\right) DET_i DET_j DET_k . DET_l} + \ldots \end{array}\right] \tag{2}$$

http://dx.doi.org/10.5772/56168

Where DET_i represents the % DET for each muscle (i, j, k, etc.) from the EMG signal during each gait cycle and delta δ_{ij} is the Kronocker delta defined in equation 3:

$$\delta_{ij} = \begin{cases} 1 & i=j \\ 0 & i \neq j \end{cases} \tag{3}$$

While for higher order of SYN (i.e. SYN_{tri}, SYN_{quad}, ...) the $\aleph$ is defined as follows:

$$\aleph_{ijkl\ldots} = \delta_{ij}\delta_{jk}\delta_{kl}\cdots \tag{4}$$

Therefore for any combination including a pair or multiple similar muscles the $\aleph_{ijkl\ldots}$ is zero. δ and $\aleph$ are used to ignore the coactivation of each muscle with itself so the result of Equation (1) represents only the coactivity of sets of two or more separate muscles. Following the strategy of the equation (2), $SYN_{n-muscle} = \left(\prod_{i=1}^{n} DET_i\right)^{1/n}$ and represents the geometric mean of the % DET of the recorded muscles.

This calculation represents the interaction of each muscle's activity with the other muscles' activity throughout a dynamic task since these muscles are all active at various times during the task. Each term in Equation 2 calculates the possible coactivation of each muscle with the other muscles in the limb. SYNERGOS basically summarizes the multidimensional correlation tensors of muscle activity into a scalar value while explicitly removing the unidimensional activity of single muscles from such tensors. Consequently, the SYNERGOS method calculates the interaction of all of the muscles, in all possible combinations. The magnitude of SYNERGOS can vary between 0 to 100 indicating the lowest and the highest level of MMA. A SYNERGOS of zero indicates that none of the muscles being measured during a task are simultaneously active regardless of the magnitude of activity in each muscle. A SYNERGOS of 100 indicates that all muscles are simoultanously active and each muscle is activated to its potentially maximum contraction level during each movement cycle (e.g., gait cycle). While theoretically possible, the index could only reach 100 if electrical stimulation was used to achieve tetanus in all monitored muscles. Values between 0 and 100 represent the average simultaneous activation scaled by the magnitudes of activity and temporal sequencing of the respective muscles. During movements a certain coactivity level among several agonist and antagonist muscles exists therefore, a SYNERGOS value between 0 and 100 will be obtained by analyzing the measured muscles.

For instance, in the current study the SYNERGOS algorithm for measuring the level of multiple coactivation for pairs of muscles (i.e., the first component in Equation 2) uses the upper triangular matrix of % DET indicated in equation (5) (where D represents % DET of each EMG signal).

$$\begin{bmatrix} D_{SO}D_{SO} & D_{SO}D_{GA} & D_{SO}D_{TA} & D_{SO}D_{VA} & D_{SO}D_{RF} & D_{SO}D_{BF} \\ & D_{GA}D_{GA} & D_{GA}D_{TA} & D_{GA}D_{VA} & D_{GA}D_{RF} & D_{GA}D_{BF} \\ & & D_{TA}D_{TA} & D_{TA}D_{VA} & D_{TA}D_{RF} & D_{TA}D_{BF} \\ & & & D_{VA}D_{VA} & D_{VA}D_{RF} & D_{VA}D_{BF} \\ & & & & D_{RF}D_{RF} & D_{RF}D_{BF} \\ & & & & & D_{BF}D_{BF} \end{bmatrix} \quad (5)$$

The delta function negates the elements of the matrix located on the diagonal (equation 6) for the EMG from the following muscles: rectus femoris (RF), tibialis anterior (TA), lateral gastrocnemius (GA), soleus (SO), vastus medialis (VM), and biceps femoris (BF).

$$\begin{bmatrix} 0 & D_{SO}D_{GA} & D_{SO}D_{TA} & D_{SO}D_{VA} & D_{SO}D_{RF} & D_{SO}D_{BF} \\ & 0 & D_{GA}D_{TA} & D_{GA}D_{VA} & D_{GA}D_{RF} & D_{GA}D_{BF} \\ & & 0 & D_{TA}D_{VA} & D_{TA}D_{RF} & D_{TA}D_{BF} \\ & & & 0 & D_{VA}D_{RF} & D_{VA}D_{BF} \\ & & & & 0 & D_{RF}D_{BF} \\ & & & & & 0 \end{bmatrix} \quad (6)$$

Finally, the technique calculates the sum of the square roots of the Equation 7 matrix elements. The outcome is averaged over the number of combinations (equation 7).

$$SYN_{bi} = \frac{1}{\binom{6}{2}} \sum_{i=1}^{6} \sum_{j=i}^{6} \sqrt{(1-\delta_{ij})DET_i DET_j} = \ldots \quad (7)$$

Other components of the SYNERGOS requires the calculation of combinations of % DET of three muscles (SYN_{tri}), four muscles (SYN_{quad}), five muscles (SYN_5), and six muscles (SYN_6) while controlling for the number of combinations ($\binom{6}{2}=15$ for two muscles, $\binom{6}{3}=20$ for three muscles, $\binom{6}{4}=15$ for four muscles, $\binom{6}{5}=6$ for five muscles, $\binom{6}{6}=1$ for six muscles).

Finally, for each subject, to obtain a single SYNERGOS index for the EMG signals during each gait speed, the root mean square of the five SYNERGOS indices obtained from the clustered EMG signals (five gait cycles per gait speed; see Recurrence Quantification Analysis) were calculated (equation 8). This single value represented the quantified MMA during each gait speed.

$$SYN_{GS,j} = \sqrt{\frac{\sum_{i=1}^{5} SYN_{i,j}^2}{5}}, \; j = 1 \; to \, number \, of \, gait \, speed \, conditions \quad (8)$$

Where $SYN_{GS,j}$ is the SYNERGOS index calculated for the jth gait speed condition and $SYN_{i,j}$ is the SYNERGOS index calculated for the data clustered in the ith gait cycle (i=1, 2, ..., 5) within the jth gait speed condition.

2.5. Statistical analysis

To analyze the efficiency of the proposed method, a restricted maximum likelihood linear mixed model was employed to identify changes in MMA measured by SYNERGOS associated with gait pattern (i.e. walk or run) and with changing gait speed. The model included three fixed effects, speed, pattern (walk or run), and speed-by-pattern interaction, and two random effects, subjects and measurement error (i.e., random within-subject variation). This analytical approach is similar to repeated measures analysis of variance in that it accounts for dependency resulting from multiple measures per subject but unlike analysis of variance does not require the same number of measures for each subject. The fixed effects were used to test the study hypotheses. The random effects were used to compute intraclass correlation coefficients (ICC) of type (2,1) (i.e., degree of consistency among measures) [43] and the corresponding standard errors of measurement (SEm) as relative and absolute reliability estimates, respectively (i.e. indicators of the consistency and precision of the SYNERGOS measure). The significance level was set at $p \leq 0.05$. The analysis was conducted by using SPSS 16.0.1 (SPSS Inc., Chicago, Illinois, USA).

3. Results

3.1. Surrogate testing

The results of the discriminant statistics (see Appendix-Shuffled Surrogate Tests of EMG). for each muscle and algorithm are shown in Table. 1. For all subjects, muscles, and gait cycle, the results of three different surrogate tests rejected the null hypotheses of equal or more determinism in surrogate data compared to the original data ($\varphi > 2$ and $p < 5\%$). The rejection of this null hypothesis indicated significant change in the nonlinear behavior of the surrogate signals (i.e. reduction of determinism) compared to the collected EMG signals which justified the application of higher order nonlinear data analysis techniques such as RQA to investigate the underlying dynamical pattern of the EMG signals specifically in SYNERGOS.

In Fig.2(a) an example of soleus EMG activity obtained during a single gait cycle (right heel strike to right heel strike) is depicted. Soleus contributes to the ankle planterflexion during body propulsion in stance phase of the gait. Muscle activity dramatically increases during midstance and peaks during the terminal stance phase with a rapid decrease in muscle activity in the pre-swing phase. The muscle remains fairly quiet during the swing phase of gait. Fig. 2(b) displays the recurrence plot (RP) of the soleus activity in which recurrent points are positioned along several parallel diagonal recurrent lines demonstrating the existence of a specific deterministic muscular activity in the soleus during the gait cycle. Fig.2(c) represents the randomized shuffling of the EMG signal using surrogate testing algorithms. The RP of the shuffled data are presented in Fig.2(d). No particular deterministic pattern can be recognized by observing several recurrent points scattered on the plot as these points do not generate long diagonal recurrent lines that would indicate determinism of the signal. The analyses of the original and surrogate signals also confirmed the results displayed in Fig.2(b) and Fig.2 (d). The reduction in % DET and increase in ApEn indicates that the surrogate data follows different dynamical patterns than the original EMG signal therefore the EMG signal included nonlinear behaviors (i.e. determinism) that were altered by the randomization of the original signal.

			SO	GA	TA	VA	RF	BF
Time Shuffled	φ_{ApEn}	Mean	37.54	37.02	24.76	38.99	30.46	27.35
		SD	6.52	7.12	7.30	7.81	7.00	3.42
	$\varphi_{\%DET}$	Mean	454.65	518.50	344.20	292.60	42.17	213.00
		SD	165.09	93.84	111.21	89.51	26.36	68.31
FT	φ_{ApEn}	Mean	42.16	40.60	32.22	43.79	24.18	25.61
		SD	7.43	7.38	12.72	8.92	5.82	4.83
	$\varphi_{\%DET}$	Mean	61.26	94.09	232.65	22.43	69.42	48.27
		SD	23.08	57.94	46.55	8.34	26.57	9.20
IAAFT	φ_{ApEn}	Mean	16.63	14.77	18.56	12.47	17.22	15.78
		SD	4.16	4.70	6.01	4.59	4.44	1.45
	$\varphi_{\%DET}$	Mean	49.24	66.33	53.88	25.84	35.58	11.03
		SD	4.95	22.98	41.35	23.47	11.35	4.57

Table 1. The values of surrogate testing for three different algorithms; φ_{ApEn} and $\varphi_{\%DET}$ represents the value of statistics calculated from ApEn and % DET of the EMG signals and surrogate data series. (Fourier transform (FT), Iterated amplitude adjusted Fourier transform (IAAFT), rectus femoris (RF), tibialis anterior (TA), lateral gastrocnemius (GA), soleus (SO), vastus medialis (VM), and biceps femoris (BF))

3.2. SYNERGOS analysis

The SYNERGOS indices during walking, running, and the whole protocol are summarized in table2.

Condition	Average	SD
Walking	17.61	11.57
Running	33.86	10.89
Overall	25.71	13.76

Table 2. The SYNERGOS indices averaged across all subjects and during walking, running, and the full protocol. The average index increased significantly during running compared to walking.

http://dx.doi.org/10.5772/56168

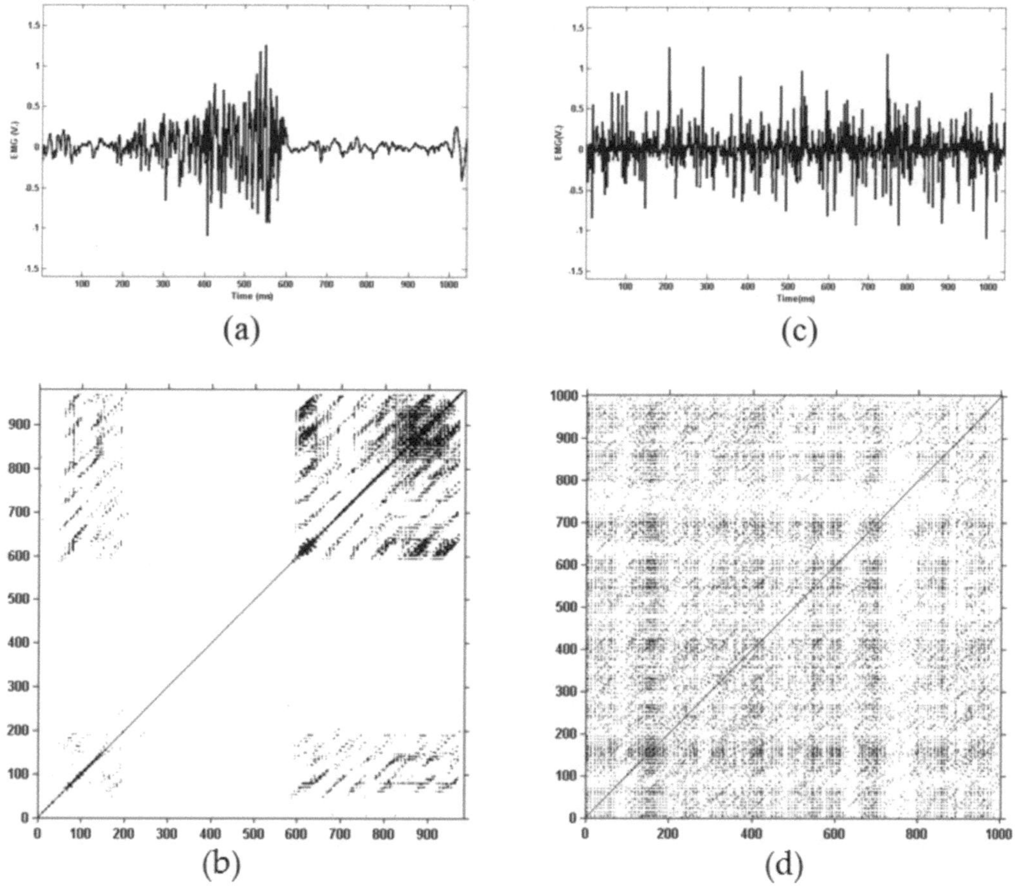

Figure 2. (a) The neuromuscular activities of soleus muscle during a gait cycle are depicted by EMG activities in in which soleus is mostly active during the propulsion of body during stance phase while showing little activity during swing phase. (b) The Recurrence plots (RP) generated based on the original data is shown in the graph (a) indicating the existence of a specific pattern in the soleus activity during the gait cycle. This pattern is depicted by several recurrent points located along particular diagonal lines which are parallel to the main diagonal line (see Appendix-RQA formulation). The outcome of the RQA also verified the existence of the aforementioned pattern (% REC = 1.98; % DET = 51.80, radius=2.86, ApEn=0.72). Figure (c) contains the randomized shuffled data of the signal shown in 1(a). Figure (d) is the RP of the randomized signal which shows no significant determinism in the shuffled data. The time delayed dimensional data in RP are randomly scattered around the main diagonal line and the recurrent points are positioned along very short length. In addition, the outcome of RQA has shown significant reduction in determinism in the randomized data (% REC = 1.99 radius=8.70, ApEn=1.46). The drastic drop in the determinism of the signal detected by decreasing % DET and increasing ApEn verified the nonlinear dynamics of the EMG signal.

As expected, the changes in the gait mode (walking vs. running) altered the activation of muscles contributing to gait. Fig.3 shows the normalized EMG activities in one of the subjects whose SYNERGOS indices increased significantly from 2.58% during the slowest walking speed to 41.56% during the fastest running speed indicating an increase in cooperation among multiple muscles.

This change was detected by a significant alteration in the SYNERGOS index with the index being significantly greater during running than during walking ($F(1,382.149) = 54.067$, $p < 0.001$) suggesting increased muscle multiple coactivity during more vigorous movements. In addition, the hypothesis that SYNEGOS could detect changes in MMA associated with slight increases of 0.045 m/s in gait speed was confirmed ($F(1,382.537) = 675.85$, $p < 0.001$). A significant interaction effect of gait speed and movement pattern ($F(1,382.082) = 48.075$, $p < 0.001$) was also detected indicating that increases in SYNERGOS values occurred at a lower rate during increases in running speed than during increases in walking speed. A high degree of reliability was detected during both walking (ICC=0.92, SEm=3.14) and running (ICC=0.91, SEm=2.71).

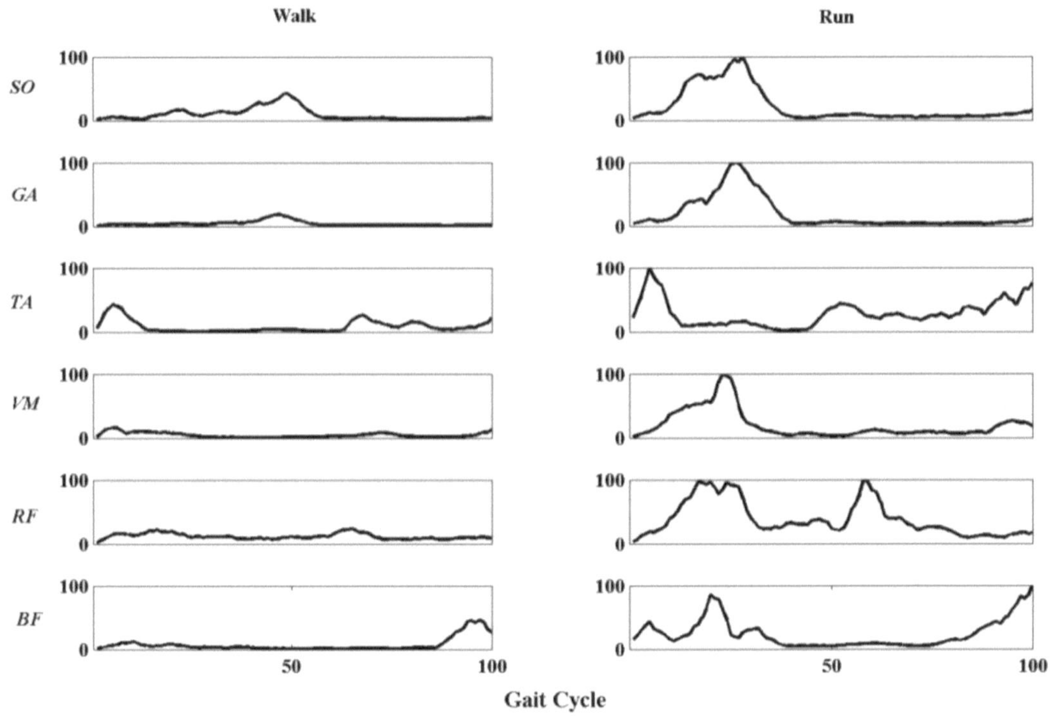

Figure 3. The EMG activity of the lower extremity muscles in soleus (SO), gastrocnemius (GA), tibialis anterior (TA), vastus medialis (VM), rectus femoris (RF), and biceps femoris (BF) comparing walking and running stage. The data are time normalized using a linear length normalization method to convert different each gait cycle into equally scaled units (each unit represents 1% of gait cycle). A gait cycle was defined as the duration between right heel strike and the next right heel strike (gait cycle = 100% of scaled unit). For demonstration purposes, the amplitude for each muscle was normalized to the maximum EMG obtained during the data collection. This maximum was always reached during running.

Fig.4 displays the 95% confidence intervals (95% CI) of SYNERGOS index across all subjects for each of the gait speeds. In addition, the final fitted model slopes both during walk and run in the SYNERGOS indices across treadmill speeds (solid lines) is depicted. The model consistently increased in response to increasing gait speed and had larger absolute values during running, indicating greater magnitude and coactivation (SYNERGOS walk 16.517 ± 3.14 vs.

SYNERGOS run = 32.84 ± 2.71). Furthermore, the fitted slopes for increases in the SYNERGOS index during walking (slope = 18.30) and running (slope=15.35) were significantly ($p<0.001$) different.

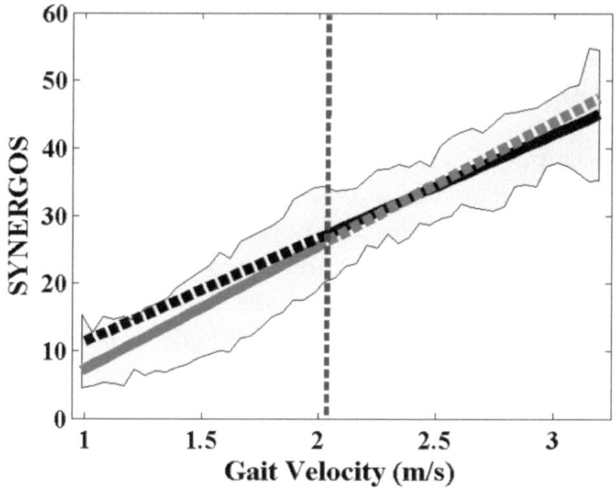

Figure 4. The shaded area indicates the 95% CI of the SYNERGOS index for each gait speed. The vertical dotted line indicates the average walk to run transition speed. The linear fit model for walk and run are shown by solid line while the extrapolation of the linear fit model into the opposite gait pattern was shown by dotted lines for the SYNERGOS indices. In both walking and running conditions the SYNERGOS indices increased consistently in response to increasing gait speed. The index had larger absolute values (>20) during running, indicating greater magnitude and activation of muscle activity, but the slope for walking (slope = 18.30) was significantly ($p<0.001$) higher than the slope in running condition (slope=15.35) indicating a greater rate of change in MMA when increasing walking speed relative to increasing running speed.

4. Discussion

We have introduced a new analysis method, SYNERGOS that provides an index for quantifying the state of muscle multiple coactivation during a given movement task and demonstrated that it could successfully discriminate between muscle coactivation patterns associated with changing gait mode and speed as a particular combination of the % DET for multiple muscles. As mentioned previously a SYNERGOS index of 100 would represent 100% contraction and simultaneous activation of all measured muscles. Such a possibility is extremely unlikely when considering any voluntary contraction but definitely would not occur during a dynamic movement as rigidity would result.

4.1. SYNERGOS considerations

Several studies investigated the effect of increasing gait speed on the neuromuscular activities of the lower extremities [22, 44-49]. These studies reported increasing average and peak EMG voltage associated with increasing speed in the soleus, gastrocnemius, tibialis anterior, vastus medialis, rectus femoris, and bicep femoris muscles [22, 44-49]. In addition, significant increases in musle cocontraction were reported during increasing gait speed [48]. The increases observed in the SYNERGOS indices are consistent with the previous studies verifying greater EMG activity during faster gait speeds.

Previous studies have indicated that the stability of the human body decreases during higher gait speed which might be correlated with higher risk of fall and injury [50-52]. Muscular cocontraction is a strategy used to stiffen the joints resulting in the reduction of kinematic degrees of freedom to enhance stability during dynamic movements that may threaten postural stability [48]. During faster movements kinematics (velocity and accelerations) and kinetics (i.e. forces, torque, and momentum) parameters alter with higher rates therefore more reliable postural and movement strategy is required to ensure relatively quicker response to the variations in the stability of the system. Thus, increasing the level of MMA provides an effective way for the CNS to reduce the numerous DOF during more demanding movements such as running to provide more stability of human body in faster gait speeds. Increasing SYNERGOS indices are compatible with the aforementioned observation of the motor control strategy.

Several methods for quantifying the coactivity of a group of muscles have been described previously, including muscle cocontraction and various linear techniques. Muscle cocontraction studies are limited to evaluation of only two antagonistic muscles at a time [53, 54]. While analysis of muscle cocontraction may be valuable for various clinical assessments, evaluation of only two muscles does not adequately represent the complex control required to evaluate full-body motion; SYNERGOS overcomes this limitation by offering the potential to represent the combination of EMG activity from all monitored muscles. Linear data analysis methods such as principal components analysis or other factorization techniques have been used to identify the time-invariant patterns of multiple muscle coactivation [2, 4-6, 19, 21, 55], but the nonlinear patterns of information embedded in EMG signals have received little attention [4, 6, 18, 56]. In contrast, SYNERGOS quantifies the changes in MMA of a potentially unlimited number of muscles within the constraints imposed by the practical considerations of the number of muscles EMG can reasonably be collected from during a given movement and analyzes the signals using a powerful nonlinear technique. The SYNERGOS method detects the changes in muscle coactivity states by accounting for both time dependent and time invariant characteristics of EMG signals assessed by % DET EMG without assuming linearity (i.e. stationarity) of EMG signals [13, 14, 16-18].

The SYNERGOS index is an overall estimation of MMA during a specific cycle. The simplicity of the single quantity will come with a price of losing some temporal aspects of muscular activation. Although SYNERGOS algorithm in the first step captures subtle changes in the temporal and magnitude characteristics of each EMG signal by using the % DET in the second step it calculates the overall MMA by averaging the muscular activities using equation (16). Therefore the single quantity cannot demonstrate the exact simultaneous multiple activities of each muscle with others in every single EMG data point. The time-unit of each SYNERGOS index can be set to the duration of the epochs. However this limitation (single SYNERGOS index per epoch) provides simplicity to monitor and track the multiple muscle activations over a longer period of time.

As the CNS likely uses optimized MMA strategies to control different movement tasks, a quantity indicating an overall multiple muscle coactivity may be valuable, particularly in clinical settings, to assess the changes in the performance of the CNS of different patient populations. After further evaluation and validation using data collected during a variety of activities from a variety of patient populations, SYNERGOS may enable clinicians to screen the effectiveness of treatments on neuromuscular activities and could potentially be used as a diagnostic tool to detect abnormal activation in the neuromuscular system.

4.2. RQA considerations

Several previous studies have investigated the application of RQA and % DET to provide insight into the state of muscle activation in various activities during both isometric and dynamic movements. These studies have demonstrated the benefits of such nonlinear techniques to study the neuromuscular activities quantified by EMG signals [13, 14, 16-18, 32]. To perform various activities, muscles are required to generate different forces to satisfy the task related goals that may result in variation of motor unit recruitment and ultimately changes in motor units synchronization [9, 10]. The great sensitivity of RQA to the subtle changes in dynamical systems has increased the use of this analysis for understanding various procedures in motor control, specifically in analyzing EMG signals [13, 16, 18, 29, 35, 40]. However, RQA should be conducted with careful selection of initial parameter settings. % DET has been shown to have high sensitivity to the interaction of noise and embedding dimension if the time lag is more than 8 samples ($\tau > 8$ samples) [29]. Therefore, the selection of the embedding dimension and time lag was conducted using False Nearest Neighbor and Mutual Information techniques for all EMG signals during each gait cycle as the artificial changes in % DET caused by noise may alter the outcome of SYNERGOS.

4.3. EMG considerations

EMG signals depict the overall presentation of action potentials from motor units. Low frequency noises such as power line noise and cable movement are removed using the current technology in EMG data collection devices [57]. Two major sources of noise that may affect the integrity of the EMG signal are baseline noises and movement artifact noise. The baseline noise is generated in electrode amplification process during data collection. In addition, skin movement artifacts are generated during dynamical movement of the muscles resulting in the relative change in the location of the electrode to the targeted muscles. These artifacts can also be generated during highly demanding movement activities in which the impulse of the forces may travel through the muscles and approach the electrodes. In this study a 10-500Hz bandwidth was used to filter the collected EMG signals during the movements. Although in more vigorous activities the corner frequency of 20Hz was shown to remove some additional noises [57], in this study the corner frequency of bandwidth was chosen based on the recommendations of International Society of Electrophysiology and Kinesiology (corner bandwidth frequency of 10 Hz) [30]. As further filtering of data might remove some portions of the 'true'

EMG signal generated by neuromuscular activation, which might result in limited exposure of actual muscular activities to the RQA, hence dismissing 'true' subtle changes in the EMG signal [16, 32] Thus no further filtering was applied on the EMG signals used in this study. Additionally the effect of noise on the % DET as the inputs of SYNERGOS was also minimized by the careful selection of initial parameters (i.e. embedding dimension, delay, and radius) to ensure the integrity of the algorithm (see "RQA consideration").

In conclusion, we have proposed a nonlinear multiple-muscle coactivation quantification tool, "SYNERGOS", that is sensitive to changes in both the magnitude and the timing of muscle activity caused by environmental or task related changes. In the future, this method may have application as a diagnostic tool for the evaluation of the therapeutic interventions in individuals with neuromuscular disorders, or those in rehabilitation settings. Further development, validation, and application of the SYNERGOS measure in clinical populations are currently being explored. Additionally, assessment of SYNERGOS's intra- and inter-day reliability is also underway.

Acknowledgements

We would like to extend our sincere thanks to all the University of Houston students who participated in the study. Additionally, we are thankful to Mr. Chris Arellano, Mr. Marius Dettmer, and Ms. Azadeh Khorram for their help with the data collection.

Apendix

RQA formulation

RQA is a nonlinear data analysis tool, that quantifies the recurrent data in the phase space trajectory of a time series data set, here EMG signals [15, 18]. For RQA analysis each time series is defined as the EMG activity recorded for each muscle during each gait cycle depicted by "$\vec{d}$":

$$\vec{d} = \left[d_1, d_2, \ldots, d_N\right]^T \tag{9}$$

Where N represents the total number of collected data points in each bin (i.e. EMG data). In our study, N decreased as the gait speed increased, owing to the shorter gait cycles. In the next step the phase space vector is calculated based on the embedding dimension (m=6) found by False Nearest Neighbor method and time delay (τ= 0.005 second equal to 5 EMG data samples) found by Mutual Information technique [33], [34]. The equation of the phase space can be constructed as [15]:

$$\hat{\vec{s}}_i = \left[d_i, d_{i+\tau}, d_{i+2\tau}, \ldots, d_{i+(m-1)\tau} \right]^T \tag{10}$$

resulting in a vector with $N_s = N - (m-1)\tau$ elements. Based on the above phase space vector a Distance Matrix (DM) is defined. The elements of the DM are the Euclidian norm of the distance of each of two generated elements of the phase space vector [13].

$$\mathbf{DM}^m_{i,j} = \left\| \vec{s}_i - \vec{s}_j \right\| \qquad \vec{s}_i \in \mathrm{R}^m \quad i, j = 1, \ldots, N_s \tag{11}$$

Here $\mathbb{R}$ indicates the real numbers. In the next step, RQA assesses the proximity of each element in the DM with other elements. This proximity is tested based on a predefined threshold radius (ε_i). In this study, the threshold radius is found by an algorithm to keep the recurrence rate less than 2 percent [18] resulting in $2 < \varepsilon_i < 10$ units of the normalized DM by the maximum element in the original DM. Next, the outcome of this assessment is converted into a binary matrix as representing the approximately close elements while 0 indicates the "not-close" elements:

$$\mathbf{R}^{m,\varepsilon_i}_{i,j} = H(\varepsilon_i - \mathbf{DM}^m_{i,j}) \tag{12}$$

In which H represents the Heaviside function defined as

$$H(x) = \begin{cases} 0 & x < 0 \\ 1 & x \geq 0 \end{cases} \tag{13}$$

Equation 12 can be summarized into equation 14 as

$$\mathbf{R}_{\mathbf{i},\mathbf{j}} = \begin{cases} 0 & dm_i \circledR dm_j \\ 1 & dm_i \cong dm_j \end{cases} \quad i, j = 1, \ldots, N_s \tag{14}$$

in which dm_i and dm_j are two elements on the DM matrix [15]. All elements compared with itself (i.e. i = j) results in the recurrence matrix element of 1. Recurrence plots which visualize the recurrence matrix can be generated based on the frequency distribution of the recurrent points (non-zero elements in recurrence matrix). To calculate the % DET the noncumulative frequency distribution of the constructed diagonal lines (recurrent points) in the Recurrence matrix is defined as

$$P^{\varepsilon}(l) = \{l_i; i=1,2,\ldots,N_l\} \tag{15}$$

Where N_l represents the number of diagonal lines with the length of l_i [17]. Due to the increase in the deterministic pattern of EMG signal resulted from increasing motor unit firing rate during more intense activities (i.e. running) N_l increased for longer diagonal lines and decreased for shorter lines. Finally, % DET was calculated based on equation (16).

$$\%DET = \frac{\sum_{l=l_{min}}^{N} l P^{\varepsilon}(l)}{\sum_{i,j}^{N} \mathbf{R}_{i,j}^{m,\varepsilon_i}} \tag{16}$$

in which l_{min} is the minimum number of recurrent point in a diagonal line required to define a line [15]. $l_{min}=1$ represents the condition generated by the tangential motion of phase space trajectory [15] that is not indicating the systematic determinism of the recorded EMG signal. In this study, $l_{min}=3$ was chosen to demonstrate the deterministic pattern of the space trajectory based on the recommendation of previous studies [16, 18]. As the denominator of the equation (16) indicates the total recurrent points, % DET measures the proportion of recurrent points that define recurrent diagonal lines longer than lmin representing the determinism or predictability of the dynamical system, i.e. EMG signal.

Shuffled Surrogate Tests of EMG

To obtain a one-tailed significance level of $\alpha = 0.05$, nineteen (M=19) surrogate data series out of 20 should reject the null hypothesis ($M = \frac{K}{\alpha} - 1$ in which K=1). The results of the surrogate testing were evaluated using a one-tail significance level because we had a directional hypothesis that predicted a reduction in the determinism of the surrogate signals after shuffling the original EMG [35, 36, 40, 42]. In the first series, temporally independent surrogate data were generated by random shuffling of the time ordering of EMG data which destroyed any time synchronization and correlation in the original data while saving statistical properties such as the mean and standard deviation [35, 38]. In this step, rejecting the null hypothesis that the EMG signals are originated from white noise is evidence of the existence of a dynamical system in the EMG signal [37]. Next, a phase randomized surrogate algorithm [37] was used to shuffle the original data by these three steps: 1) determining the Fourier transformation of the EMG signals 2) randomization of the phase of Fourier transform 3) applying the inverse Fourier transform to obtain a surrogate time series. The goal of this test is to reject the null hypothesis that the EMG signal has a linearly correlated Gaussian noise pattern. Iterated amplitude adjusted Fourier transform (IAAFT) was the third algorithm to generate surrogate data series [36, 37, 39]. IAAFT algorithm generates surrogate data, which resemble the rank ordering and power spectrum of the original EMG signals. Rejecting the null hypothesis by using IAAFT algorithm can be an indicator of deterministic chaos in the original time series

[36, 37, 39, 40], therefore the latter algorithm has the advantage of demonstrating the nature of nonlinearity in the signal.

To test the null hypotheses, discriminating statistics were applied to investigate the changes in the dynamical pattern of surrogate data. These statistics should be sensitive to higher order nonlinearity of the signal [36, 37]. In this study, the null hypotheses were generated based on the changes in the approximate entropy (ApEn) and % DET of the surrogate data. ApEn is a single quantity by which the regularity of a signal can be measured [58, 59]. ApEn has been shown to classify underlying complexity of the signals while no significant changes in frequency and amplitude parameters were detected [40-42]. ApEn rages from 0 to 2 for completely predictable signals (i.e. sine wave) to white Gaussian noise respectively. A value of ApEn=2 indicates complete uncertainty in prediction of future behavior of a dynamical system. Therefore, in surrogate testing the expected outcome is a significant increase in ApEn value while a significant drop in % DET as a result of random shuffling procedure [35, 38].

ApEn value for both original EMG signals and surrogate data were calculated by applying the parameter settings of embedding-dimension of m=2 and r= 0.2 × standard deviation of the signal. In addition, after conducting the RQA analysis on the original EMG signals, a Matlab script was used to perform the RQA on the surrogate data using the same parameter settings (m=6 and τ= 0.005 second). The script increased the radius to obtain similar level of % REC (the percentage of recurrent points in the recurrence plot graphs) for each set of muscles per gait cycle and the % DET was calculated base on the modified radius.

Finally, the ApEn and % DET of surrogate data were statistically compared to the ApEn and % DET of original EMG signal by defining the following statistics [37, 40]:

$$\varphi_i = \left| Q_{original} - \bar{\mu}(surrogate)_i \right| / SD_{(surrogate)_i} \qquad i = 1 \; to \; n \tag{17}$$

Where n is the number of muscles and $Q_{original}$ indicates ApEn or % DET statistic from original EMG for each muscle per gait cycle. $\bar{\mu}_{(surrogate)_i}$ and $SD_{surrogate}$ denote the average and standard deviation of computed ApEn and % DET of the surrogate series. φ_i indicates the amount of change in the ApEn and % DET of the original data in the scale of standard deviations. To reject the null hypothesis a minimum $\varphi_i > 2$ is required to obtain a 5% significance level (normality assumed) [39].

Nonlinear data analysis techniques are capable of revealing subtle changes in dynamical systems that may be ignored during linear data analysis. However they require more sophisticated analysis procedures and are generally more time consuming and costly, therefore the application of such techniques should be justified especially during clinical measurements. In the current study, three algorithms were used to test the state of nonlinearity in the EMG signals. The first two algorithms (time shuffled and FT) confirmed the fact that the recorded EMG signals contain higher order nonlinear dynamics. The use of the third surrogate testing method (i.e. IAAFT algorithm) expands our understanding from the nature of the dynamical nonlinearity. In our investigation, the existence of deterministic patterns measured by % DET is a key to the SYNERGOS equation. Therefore the use of third surrogate algorithm, IAAFT was justified. In previous studies amplitude adjusted Fourier transform (AAFT) algorithms were used to investigate the nature of the EMG signal [40] however it has been argued that for short and highly correlated data series the AAFT algorithm may result in flatness of power spectrums [36] therefore IAAFT algorithm was introduced to overcome such a bias by iteratively correcting the deviations in the power spectrum. [36, 39].

Author details

Amir Pourmoghaddam, Daniel P O'Connor, William H Paloski and Charles S Layne

The Center for Neuromotor and Biomechanics Research, Department of Health and Human Performance, University of Houston, Houston, TX, USA

References

[1] Bernstein, N. A. Coordination and Regulation of Movement(1967). New York: Pergamon Press. 196.

[2] Cheung, V. C, Avella, A. d, & Bizzi, E. Adjustments of motor pattern for load compensation via modulated activations of muscle synergies during natural behaviors. J Neurophysiol, (2009). , 1235-1257.

[3] Rosenbaum, D. A. Human Motor Control(1990). Academic Press.

[4] Ting, L. H, & Macpherson, J. M. A limited set of muscle synergies for force control during a postural task. J Neurophysiol, (2005). , 609-613.

[5] Torres-oviedo, G, Macpherson, J. M, & Ting, L. H. Muscle synergy organization is robust across a variety of postural perturbations. J Neurophysiol, (2006). , 1530-1546.

[6] Wang, Y, et al. Muscle synergies during voluntary body sway: combining across-trials and within-a-trial analyses. Exp Brain Res, (2006). , 679-693.

[7] Layne, C. S, et al. Alterations in Human neuromuscular activation during overground locomotion after long-duration spaceflight. Journal of Gravitational Physiology, (2004). , 1-16.

[8] Sekine, M, et al. Fractal dynamics of body motion in patients with Parkinson's disease. J Neural Eng, (2004). , 8-15.

[9] Del SantoF., et al., Recurrence quantification analysis of surface EMG detects changes in motor unit synchronization induced by recurrent inhibition. Exp Brain Res, (2007)., 308-315.

[10] Del SantoF., et al., Motor unit synchronous firing as revealed by determinism of surface myoelectric signal. J Neurosci Methods, (2006)., 116-121.

[11] Farina, D, et al. Nonlinear surface EMG analysis to detect changes of motor unit conduction velocity and synchronization. J Appl Physiol, (2002)., 1753-1763.

[12] Felici, F, et al. Linear and non-linear analysis of surface electromyograms in weightlifters. Eur J Appl Physiol, (2001)., 337-342.

[13] Filligoi, G, & Felici, F. Detection of hidden rhythms in surface EMG signals with a non-linear time-series tool. Med Eng Phys, (1999)., 439-448.

[14] Liu, Y, et al. EMG recurrence quantifications in dynamic exercise. Biol Cybern, (2004)., 337-348.

[15] Marwan, N, et al. Recurrence plots for the analysis of complex systems. Phys Rep, (2007)., 237-329.

[16] Webber, C. L, Jr, M. A, & Schmidt, J. M. Walsh, Influence of isometric loading on biceps EMG dynamics as assessed by linear and nonlinear tools. J Appl Physiol, (1995)., 814-822.

[17] Marwan, N. Encounters With Neighbors- Current Developments Of Concepts Based On Recurrence Plots And Their Applications, in Institut für Physik und Astronomie(2003). University of Potsdam.

[18] Webber, C. L, & Jr, J. P. Zbilut, Recurrence quantification analysis of nonlinear dynamical systems, in To appear in: Riley MA, Van Orden G (eds) Tutorials in contemporary nonlinear methods for the behavioral sciences., (Chapter 2, (2005)., 26-94.

[19] Krishnamoorthy, V, et al. Muscle synergies during shifts of the center of pressure by standing persons: identification of muscle modes. Biol Cybern, (2003)., 152-161.

[20] Latash, M. L, & Anson, J. G. Synergies in health and disease: relations to adaptive changes in motor coordination. Phys Ther, (2006)., 1151-1160.

[21] Latash, M. L, Scholz, J. P, & Schoner, G. Motor control strategies revealed in the structure of motor variability. Exerc Sport Sci Rev, (2002)., 26-31.

[22] Sasaki, K, & Neptune, R. R. Differences in muscle function during walking and running at the same speed. J Biomech, (2006)., 2005-2013.

[23] Hortobagyi, T, et al. Interaction between age and gait velocity in the amplitude and timing of antagonist muscle coactivation. Gait Posture, (2009)., 558-564.

[24] Osternig, L. R, et al. Co-activation of sprinter and distance runner muscles in isokinetic exercise. Med Sci Sports Exerc, (1986)., 431-435.

[25] Craig, C. L, et al. International physical activity questionnaire: 12-country reliability and validity. Med Sci Sports Exerc, (2003). , 1381-1395.

[26] Crenna, P, et al. Impact of subthalamic nucleus stimulation on the initiation of gait in Parkinson's disease. Exp Brain Res, (2006). , 519-532.

[27] Tricon, V, et al. Balance control and adaptation of kinematic synergy in aging adults during forward trunk bending. Neurosci Lett, (2007). , 81-86.

[28] Hreljac, A, et al. When does a gait transition occur during human locomotion? Journal of Sports Science and Medicine, (2007). , 36-43.

[29] Hasson, C. J, et al. Influence of embedding parameters and noise in center of pressure recurrence quantification analysis. Gait Posture, (2008). , 416-422.

[30] Merletti, R, & Torino, P. d. Standards for Reporting EMG Data. Journal of Electromyography and Kinesiology, (1997). p. I-II.

[31] Van Boxtel, A. Optimal signal bandwidth for the recording of surface EMG activity of facial, jaw, oral, and neck muscles. Psychophysiology, (2001). , 22-34.

[32] Buzzi, U. H, et al. Nonlinear dynamics indicates aging affects variability during gait. Clin Biomech (Bristol, Avon), (2003). , 435-443.

[33] Kennel, M. B, Brown, R, & Abarbanel, H. D. I. Determining embedding dimension for phase-space reconstruction using a geometrical construction. Physical Review A, (1992). , 3403.

[34] Fraser, A. M, & Swinney, H. L. Independent coordinates for strange attractors from mutual information. Phys Rev A, (1986). , 1134-1140.

[35] Morana, C, et al. Recurrence quantification analysis of surface electromyographic signal: sensitivity to potentiation and neuromuscular fatigue. J Neurosci Methods, (2009). , 73-79.

[36] Schreiber, T, & Schmitz, A. Surrogate time series. Physica D: Nonlinear Phenomena, (2000). , 346-382.

[37] Theiler, J, et al. Testing for nonlinearity in time series: the method of surrogate data. Physica D: Nonlinear Phenomena, (1992). , 77-94.

[38] Riley, M. A, Balasubramaniam, R, & Turvey, M. T. Recurrence quantification analysis of postural fluctuations. Gait Posture, (1999). , 65-78.

[39] Nagarajan, R. Surrogate testing of linear feedback processes with non-Gaussian innovations. Physica A: Statistical Mechanics and its Applications, (2006). , 530-538.

[40] Vaillancourt, D. E, Larsson, L, & Newell, K. M. Time-dependent structure in the discharge rate of human motor units. Clin Neurophysiol, (2002). , 1325-1338.

[41] Vaillancourt, D. E, & Newell, K. M. The dynamics of resting and postural tremor in Parkinson's disease. Clin Neurophysiol, (2000). , 2046-2056.

[42] Vaillancourt, D. E, Slifkin, A. B, & Newell, K. M. Regularity of force tremor in Parkinson's disease. Clin Neurophysiol, (2001). , 1594-1603.

[43] Mcgraw, K. O, & Wong, S. P. Forming inferences about some intraclass correlation coefficients.. Psychological Methods, (1996). , 30-46.

[44] Cipriani, D. J, Armstrong, C. W, & Gaul, S. Backward walking at three levels of treadmill inclination: an electromyographic and kinematic analysis. J Orthop Sports Phys Ther, (1995). , 95-102.

[45] Lange, G. W, et al. Electromyographic and kinematic analysis of graded treadmill walking and the implications for knee rehabilitation. J Orthop Sports Phys Ther, (1996). , 294-301.

[46] Nymark, J. R, et al. Electromyographic and kinematic nondisabled gait differences at extremely slow overground and treadmill walking speeds. J Rehabil Res Dev, (2005). , 523-534.

[47] Stoquart, G, Detrembleur, C, & Lejeune, T. Effect of speed on kinematic, kinetic, electromyographic and energetic reference values during treadmill walking. Neurophysiol Clin, (2008). , 105-116.

[48] Schmitz, A, et al. Differences in lower-extremity muscular activation during walking between healthy older and young adults. J Electromyogr Kinesiol, (2009). , 1085-1091.

[49] Bovi, G, et al. A multiple-task gait analysis approach: kinematic, kinetic and EMG reference data for healthy young and adult subjects. Gait Posture, (2011). , 6-13.

[50] England, S. A, & Granata, K. P. The influence of gait speed on local dynamic stability of walking. Gait Posture, (2007). , 172-178.

[51] Espy, D. D, et al. Independent influence of gait speed and step length on stability and fall risk. Gait Posture, (2010). , 378-382.

[52] Kang, H. G, & Dingwell, J. B. Effects of walking speed, strength and range of motion on gait stability in healthy older adults. J Biomech, (2008). , 2899-2905.

[53] Gorassini, M. A, et al. Changes in locomotor muscle activity after treadmill training in subjects with incomplete spinal cord injury. J Neurophysiol, (2009). , 969-979.

[54] Falconer, K, & Winter, D. A. Quantitative assessment of co-contraction at the ankle joint in walking. Electromyogr Clin Neurophysiol, (1985). , 135-149.

[55] Tresch, M. C, Saltiel, P, & Bizzi, E. The construction of movement by the spinal cord. Nat Neurosci, (1999). , 162-167.

[56] Stergiou, N, et al. Innovative Analyses of Human Movement(2003). Human Kinetics Publishers.

[57] De Luca, C. J, et al. Filtering the surface EMG signal: Movement artifact and baseline noise contamination. J Biomech, (2010). , 1573-1579.

[58] Pincus, S. M. Approximate entropy as a measure of system complexity. Proc Natl Acad Sci U S A, (1991). , 2297-2301.

[59] Pincus, S. M, Gladstone, I. M, & Ehrenkranz, R. A. A regularity statistic for medical data analysis. J Clin Monit, (1991). , 335-345.

Chapter 8

How Deep Should You Squat to Maximise a Holistic Training Response? Electromyographic, Energetic, Cardiovascular, Hypertrophic and Mechanical Evidence

Gerard E. McMahon, Gladys L. Onambélé-Pearson, Christopher I. Morse, Adrian M. Burden and Keith Winwood

Additional information is available at the end of the chapter

http://dx.doi.org/10.5772/56386

1. Introduction

Skeletal muscle possesses the ability to change its structural and mechanical characteristics in response to its external environment (i.e. it is adaptable). The exact nature of such adaptations is manipulated by, amongst other things, the mechanical stimulus provided to the said muscle. Resistance exercise is an example of one such stimulus, and is used in a variety of settings, such as athletic performance, general health and fitness, injury prevention and rehabilitation. It is also now commonplace for resistance exercise to be used to offset the debilitating effects of illness, disease and sarcopenia (the latter being a term used to describe the age-related loss in muscle mass, which is also accompanied by increased fatty tissue infiltration and the ensuing decrement in muscle 'quality'). The objectives of the resistance exercise protocol therefore, will vary due to the unique nature of each setting, and therefore should be optimised in order to bring about a specific and desirable set of adaptations. Frequent adaptations that are sought from resistance exercise regimes include an increase in muscle cross-sectional area (CSA) and strength [1], alterations to muscle architecture (spatial arrangement of muscle fibres within a muscle [2]), and greater maximal activation of the musculature [3].

Muscle activation has been widely assessed using surface electromyography (SEMG), and in many cases is expressed as a relative level (%) of maximal voluntary contraction (or MVC). It comprises the sum of the electrical contributions made by the active motor units in proximity to the measurement site. The global characteristics of the surface EMG, such as its amplitude and power spectrum, depend on the membrane properties of the muscle fibres as well as on the timing of the single fibre action potentials. Thus the surface EMG reflects both peripheral and central properties of the neuromuscular system [4]. For many muscles, optimal firing rate, which is that elicited by a maximal voluntary effort, is sufficient to generate a fused tetanus in individual motor units. In predominantly fast-twitch muscles (e.g. biceps brachii), this firing rate is ~30Hz whereas in predominantly slow-twitch muscles (e.g. soleus), this firing rate is ~10Hz [5]. This electromyographic signature is warranted in order for the muscle to express its maximal force generating capabilities, and there have been many studies carried out that have reported a significant increase in agonist SEMG recordings following a resistance training program in both males and females, and in the young as well as the elderly [3, 6-12]. As mentioned previously, muscle adapts in a specific manner to the stimulus provided, and in the case of the aforementioned studies, increases in agonist muscle activation has been shown to be specific to the mode of muscular contraction employed during the resistance training period, and has been fairly well characterised. It is however unclear whether chronic changes in the magnitude of the EMG signal occur with training.

One aspect of resistance training that is scarcely reported in the literature is the acute (and/ or chronic) responses to resistance training programs whereby the length of the muscle when it is loaded is being manipulated. Acutely, it has been demonstrated that there are significantly different responses to exercising at different joint-angles (and thus different muscle lengths). De Ruiter et al. [13] showed that during isometric MVC exercise at 30°, 60°, and 90° of knee flexion, maximal activation of the knee extensors was significantly greater at 90° than the other two angles, despite having identical torque production as 30° (90°; 199±22Nm, 30°; 199±29Nm) and significantly lower torque production than 60° (298±41Nm). A subsequent study [14] found that maximal muscle oxygen consumption was reached significantly later, and was on average ~60% less at 30° compared to 60° and 90° knee flexion. Furthermore, Hisaeda et al.[15] found that when performing isometric contractions at 50% MVC to failure at either 50° or 90° of knee flexion, endurance time was significantly shorter at 90° than 50°. This effect was present both when the exercise was performed with the local circulation occluded and not occluded, thereby highlighting local events as being key to the performance of the musculature at discrete knee angles (or muscle lengths). In addition to this, the slope of the iEMG-time to fatigue regression was significantly greater in the 90° condition compared to 50°. It is proposed that one of the reasons for an increase in oxygen consumption at longer muscle lengths (or more flexed joint angles) is that to produce the same external torque, the internal mechanical stress must be higher at more flexed angles (90°) compared to extended angles (30° or 50°) because the moment arm of the in-series elastic component (i.e. the distance between the tendon and the joint centre of rotation, a factor which impacts on the forces required at the muscle) is shorter [16] at more flexed angles. The above studies provide compelling evidence of the link between the muscle length during a bout of resistance exercise and the acute impact on muscle activation levels, energetic provision, fatigability, as well as torque production. It has therefore been important to determine the nature of the acute effects of length-specific training because it is the accumulation of the acute responses that ultimately are reflected in the chronic muscle adaptations (known as the repeated bout effect).

Previous investigations have also identified the link between muscle length (or joint-angle) and gains in strength and/ or levels of muscle activation following more extended periods of resistance training [17-21]. Briefly, these studies have shown that significantly greater increases in isometric strength are attained when tested at the training length or position, and that these changes in strength are accompanied by significantly greater activation of the muscle at the training position. Furthermore, several studies have outlined that at shorter muscle lengths, the phenomenon of length-specific adaptations are more marked compared to those at longer muscle lengths [19, 21]. For example, performing resistance training at a shorter muscle length results in increases in strength at, and close to the training muscle length, whereas training at longer muscle lengths results in strength increases at, and around a larger range of muscle lengths. However, all of the above data is provided via controlled isometric (static) contractions, when resistance training programs for most individuals are predominantly of a dynamic nature, and therefore warrants further research to extend the knowledge in this area. Therefore the aims of the body of work presented for the first time here were:

1. To describe the acute differences in activation of the Vastus Lateralis (VL) muscle whilst performing dynamic resistance exercise over relatively short muscle lengths compared to long muscle lengths; here comparisons were carried out a) where the external 'perceived' workload is matched, and b) when the internal workload is systematically matched between the two training modalities. 2. To describe the changes in oxygen consumption and cardiovascular responses during these exercise protocols. 3. To identify any link between the acute responses to loading at shorter vs longer muscle lengths; and the more chronic adaptations on VL muscle activation following 8 weeks of length-specific resistance training and 4 weeks detraining.

2. Methods

2.1. Acute study

Ten males (23±3 years, 1.79±0.06m, 73.4±8.4Kg) gave written informed consent to take part in the study. All procedures and experimental protocols were approved by the Ethics Committee at the Manchester Metropolitan University. Exclusion criteria for participation in the study were the presence of any known musculoskeletal, neurological, inflammatory or metabolic disorders or injury. Participants were physically active, involved in recreational activities such as team sports, and had either never taken part in intensive (more than two hours a week) lower limb resistance training or not within the previous 12 months. Participants attended the laboratory for a total of five occasions. The first visit included demonstration of the appropriate squat technique for a standard barbell back squat, and familiarisation of the exercise protocol and testing equipment. The following week participants returned on four occasions, firstly to record their one repetition maximum over each range-of-motion, which was defined as the maximum amount of external weight (Kg) that could be lifted in a controlled manner through the entire range-of-motion, and their MVC on an isokinetic dynamometer (Cybex, Phoenix Healthcare Products, UK) at 50° and 90° of knee flexion. The time-line of the sessions was as follows: Day 1; 1RM & MVC, Day 2; Rest, Day 3; Protocol 1, Day 4; Rest, Day 5; Protocol 2, Day

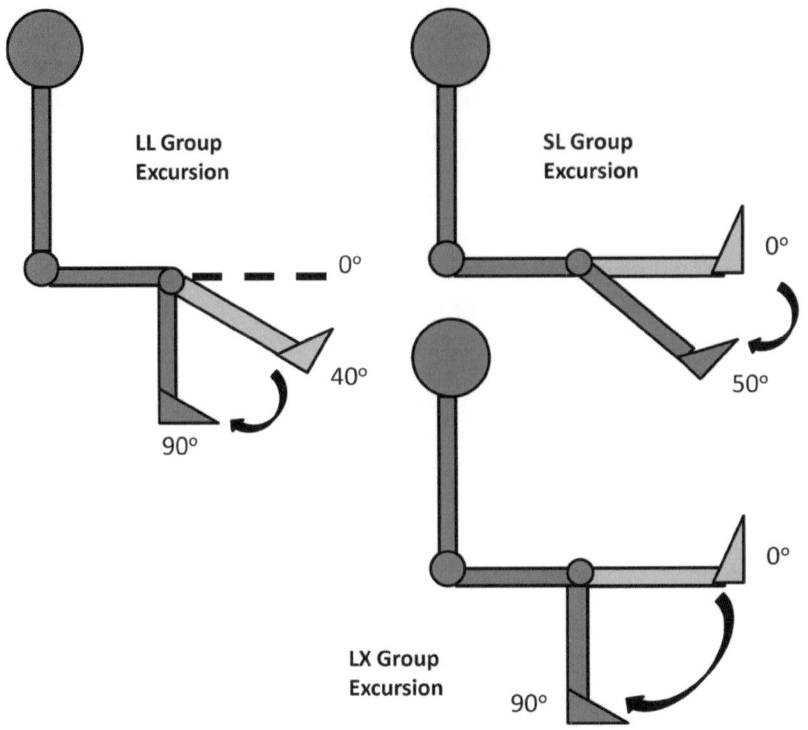

Figure 1. Diagram showing the various knee-joint ranges-of-motion used in the training protocols with a view to describe both acute and chronic training responses

6; Rest, Day 7; Protocol 3. During each of the resistance exercise protocol days, the participants were randomly allocated to perform the resistance exercise session of one of the three designated ranges-of-motion. During each of the resistance exercise sessions, all acute variables (EMG, VO_2, heart rate, blood pressure) were measured.

Exercise Protocols; Each exercise protocol involved performing exercise over one of three ranges-of-motion (Figure 1). The three ranges-of-motion were; 0-50° knee flexion (shorter muscle lengths, SL), 40-90° knee flexion (longer muscle lengths, LL) and 0-90° knee flexion (complete range-of-motion incorporating shorter and longer muscle lengths, LX). A goniometer was attached to the knee joint centre of rotation, from which the investigator confirmed each angle was met during exercise performance. Each exercise session required participants to perform one set of five repetitions back squats at an absolute load of 20Kg, 40Kg and finally 60Kg. Sets were interspersed by two minutes of recovery. Following a further ten minutes rest, each participant performed a further set of five back squats at 40%, 60% and 80% 1RM, interspersed by two minutes of rest.

Electromyography; A pair of self-adhesive Ag-AgCl electrodes 15 mm in diameter (Neuroline 720, Ambu, Denmark), were placed on clean, shaved, and previously abraded skin, in a bipolar configuration with an inter-electrode distance of 20 mm. The electrodes were placed at 50% of femur length and 50% of muscle width of the *Vastus Lateralis* muscle (VL). The reference electrode (Blue sensor L, Ambu, Denmark) was placed on the lateral tibial condyle. The raw EMG signal was amplified and bandpass filtered between 10-500 Hz (MP100, Biopac Systems Inc., USA) with a 50Hz notch filter, and sampled at 2000 Hz. All EMG and torque signals were displayed in real time in AcqKnowledge software (Biopac Systems Inc., USA) via a PC (iMac, Apple Inc., USA). The root mean square (RMS) EMG activity was averaged for a 500ms period which coincided with the plateau of peak torque of all analysed muscle contractions.

Oxygen Consumption (VO_2); Gases for VO_2 consumption were collected using standard Douglas Bag techniques. Prior to the beginning of each set of exercise, a clip was placed on the nose of the participant, the Douglas bag mouthpiece was inserted into the mouth and the valve on an empty bag subsequently opened. After the set of exercise was completed, 30 seconds were allowed to elapse before the valves were closed. This was to allow for any excess post-exercise oxygen consumption during the immediate recovery period. A separate Douglas bag was used for every set of exercise completed. Each bag was analysed using a gas analysis program (Servomex 5200 Multiuse, Crowborough, UK) and was used to calculate the $FECO_2$ and FEO_2 percentages. For these calculation, the data from Gas which had been evacuated for 60 s with a flow rate of 2.1 L/min, the total gas volume which was obtained using a Harvard Dry Gas vacuum (NB. the flow rate (2.1 L) was added to the final figure to give the VE stpd (L/ min^{-1})), the time period in which the Douglas bag was open (secs), load (kg) and subjects' heart rate were all inserted into the gas analysis programme. The VO_2 ($ml/kg^{-1}/min^{-1}$) was also recorded.

Heart rate & Blood Pressure; Heart rate and blood pressure were recorded at rest in the supine position before the onset of exercise using a standard heart rate monitor (Polar, UK) and electronic blood pressure monitoring device (Panasonic Diagnostec, UK). These parameters were also measured immediately post-exercise, after every set of exercise. Rate of perceived exertion (RPE) was also recorded following the conclusion of each individual set of exercise.

2.2. Chronic resistance exercise program study

Thirty two activity-matched participants were allocated to a training group – SL (shorter muscle length 0-50°; 6 males, 4 females; aged 19±2.2 years, 1.76±0.15m, 75.7±13.2Kg), LL (longer muscle length; 5 males, 6 females 40-90°; 21±3.4 years, 1.75±0.14m, 74.9±14.7Kg) or LX (Whole range of motion, 6 males, 5 females 0-90°;19.2±2.6 years, 1.71±0.11m, 73.8±14.9Kg). Ten participants (6 males and 4 females; 23±2.4 years, 1.76±0.09m, 77.9±13.1Kg) were assigned to the non-training control group (Con), and continued their normal habitual activity throughout the study period. A One-way ANOVA revealed that the population was homogeneous at baseline for all parameters of interest ($P>0.05$). All groups were assessed at baseline (week 0), post-training (week 8), after two weeks of detraining (week 10) and following a further two weeks of detraining (week 12).

Electromyography; Preparation of EMG site, measurement and assessment of EMG were as described in the previous section. In addition to these measurements, EMG of the biceps femoris was also recorded during graded maximal contractions in order to assess antagonist muscle co-activation.

Resistance Training Program (RT); RT was carried out 3 days per week for 8 weeks and ceased during the 4 week detraining period. RT included performing 3-4 sets of 8-12 reps (depending on the stage of the training program) of exercises designed to overload the knee extensors muscle group. Exercises included the barbell back squat, leg extension, leg press, Bulgarian split squat, and forward lunge. 1RMs were assessed and recorded every two weeks to progress the exercise loads.

Muscle size measurements; VL muscle widths were measured using B-mode ultrasonography (AU5, Esaote Biomedica, Italy) at 25%, 50% and 75% of femur length. The ultrasound probe was held in the transverse plane and used to locate the borders of either side of the VL muscle. Each of these junctures was marked on the skin and the distance between them measured. In addition, at each of the aforementioned sites, thigh girths were also measured using standard anthropometric techniques. All data is presented as mean ± standard deviation (S.D.).

Muscle strength measurements; Throughout the training program, 1RM of the knee extensors systematically monitored on a knee extension machine (Technogym, Bracknell, UK).

3. Results

3.1. Acute responses

Muscle Activation; As expected *Vastus lateralis* activation increased linearly with absolute external load, with activation being significantly greater ($P<0.05$) when lifting 40Kg compared to 20Kg, and also when lifting 60Kg compared to 40Kg ($P<0.05$) and 20Kg ($P<0.001$). When comparing activation between ranges-of-motion as a percentage of MVC, activation of the muscle was significantly ($P<0.05$) less at SL (59±6%, 63±7%) compared to LL (73±7%, 77±5) and LX (70±7%, 75±6%) at 40Kg and 60Kg loads respectively (Figure 2A). During relative loading, performing exercise at 60% 1RM did not increase activation compared to 40% 1RM ($P>0.05$), though activation was increased at 80% 1RM compared to 60% ($P<0.05$), and 40% ($P<0.001$). There were no significant differences in activation at 40% and 60% 1RM between the three ranges-of-motion ($P>0.05$), whilst at 80% 1RM, VL activation was significantly greater during exercise in LL and LX compared to SL (Figure 2B; $P<0.05$). It is notable that these effects were similar for all two 'long muscle' training protocols so that there were no significant differences between the longer muscle length ROM and the complete ROM under any loading conditions ($P>0.05$).

Oxygen Consumption (VO_2); There was no significant changes in VO_2 between any of the absolute loading conditions or between any ROM ($P>0.05$). Furthermore, in the relative loading conditions, mean VO_2 was significantly greater at 80% 1RM compared to 40% 1RM (6.4±0.9 $ml/kg^{-1}/min^{-1}$ vs. 9.93±1.3 $ml/kg^{-1}/min^{-1}$, $P<0.05$). VO_2 was greater at 40% and 60% 1RM in LL and LX than SL, however there were no significant differences between these ROMs. At 80% 1RM there was a significantly greater VO_2 (Figure 3) in the LL ROM compared to SL ($P<0.05$),

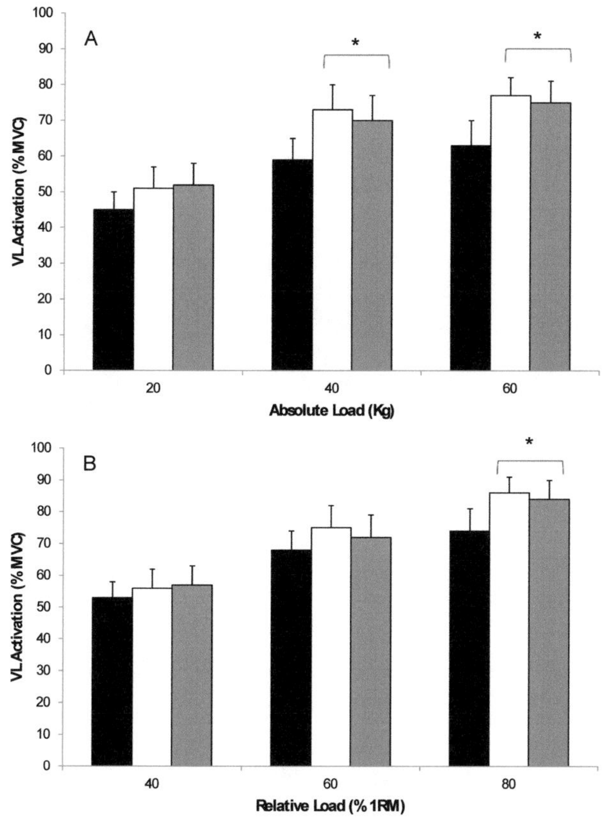

Figure 2. Vastus Lateralis activation in SL (black bars), LL (white bars) and LX (grey bars) following varying magnitudes of absolute and relative loading. * Significantly different to SL

however there were no significant differences between LL and LX, or SL and LX at this loading intensity (P>0.05).

Heart rate & Blood Pressure; There was a significantly greater (P<0.05) mean heart rate difference between LL (139±10 beats per minute) and LX (136±11bpm) compared to SL (118±12bpm) in both absolute and relative loading conditions, with no difference between LL and LX (P>0.05). Mean systolic blood pressure yielded no significant differences (P>0.05) between the three ROMs under relative loading conditions, however LX (148±8 mmHg) mean systolic blood pressure was significantly greater than both SL (138±6 mmHg) and LL (135±8 mmHg) following loading under absolute loads (P<0.05).

3.2. Prolonged resistance training responses

Agonist (VL) Muscle Activation; Figures 4 and 5 shows absolute (i.e. raw RMS_EMG signal) and relative (i.e. RMS_EMG normalised for values at baseline) changes in muscle activation at baseline and post-training. At week 8, absolute maximal agonist activation did not appear

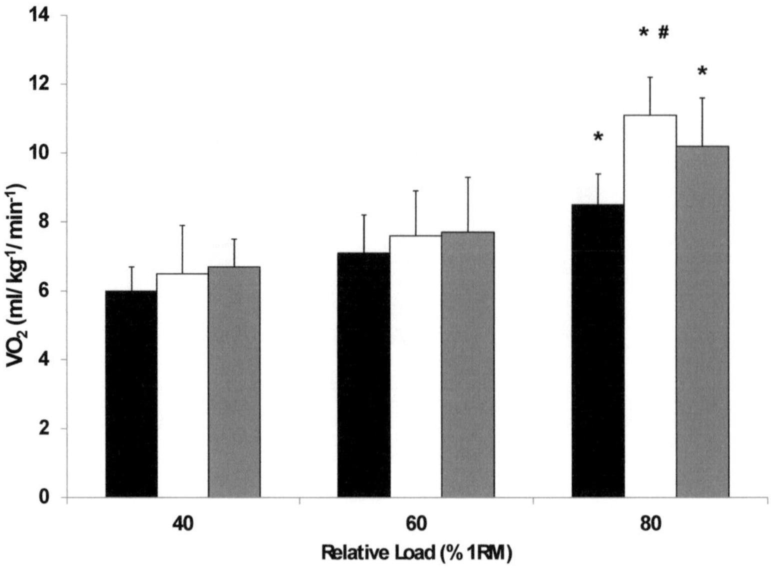

Figure 3. Oxygen consumption (VO_2) during relative loading in SL (black bars), LL (white bars) and LX (grey bars). * Significantly different to 40% 1RM. # Significantly different to SL.

to increase significantly in chronic response to the training protocols, with no significant difference between training groups at any knee angle (P>0.05, Figure 4). However, on further investigation, it was found that in fact, post-training there was a significant relative increase in activation at 50° (23±15%, P<0.05), 70° (26±15%, P<0.01) and 90° (16±13%, P<0.05) in the LX group and at 70° (24±9%, P<0.01) and 90° (25±9%, P<0.01) in LL group. In the SL group there was no significant change at 50°, although there were significant (P<0.05) reductions in VL activation at both 70° (-15±6%) and 90° (-13±5%). Following detraining, muscle activation at 70° decreased at week 10, and levelled off for the remainder of the detraining period (week 12) in both LL and LX groups with no significant changes compared to week 8. In the SL group, activation reduced at both weeks 8, 10 and 12 compared to baseline, however despite larger decrements in this group, there was no significant differences between all three training groups (Figure 6, P>0.05).

Muscle widths and thigh girths; Changes in muscle widths are shown in Table 1. At week 8, VL muscle widths had increased significantly at all three measurement locations in all training groups compared to baseline (P<0.001). Following the first period of detraining at week 10, the SL group had returned to baseline values at all three measurement sites (P>0.05), however both LL and LX groups retained adaptations at this juncture relative to baseline (P<0.01). At week 12 LX group had returned to baseline levels at 25% and 50% width but still remained significantly hypertrophied at 75% femur length compared to baseline (P<0.05). The LL group retained their significant gains in muscle width at all three sites for the duration of detraining (P<0.01). There were no significant (P>0.05) mean relative changes between training groups post-training or following detraining at 25% and 50% femur length (SL; 12±13%, LL; 11±7%, LX; 13±11%). However, LL and LX groups had a greater significant (P<0.05) relative increase in muscle width at week 10 (LL; 26±13%, LX; 21±9%) compared to SL (13±8%) at 75% femur length. This was also the case at week 12, however only LL group was significantly greater (P<0.05) than SL group at this measurement site. Thigh girths increased following training at week 8 in all training groups and at all sites (mean over three sites SL; 3±2%, LL; 4±3%; LX; 4±2%), however this was not significantly different to baseline values (P>0.05) with no differences between groups. Thigh girths also did not differ significantly at weeks 10 or 12 compared to baseline or between groups.

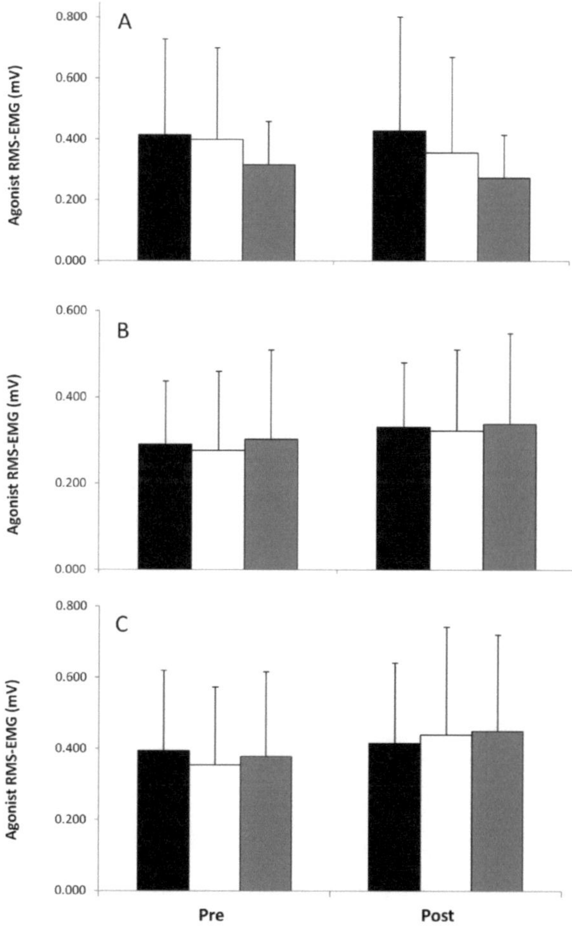

Figure 4. Absolute Changes in VL activation at baseline (pre) and week 8 (post) training at 50° (black bars), 70° (white bars) and 90° (grey bars) knee flexion in A) SL, B) LX and C) LL groups.

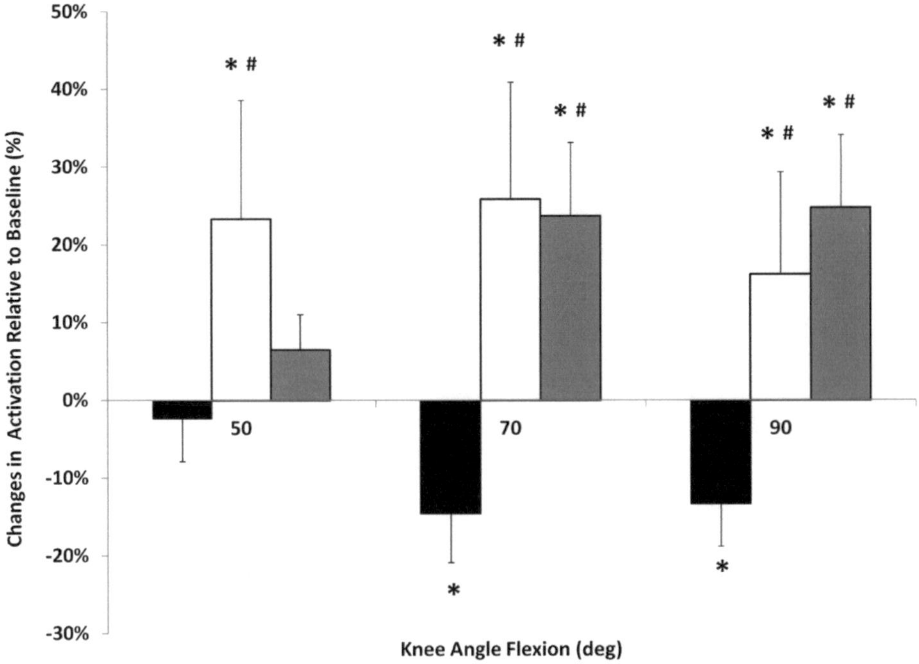

Figure 5. Relative changes in VL activation at week 8 at three knee joint-angles in SL (black bars), LX (white bars) and LL (grey bars). * Significantly different to baseline. # Significantly different to SL group.

Group	% Femur Length	Baseline (cm)	Week 8 (cm)	Week 10 (cm)	Week 12 (cm)
SL	25	12.7±2.3	13.9±2.0*	13.2±1.8	12.9±1.6
	50	12.8±2.7	14.2±2.5**	13.6±1.9	13.3±1.9
	75	9.6±2.2	11.0±1.9*	10.1±1.2	9.6±1.1
LL	25	14.0±1.3	15.3±1.6**	15.6±1.1**	15.3±0.9**
	50	13.8±1.6	15.6±2.0**	15.8±1.5**	15.4±1.3**
	75	9.4±1.8	11.4±1.4**	11.5±1.2**	11.1±1.3**
LX	25	12.2±2.7	14.2±1.9**	13.0±2.0**	12.4±1.8
	50	12.1±2.6	14.3±2.3**	13.1±2.0**	12.3±2.0
	75	8.2±2.2	10.6±1.5**	9.6±1.6**	8.8±1.2*

Table 1. Changes in Vastus Lateralis muscle width at each measurement site throughout training and detraining. * Significantly different to baseline ($P<0.05$) ** Significantly different to baseline ($P<0.01$)

http://dx.doi.org/10.5772/56386

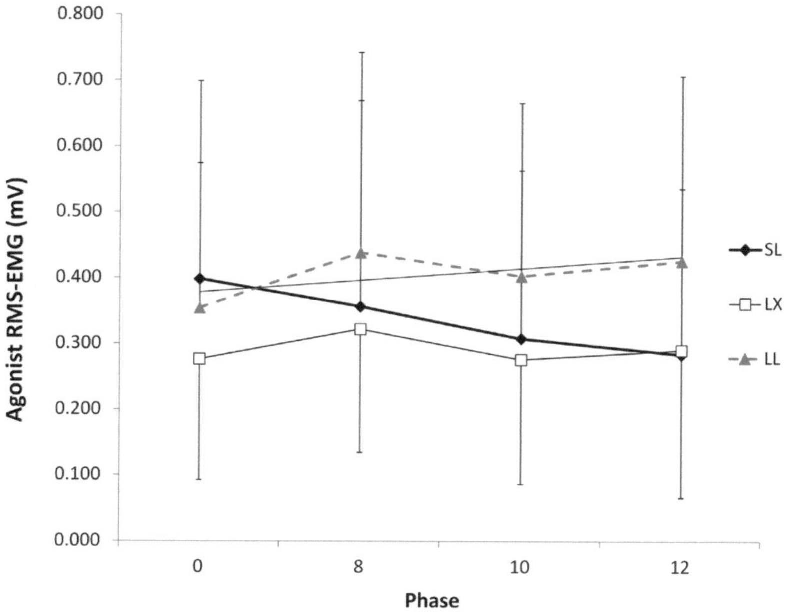

Figure 6. Absolute changes in VL activation throughout training and detraining periods at 70° knee flexion. No significant were detected between phases or training groups (P>0.05).

Strength measures; 1RM in knee extension did not increase significantly compared to baseline until week 4 of the training program (data pooled, P<0.05) with each training group making similar increments in weight (SL; 11±4%, LL; 9±5%, LX 12±5%). There were further significant increases at week 6 (mean of groups 16±6%, P<0.01) and week 8 (mean of groups 22±8%, P<0.001), with no significant difference in the rate of relative increase in 1RM between groups (P>0.05). When muscle activation was normalised against torque at week 8 (Figure 7) as a marker for muscle efficiency, both LL and LX groups showed significantly better improved muscle efficiency compared with SL (P<0.01) at 90° of knee flexion, however there were no differences in muscle activation per unit torque at 50° or 70° following training (P>0.05). LL and LX were not significantly different to each other in terms of the degree of muscle efficiency increase.

4. Discussion

Resistance training presents a medium through which muscular function can be enhanced. In order to devise an appropriate and effective resistance training program tailored with functional and structural enhancement objectives, it is necessary to understand the responses to both an acute bout of exercise, and the adaptations to exercise over a prolonged period of training. An important aspect for muscular performance is the degree to which the muscle can be activated. Previous work using isometric contractions of the knee extensors, has demonstrated that the magnitude of maximal muscle activation is dependent on the joint-angle (and thus muscle-length) used during exercise, even when external torque produced is maintained at a similar level at the different joint angles [13]. This earlier study showed that activation of the quadriceps is significantly greater at 90° knee flexion compared to both 30° and 60°, despite isometric MVC torque being significantly less than 60° and identical to 30°. In the current study, unlike previous research, our participants exercised dynamically over a range-of-motion that was predominantly over shorter muscle lengths (0-50°), longer muscle lengths (40-90°) or over both short and long muscle lengths (0-90°) during exercise using absolute and relative loading patterns. During absolute loading, weight lifted increased in a graded manner, and was reflected by significantly increased muscle activation between each absolute load in the training groups. This result was a more easily predicted outcome and reflects one of the fundamental properties of the neuromuscular system, i.e. the size principle [22], where a greater number of motor units are recruited in order to meet the increasing demands of force production. When exercising over longer muscle lengths (LL) and the complete ROM (LX), muscle activation was significantly greater during absolute and relative loading compared to shorter muscle lengths (SL). So why would a muscle exhibit greater activation whilst moving the same external weight but at different muscle lengths? By moving through a range of muscle lengths or joint-angles, the moment arm of the in-series elastic component (i.e. the tendon) also changes. As the amount of force needed to lift an external load (F) is $F = f \times d$, where f is the internal force produced by the muscle and d is the length of the moment arm, when d is greater f will be smaller and vice versa, and therefore when the external force produced is the same but the moment arm (d) is smaller, the contribution from internal muscle force production increases. An example of this experienced in daily living is the increased difficulty in rising from a low seat position compared to a higher seated position. It has been demonstrated previously that when the joint-angle in the knee extensors is at 90° flexion (such as the end of LL and LX group ROM), the moment arm is considerably shorter [16] than when at 50° (the end of SL ROM). Therefore when exercising at 90°, internally the muscle must produce a greater amount of contractile force to overcome the external weight than that required at 50° knee angle. Again due to the overloading principle of training response, a larger number of motor units will have needed to be recruited to match the force demands at the longer muscle lengths, reflected by the increase in RMS-EMG activity of the VL muscle. In support of this hypothesis, Kubo et al. [21] trained the knee extensors isometrically at either 50° or 100° of knee flexion. Based on their MVC and EMG recordings, they estimated that the internal force on the quadriceps muscles was 2.3 times greater at longer muscle lengths (i.e. 100°) than at shorter lengths. A further variable that must be considered is the influence of changing muscle lengths on the force-length relationship of muscle (for review see [23]). In short, when one alters the length of a muscle, the basic contractile units of individual muscle fibres, known as sarcomeres, also change length. The ability of sarcomeres (and thus muscle) to exert force is determined mainly by actin and myosin filaments interaction and cross-bridge formation. As sarcomere (or muscle) lengths increase, cross-bridges number and force is increased up to an optimal length. Beyond this length (i.e. with further lengthening), decreases cross-bridges formation and force are seen (NB. The caveat here is lies with contractile speed, and preceding type and degree of muscle contraction [24]. If longer muscle lengths are less optimal for force production and cross-bridge formation than shorter muscle lengths, then greater motor unit recruitment will be necessary to overcome the external resistance. Therefore the two factors likely for greater activation in LL and LX compared to SL may be due to the greater internal mechanical stress on the muscle because of a shorter moment arm, and/ or the length of the muscle reducing cross-bridge formation and force production per sarcomere, all other things (contraction type, speed and history) being equal.

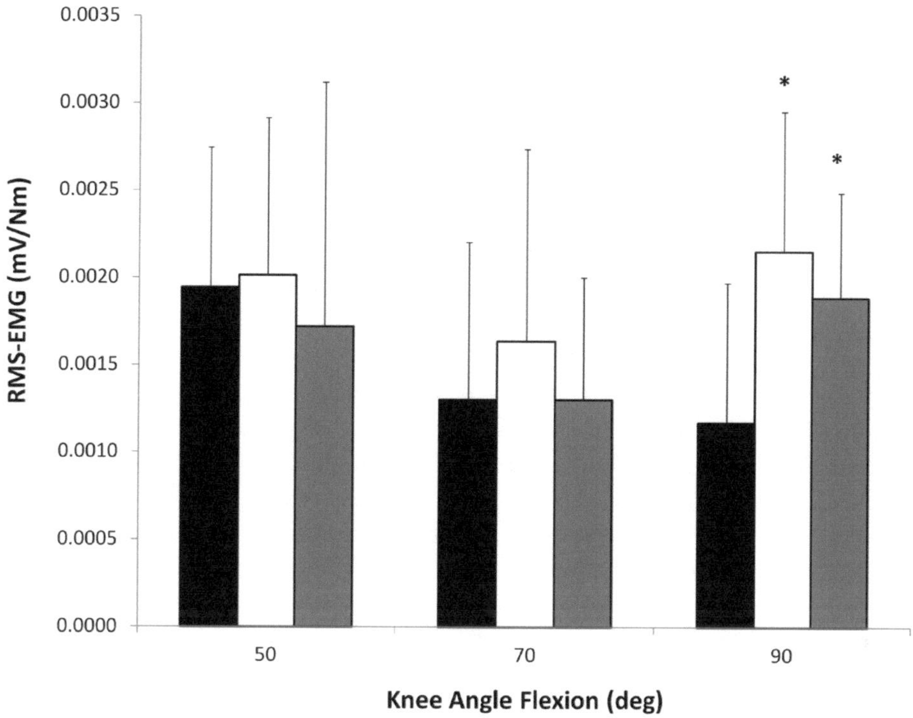

Figure 7. Vastus Lateralis muscle efficiency (i.e. activation per unit of torque) at week 8 at three joint-angles in SL (black bars), LL (white bars) and LX (grey bars). * Significantly different to SL (P<0.05). N.B. there were no between group differences at baseline.

In the current study, oxygen consumption (VO_2) was shown to be significantly greater at 80%1RM compared to 40% 1RM, and also significantly greater in both the LL and LX ROMs compared to SL ROM at 80% 1RM loading. VO_2 is used in exercise physiology to provide valuable information, such as an indicator of energy expenditure. Oxygen is 'consumed' by the working muscle during oxidative phosphorylation in order to produce, maintain and/ or replenish the energy used during the many different processes involved with muscular contraction. Therefore if a particular form of exercise requires the use of greater volumes of oxygen, this indicates that the system is working harder in order to meet the demands. It has been demonstrated previously in humans that oxygen consumption increases with work intensity during constant isometric loading of the knee extensors [13, 14], and this is reflected by the increased VO_2 at 80% 1RM compared to 40% 1RM, where although performing the same ROMs, participants were exerting greater force, requiring more energy to supply muscular contraction. The relative VO_2 levels are much lower than normally encountered during aerobic exercise for example, due to the shorter duration of exercise bouts and greater contribution to energy supply from anaerobic sources such as ATP-PCr system and glycolysis. Of more interest in the present study was the fact that both LL and LX ROMs had significantly greater VO_2 compared to SL at 80% 1RM. Previous research using near-infrared spectroscopy has demonstrated that during isometric exercise of the knee extensors, VL muscle VO_2 is significantly increased at longer muscle lengths (60° and 90°) compared to shorter muscle lengths (30°). This was even despite the fact that MVC torque relative to the maximum torque capacity (MTC) tended to be greater (~85% of MTC) at 30° compared to both 60° and 90° (~75% MTC). A subsequent study by Kooistra et al. [14] demonstrated that knee extensor muscle activation and VO_2 were significantly less, and time to VO_{2max} significantly longer at the same relative torque levels at 30° compared to 60° and 90°. An additional indication of the increased stress at longer muscle lengths was the observation that at 80% 1RM, although covering almost half the ROM of LX, LL group showed a trend (though not statistically significant) to consuming greater volumes of oxygen. This suggests that the energetic cost of constantly working at longer muscle lengths is at least just as, if not more demanding than, alternating between longer and shorter muscle lengths even when over a relatively large ROM. With significantly higher heart rates in both LL and LX groups (and also greater blood pressure in LX) compared to SL during exercise, the results also suggest that the cardiovascular system was also under greater stress at longer muscle lengths. Taken into consideration with both the aforementioned differences between the LL and LX groups compared to SL with regards muscle activation and oxygen consumption, it appears that performing exercise over predominantly longer muscle lengths (or incorporating longer muscle lengths into a full ROM) present a more potent stress to both neuromuscular and cardiovascular systems than performing exercise over mainly shorter muscle lengths. So what factors are present that would require greater oxygen consumption at longer muscle lengths? First of all, as mentioned previously, there are a number of processes that occur in order for a muscle to contract and produce force. One such process has been termed excitation-contraction coupling, where an action potential induces the release of calcium ions (Ca^{2+}) from the muscle membrane (sarcoplasmic reticulum) and these ions interact with the thin filaments of a sarcomere, allowing muscle contraction to occur. Ca^{2+} ions are then transported back into the sarcoplasmic reticulum for storage, allowing the muscle to relax. These processes are ATP-dependent (i.e. energy consuming) and as energy is consumed during activation, the amount of energy is measured as heat [25]. Therefore if greater activation of the muscle is occurring at longer muscle lengths, the possibility exists that the energy cost of this activation is also greater, and that this mechanism requires greater oxygen consumption to supply the energy. In addition, potentiation is force enhancement following muscle contraction, and is dependent on the contractile history. Place et al.[26] showed that following fatiguing contractions in the quadriceps muscles at either shorter (35°) or longer (75°) muscle lengths, peak twitch potentiation and doublet force were significantly greater at shorter muscle lengths, which may also allow for a reduction in energy cost as activation may be reduced.

Secondly, we have already discussed the likelihood that due to the internal architecture of muscles and tendons, that the length of the moment arm will dictate that greater muscle force will have to be produced at longer muscle lengths compared to shorter muscle lengths. Production of the additional force through recruitment of more motor units would mean that more of the contractile machinery would be used and be consuming energy, as muscular contraction from cross-bridge cycling also requires ATP [27, 28]. Therefore the additional oxygen consumption observed at longer muscle lengths may be the result of both the energetic requirements of muscle activation and the increased energetic requirements of force production. This hypothesis is consistent with the fact that endurance performance is significantly reduced with time to fatigue at longer muscle lengths compared to shorter muscle length, regardless of of the intensities of loading and circulatory conditions [15, 26, 29]. Consistent with an increased oxygen demand, would be an increase in heart rate which was observed between the groups.

When exercise is performed on a regular basis, the above acute responses to a bout of exercise will eventually result in long-term adaptations (i.e. repeated bout effect), which will allow the body to complete the same exercise bout as before but with relatively less disturbance to homeostasis. During the resistance training program, the three groups performed exercise over the same range-of-motion as during the acute bouts (i.e. SL, LL and LX), with the only differences being the degree of loading. SL and LX exercised at 80% 1RM, whereas LL exercised at 55% 1RM, where this was to allow the length of muscle excursion (50°) and the internal muscle forces to be as similar as possible during resistance training between SL and LL. Following 8 weeks of resistance training, absolute changes in muscle activation did not increase significantly at any of the angles tested (50°; shorter lengths, 70° more optimal lengths, 90° longer lengths) during an isometric MVC. There have been conflicting reports throughout the literature concerning the possible increase in agonist activation following resistance training, as there have been studies published that have reported significant changes [3, 6-12], whereas some have not [30-33]. However, comparing longitudinal changes in agonist EMG both within and between studies can prove difficult due to methodological differences [34]. In one length-specific resistance training study, Thepaut-Mathieu et al. [19] reported an increase in iEMG-force relationships at the specific joint angles used during training. These findings were also supported by Kubo et al. [21] who found that iEMG of the quadriceps (rectus femoris, vastus lateralis and vastus medialis) increased significantly in groups that trained at either shorter or longer muscle lengths, with no differences between the groups at any of the joint-angles tested. In the current study there were also no significant differences in maximal activation levels between groups and muscle lengths. However, one of the main findings from the current study was the significant relative increases in activation at all muscle lengths in LX, at longer muscle lengths in LL, and significant decreases in activation at longer muscle lengths in SL. This is further evidence of the muscle length (or joint-angle) specificity phenomenon following resistance training. Whereas a previous study [21] found that relative quadriceps iEMG increased at all measured knee angles (40-110°) following 12 weeks of isometric resistance training at shorter muscle lengths, our results show a decrease in activation at longer muscle lengths occurred following training at shorter muscle lengths. Interestingly from the study of Kubo et al. [21] was the fact that although iEMG increased within the range of ~25-45% over all testing angles (40-110°) following training at shorter muscle lengths, MVC only significantly increased between 40-80° in this group. Previous work from our laboratory has shown that MVC torque did not change significantly at longer muscle lengths following a period of resistance training at shorter muscle lengths [35], and results from the current investigation show that this could be in part be mediated by a reduction in maximal activation at these lengths. Further evidence of muscle-length specificity was the fact that only LX group, who covered an entire ROM, actually demonstrated a significant relative increase in activation at each angle tested, and also that LL only showed significant relative increases in activation at longer muscle lengths (lengths where the majority of training would have taken place). In order to allow us to describe the impact of changes in activation on strength changes, we have shown that there was significantly greater muscule efficiency (EMG per unit of torque) at longer muscle lengths (i.e. in LL and LX) compared to SL, following the 8-week training program. Changes in torque generating capacity are not accounted for solely, or at times at all by increased muscle activation. Changes in muscle architecture, morphology and/ or muscle specific tension are just a few of the many other factors that can impact a muscle's ability to produce force following resistance training as well as neural adaptations (for review see [34]). However in this case, there appears to be a relationship between the increased activation of the VL muscle and the changes in torque production following resistance training in LL and LX at longer muscle lengths.

As indicated above, one of the other factors influencing changes in torque or force production following resistance exercise is muscle morphology, such as size. There is a strong positive relationship between the size of a muscle and the force it is able to exert [1]. In the current study, all of the three training groups increased the size of the VL muscle at proximal (25%), central (50%) and distal (75% of femur length) measurement sites at week 8. However in the SL group, the muscle size increment was more significant centrally rather than at proximal and distal sites of the VL, whereas both LL and LX had fairly equal distribution of size increment along the length of the muscle. Firstly, this information suggests that the resistance training program was effective in increasing muscle size, which is a well established characteristic of resistance training. Secondly, the results also suggest that the ROM involved during resistance training (i.e. the muscle lengths used) may produce region specific variations in muscle growth. Our laboratory has provided more conclusive evidence that muscle size increments at distal regions are enhanced to a greater degree immediately following resistance training at longer muscle lengths [35], however in the current study this was only apparent following two weeks of detraining, although these were still present following a total of four weeks detraining. The region specific variation in muscle size has been previously documented throughout literature (e.g. [31]), and is probably due to the unique way in which forces are transmitted along the length of a muscle when exercised at different lengths. Forces in muscles are transmitted both serially and in parallel [36], and when training at longer muscle lengths, there may be a more pronounced parallel transmission of force at distal regions of the muscle, providing a stimulus for growth in this location. In terms of muscle growth, force production and muscle stretch are potent stimulators of muscle protein synthesis, with a combination of both having an additive effect [37]. In vitro experiments have shown that when muscle cells are stretched to longer lengths, there is a marked increase in protein synthesis and growth factor mRNA [38]. The LL and LX groups when performing exercise at longer muscle lengths would have experienced a larger degree of muscle stretch compared to SL, and would have also been simultaneously producing force. In addition, because LX group worked at an intensity of 80% 1RM, peak force generation would also have been greater in this group. This is supported by the mean relative increase in VL muscle width being greatest in this group at all measurement sites, although due to the variation between subjects, this was not statistically significant. It is encouraging that despite the greater absolute force generations in LX compared to LL, the LL group (who remained at longer muscle lengths throughout each training session, and therefore muscle stretch would probably have persisted compared to LX group who worked between shorter and longer muscle lengths), these two groups exhibited similar muscle hypertrophy responses. What is more, yet another encouraging aspect of LL training was the fact that at week 10, VL muscle widths were significantly greater in LL and LX at all measurement sites compared to baseline, whereas the SL group had returned to baseline values. Following a further two weeks of detraining, LX group muscle widths only remained significantly greater than baseline values at 75% femur length, whereas LL group retained post-training increments in muscle width at all measurement sites for the entirety of the detraining period. Therefore not only does training at longer muscle lengths possibly confer more beneficial adaptations following training, but it also appears to allow retention of these adaptations for a longer period of time. This is a positive finding from the current study, in that following any periods on illness, injury or tapering that occur to the individual, longer-term retention of the benefits of the preceding resistance exercise will minimise the impact of such deleterious events.

5. Conclusion

Performing resistance training over predominantly longer muscle lengths compared to shorter muscle lengths produces stepwise degrees of acute muscular, energetic and cardiovascular responses, which then culminate to differential magnitudes of chronic training as well as detraining adaptations. As a progression to the earlier research evidence from isometric exercise in terms of both acute [13, 14] and chronic [21] muscle length-specific training, the current study is the first to systematically show that dynamic exercise at longer muscle lengths also results in greater activation and oxygen consumption. The nature of the acute responses suggests that the muscle is more physiologically stressed at longer muscle lengths. Following a prolonged period of resistance training (i.e. an accumulation of training bouts), we show that long-length trained muscle exhibits relatively greater muscle activation, neuromuscular efficiency and hypertrophy compared with its short-length trained counterpart. Similarly with detraining, long-length training was associated with a greater retention of improvements in muscle characteristics. It is likely that in this case also, the more beneficial size increments in particular, were the result of greater physiological stress, a result of the combined effects of smaller moment arm and enhanced muscle stretch. These findings have implications for athletic, elderly, or post-operative populations to name but a few end users.

Author details

Gerard E. McMahon, Gladys L. Onambélé-Pearson*, Christopher I. Morse, Adrian M. Burden and Keith Winwood

*Address all correspondence to: g.pearson@mmu.ac.uk

Institute for Performance Research, Department of Exercise & Sport Science, Manchester Metropolitan University, Crewe, UK

References

[1] Maughan, R. J, Watson, J. S, & Weir, J. Strength and cross-sectional area of human skeletal muscle. The journal of physiology, (1983). , 37-49.

[2] Kawakami, Y, et al. Training-induced changes in muscle architecture and specific tension. European Journal of Applied Physiology and Occupational Physiology, (1995). , 37-43.

[3] Moritani, T, & Devries, H. Neural factors versus hypertrophy in the time course of muscle strength gain. American Journal of Physical Medicine, (1979). , 115.

[4] Farina, D, Merletti, R, & Enoka, R. M. The extraction of neural strategies from the surface EMG. Journal of Applied Physiology, (2004). , 1486-1495.

[5] Motor-unit, B, B. F. W. J. J. R. B. -R. discharge rates in maximal voluntary contractions of three human muscles. J Neurophysiol, (1983). , 1380-1392.

[6] Häkkinen, K, et al. Neuromuscular adaptations during bilateral versus unilateral strength training in middle-aged and elderly men and women. Acta Physiologica Scandinavica, (1996). , 77-88.

[7] Narici, M, et al. Changes in force, cross-sectional area and neural activation during strength training and detraining of the human quadriceps. European Journal of Applied Physiology and Occupational Physiology, (1989). , 310-319.

[8] Häkkinen, K, et al. Neuromuscular adaptations during concurrent strength and endurance training versus strength training. European journal of applied physiology, (2003). , 42-52.

[9] Komi, P, et al. Effect of isometric strength training on mechanical, electrical, and metabolic aspects of muscle function. European Journal of Applied Physiology and Occupational Physiology, (1978). , 45-55.

[10] Häkkinen, K, & Komi, P. V. Electromyographic changes during strength training and detraining. Medicine and science in sports and exercise, (1983). , 455.

[11] Reeves, N. D, Maganaris, C. N, & Narici, M. V. Plasticity of dynamic muscle performance with strength training in elderly humans. Muscle & nerve, (2005). , 355-364.

[12] Higbie, E. J, et al. Effects of concentric and eccentric training on muscle strength, cross-sectional area, and neural activation. Journal of Applied Physiology, (1996). , 2173-2181.

[13] De Ruiter, C. J, et al. Knee angle-dependent oxygen consumption during isometric contractions of the knee extensors determined with near-infrared spectroscopy. Journal of Applied Physiology, (2005). , 579-586.

[14] Kooistra, R, et al. Knee extensor muscle oxygen consumption in relation to muscle activation. European journal of applied physiology, (2006). , 535-545.

[15] Hisaeda, H, et al. Effect of local blood circulation and absolute torque on muscle endurance at two different knee-joint angles in humans. European journal of applied physiology, (2001). , 17-23.

[16] Krevolin, J. L, Pandy, M. G, & Pearce, J. C. Moment arm of the patellar tendon in the human knee. Journal of biomechanics, (2004). , 785-788.

[17] Lindh, M. Increase of muscle strength from isometric quadriceps exercises at different knee angles. Scandinavian journal of rehabilitation medicine, (1979). , 33.

[18] Gardner, G. W. Specificity of strength changes of the exercised and nonexercised limb following isometric training. Res Q, (1963). , 98-101.

[19] Thepaut-mathieu, C, Van Hoecke, J, & Maton, B. Myoelectrical and mechanical changes linked to length specificity during isometric training. Journal of Applied Physiology, (1988). , 1500.

[20] Kitai, T, & Sale, D. Specificity of joint angle in isometric training. European Journal of Applied Physiology and Occupational Physiology, (1989). , 744-748.

[21] Kubo, K, et al. Effects of isometric training at different knee angles on the muscle-tendon complex in vivo. Scandinavian Journal of Medicine & Science in Sports, (2006). , 159-167.

[22] Henneman, E, Somjen, G, & Carpenter, D. O. Functional significance of cell size in spinal motoneurons. Journal of Neurophysiology, (1965). , 560-580.

[23] Rassier, D, & Mac, B. Intosh, and W. Herzog, Length dependence of active force production in skeletal muscle. Journal of Applied Physiology, (1999). , 1445.

[24] RC, O.G.B.S.W., Effects of voluntary activation level on force exerted by human adductor pollicis muscle during rapid stretches. Pflugers Arch, 2004 448(4): p. 457-61.

[25] Homsher, E, et al. Activation heat, activation metabolism and tension-related heat in frog semitendinosus muscles. The journal of physiology, (1972). , 601-625.

[26] Place, N, et al. Twitch potentiation is greater after a fatiguing submaximal isometric contraction performed at short vs. long quadriceps muscle length. Journal of Applied Physiology, (2005)., 429-436.

[27] Huxley, A. F. Muscle structure and theories of contraction. Progress in biophysics and biophysical chemistry, (1957)., 255-318.

[28] Huxley, A. F, & Simmons, R. M. Proposed mechanism of force generation in striated muscle. Nature, (1971)., 533-538.

[29] Ng, A. V, et al. Influence of muscle length and force on endurance and pressor responses to isometric exercise. Journal of Applied Physiology, (1994)., 2561-2569.

[30] Garfinkel, S, & Cafarelli, E. Relative changes in maximal force, EMG, and muscle cross-sectional area after isometric training. Medicine & Science in Sports & Exercise, (1992)., 1220.

[31] Narici, M, et al. Human quadriceps cross sectional area, torque and neural activation during 6 months strength training. Acta Physiologica Scandinavica, (1996)., 175-186.

[32] Weir, J, et al. The effect of unilateral eccentric weight training and detraining on joint angle specificity, cross-training, and the bilateral deficit. The Journal of orthopaedic and sports physical therapy, (1995)., 207.

[33] Aagaard, P, et al. Increased rate of force development and neural drive of human skeletal muscle following resistance training. Journal of Applied Physiology, (2002)., 1318-1326.

[34] Folland, J. P, & Williams, A. G. The Adaptations to Strength Training: Morphological and Neurological Contributions to Increased Strength. Sports Medicine, (2007). , 145-168.

[35] McMahon, G, et al. Impact of range-of-motion during ecologically valid resistance training protocols, on muscle size, subcutaneous fat and strength. Journal of Strength & Conditioning Research, (2013). In Press).

[36] Huijing, P, & Jaspers, R. Adaptation of muscle size and myofascial force transmission: a review and some new experimental results. Scandinavian Journal of Medicine & Science in Sports, (2005)., 349-380.

[37] Goldspink, G. Changes in muscle mass and phenotype and the expression of autocrine and systemic growth factors by muscle in response to stretch and overload. Journal of Anatomy, (1999)., 323-334.

[38] Goldspink, D. F, et al. Muscle growth in response to mechanical stimuli. American Journal of Physiology- Endocrinology And Metabolism, (1995)., E288-E297.

Chapter 9

Surface Electromyography in Sports and Exercise

Hande Türker and Hasan Sözen

Additional information is available at the end of the chapter

http://dx.doi.org/10.5772/56167

1. Introduction

Exercise is constantly gaining popularity. It has been widely used especially in the fields of sports performance and rehabilitation [1].

Performance and ability tests enable the success in education of sports and exercise. Various exercise equipments are used in test protocols that are developed for this goal. The reason to use various kinds of exercise equipments for performance measurement is that every equipment and protocol cause different responses in human body. The cause for evolution of different physiological responses is about the different shapes and densities of different muscles. In this very respect, the electromyographic measurements gain great importance.

Electromyographic studies help us understand the location of the problem in the system of movement. The problem may be localized to the peripheral nervous system or the muscle itself and sometimes may also be at the neuromuscular juntion. This diagnostic tool is therefore very valuable in the differential diagnosis of nerve and muscle diseases [2]. Electromyography is also used in morphological analysis of the motor unit [3. It is important to snychronize the systems that supply cinematic data with electromyography to determine the period when different muscles join the muscle movement. These systems use cameras, electrogoniometers and other registration tools with their programs in order to give us information about position, speed and acceleration measurements. Additionaly, the study can be completed with podometer and power platform as power analysis systems and this is called the kinetic system. Surface EMG (sEMG) is an important tool of biomechanical analysis and a very important part of this system. [4,5]. It helps to understand the role of a muscle in a spesific movement [6,7]

Surface EMG has increasing importance in sports and occupational medicine and in ergonomic studies [8,9]. It can also establish dynamic analysis and therefore is important in sports [10,11]. The utilization of muscles in a right and economical fashion helps improve activity and prevents the risk of injury. The most important points to achieve healthy training are the follow up of development and performing corrections where necessary [5,12,13]. The electromyographical analysis can determine muscle activation and fatigue and thus helps achieve development of performance [9].

Muscle activation is a result of the effort of muscle but the relationship between EMG activity and effort is only qualitative [5].

Surface EMG in current sports studies also deals with determination and descriptions of the muscle types [14,15].

2. Muscular system

Muscles are designed to exert force in order to move the body. Skeletal system and muscles are connected to each other by tendons. Combination of muscle and bone is brought about by the tendon intermeshing with the skeletal periosteum sheath. Tendons are the strong connective tissue composed of three layers. And this extends the length of all the muscle and collagen protein. Epimysium, perimysium and endomysium are the connnective tissues forming each tendon. There are three types of muscle tissue in the body, they are smooth, cardiac and skeletal muscles [16,17]. Specific anatomical features that affect the length of muscle fiber, muscle fiber type and muscle compartments may differ between muscles. EMG signals may be affected by them and therefore EMG recordings and interpretation of them must take anatomical differences into account [18,19].

2.1. Muscle types

2.1.1. Smooth muscle

Smooth muscle is found in the digestive tract, surrounds the blood vessels, airways and respiratory systems. Smooth muscle is innervated by the autonomic nervous system such as cardiac muscle and therefore we do not have voluntary control over its contractions [20,17].

2.1.2. Cardiac muscle

Cardiac muscular system is located in the heart tissue and has striped appearance under light microscopy. The same striations are also found in skeletal muscle and indicate the presence of different proteins required for muscle contraction [21,17].

2.1.3. Skeletal muscle

Skeletal muscular system has the only muscle type that can be voluntarily contracted and skeletal muscle has active elements forming the movement. The human body consists of more than 600 muscles [21,17]. The functions of the muscular system are movement of blood and food within the body, the ability to stop the body moving, to store oxygen and nutrients such as glycogen for energy production and, through the energy production reactions, to produce

http://dx.doi.org/10.5772/56167

heat to help maintain body temperature [17]. Skeletal muscle converts chemical energy to mechanical and heat energy. Skeletal muscle uses adenosine triphosphate (ATP) as fuel during electrical, mechanical and chemical events. This process, called action potential begins with an electrical impulse from the brain [22,23]. This initiates a chain of biochemical reactions that ends in the burning of adenosine triphosphate, the fuel for muscle contraction. Its use results in the forces that move the limbs and generate heat. Electrodes attached to a muscle group record the electrical activity accompanying contraction; the name of this recording process is electromyography (EMG) [23].

2.2. The Motor Unit Action Potential (MUAP)

Motor units are the functional assets of the neuromuscular system. Each motor unit consists of a single motoneuron and the muscle fibers supplied by its axonal branches [24,25]. Once a motoneuron discharges, action potentials are generated at its neuromuscular junctions and then propagate along all the muscle fibers, toward the tendon regions. The summation of these potentials is termed motor unit action potentials and is responsible for the muscle contraction [25]. MUAP is the sum of the extracellular potentials of muscle fiber action potentials of a motor unit [3]. The waveform is determined by the natural properties of the relationship between muscle fibers. [24,3]. The extracellularly recorded MUAP, recorded along the length of the muscle fibers and away from the endplate region, has a triphasic waveform. The initial positive deflection represents the action potential propagating towards the electrode. As the potential passes in front of the electrode the main positive-negative deflection is recorded. When the action potential propagates away from the electrode the potential returns to the baseline. Slight repositioning of the electrode causes major changes in the electrical profile of the same motor unit. Therefore, one motor unit can give rise to MUAPs of different morphology at different recording sites. If the electrode is placed immediately over the endplate area, the initial positive deflection will not be recorded and the potential will have a biphasic waveform with an initial negative deflection [3]. All the muscle fibers of a motor unit work in unison; that is, all are discharged nearly synchronously upon the arrival of a nerve impulse along the axon and through its terminal branches to the motor end plates. A MUAP is recorded by a needle electrode. The recorded motor unit action potential can be derived from action potentials of a small number of muscle fibers, a moderate number of muscle fibers, or a great majority of muscle fibers belonging to the motor unit [26].

2.3. Types of muscle action

Among the variety of types of muscle action are the isometric, concentric and eccentric; all three forms occur during the actions seen in sport and exercise performance [27]. When there is no change in muscle length during muscle activation, the action is called isometric. Isometric action occurs when an athlete tries to leg-press a heavy load by flexing the quadriceps muscles, but cannot move the weight-stack in spite of a maximum effort. The muscle produces force, but it is insufficient to overcome the mass of the weight stack; hence, the overall muscle length does not shorten. Isometric muscle action occurs when the muscle contracts without moving, generating force while its length remains static. Isometric muscle actions are demonstrated in

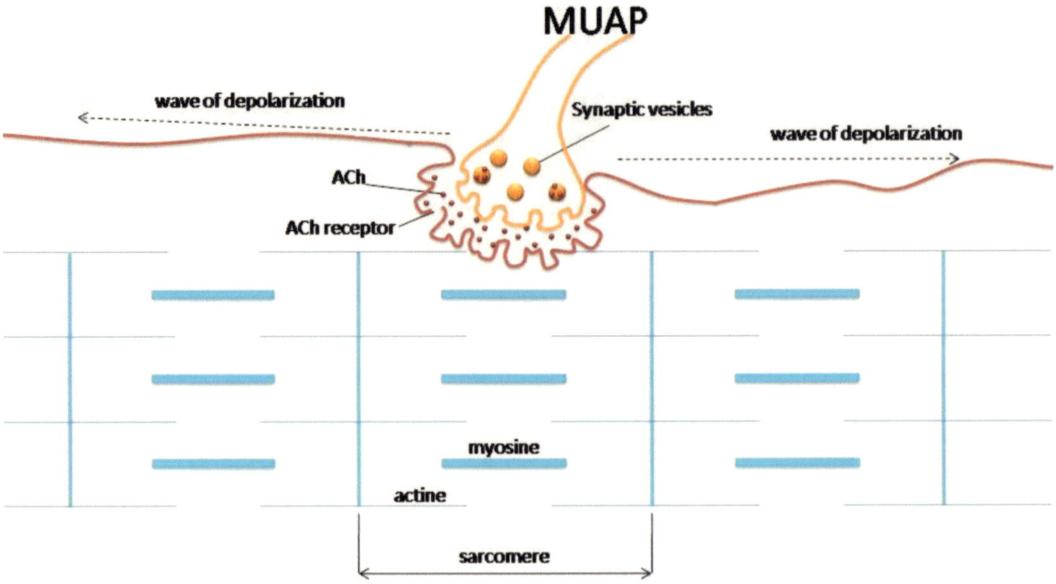

Figure 1. When a skeletal muscle fiber is activated by a MUAP, a wave of electrical depolarization travels along the surface of the fiber (drawn by Sözen H.).

an attempt to lift an immovable object or an object that is too heavy to move. The muscle fibers contract in an attempt to move the weight, but the muscle does not shorten in overall length because the object is too heavy to move [28,23,29]. Concentric muscle action occurs when the muscle force exceeds the external resistance, resulting in joint movement as the muscle shortens. Concentric action occurs when a muscle is active and shortening; for example, during the biceps curl the biceps shortens and exerts enough force to lift the barbell [23,29]. Eccentric muscle action occurs when the external resistance exceeds the force supplied by the muscle, resulting in joint movement as the muscle lengthens; for example, when lowering the barbell the biceps exerts force to ensure the movement is controlled. This is often referred to as the negative portion of the repetition. Even though the fibers are lengthening, they are also in a state of contraction, permitting the weight to return to the starting position in a controlled manner. During an eccentric action, an activated muscle is forced to elongate while producing tension [27,23,29].

3. Electromyography

Electromyography is the electrodiagnostic study of muscles and nerves. The test includes two components: Nerve conduction studies (NCS) and electromyogram (EMG). Nerve conduction studies measure how well and how fast the nerves can send electrical signals [30]. NCS can be defined as the recording of a peripheral neural impulse at some location distant from the site where a propagating action potential is induced in a peripheral nerve [2]. Nerve conduction studies provide unique quantitative information about neurological function in patients with a variety of neuromuscular disorders [31]. A nerve is stimulated at one or more sites along its course and the electrical response of the nerve is recorded. EMG testing involves evaluation of the electrical activity of a muscle and is one of the fundamental parts of the electrodiagnostic medical consultation. It is both an art and a science. It requires a thorough knowledge of the anatomy of the muscles being tested, machine settings and the neurophysiology behind the testing [2]. Obtaining the information produced by active muscle provides information about the activities of motor control centers [30,26]. This can be achieved invasively, by wires or needles inserted directly into the muscles, or noninvasively, by recording electrodes placed over the skin surface overlying the investigated muscles. The use of this latter modality is preferable in healthy voluntary sedentary subjects and in athletes, despite its limitations and drawbacks. To mention just a few of them, single-channel sEMG signals provide average information on the activity of many concurrently active motor units, the reproducibility of the results is often difficult, and standard recording procedures are still confined to few laboratories, therefore limiting comparisons among results obtained by clinical researchers [26]. EMG signal recordings used for years in bio-engineering, occupational- and sports medicine, physiotherapy, sports biomechanics, and also eventually for trainers and coaches [19,32]. Since the end of the 1960s there has been a development in miniaturized telemetric devices for monitoring complex human movements remotely. Especially for kinesiological purposes, the telemetric devices have recently been changed from two-channel registrations to eight or more-channel systems [32]. EMG is a seductive muse because it provides easy access to physiological processes that cause the muscle to generate force, produce movement, and accomplish the countless functions that allow us to interact with the world around us. The current state of surface EMG is enigmatic. It provides many important and useful applications, but it has many limitations that must be understood, considered, and eventually removed so that the discipline is more scientifically based and less reliant on the art of use. To its detriment, EMG is too easy to use and consequently too easy to abuse [5]. Electromyographic recordings are performed with intramuscular needle electrodes. However, surface electrodes are used in the study of sports science. Most of the issues affecting this modality have already been covered. Electrodes are almost always sited along the body of the muscle in question, with locations one-third and two-thirds along the length being the norm, As mentioned earlier, small pre-amplifiers are often used in order to improve signal-to-noise ratios, especially since telemetry of signals is increasingly used in order to maintain ecologically valid movement patterns [30,33,1,34]. Once the signal is filtered and amplified, some form of rectification of the signal is usually applied. As with other indices, examination of the raw signal waveform is interesting but offers little in the way of empirically analyzable data. Accordingly, and since the signal is made up of both positive and negative potentials, signals may be rectified by either ignoring all negative signals or reversing their polarity so that all signals are positive. Further signal conditioning may involve totaling activity across a regular time base, resetting counters to zero in order to provide an integrated signal. Analysis may look at amplitude or, more rarely, frequency. Increasingly, however, signal patterns are compared across two or more conditions. Thus, investigators may contrast "at rest" with active patterns, or use an increase from baseline measure, or contrast signals obtained under different execution conditions such as variations in speed. Subsequent treatments of data are increasingly complex, with the application of spectral analysis techniques to tease out underlying trends or collective patterns in the data. In this way, EMG data are making a full contribution to the comparatively new approaches within motor control, such as dynamical systems [33].

A key ingredient of strengthening protocols is *training intensity*, defined as the percentage of maximal voluntary force exerted [35]. EMG is commonly used to measure the level of muscle activation and provides a rough estimate of exercise intensity for specific muscles involved in the movement [36,35]. EMG signal has many contributions for finding the human body muscle functions [37]. EMG is the recording of the electrical activity of muscles, and therefore constitutes an extension of the physical exploration and testing of the integrity of the motor system [38].

Electromyographic analysis can provide information as to the relative amount of muscular activity an exercise requires, as well as the optimal positioning for the exercise [39]. Electrophysiological techniques enable us to relatively easily obtain very valuable information about neuromuscular activity [40]. Two techniques are usually used in clinical situations: neurography and needle EMG. The former allows the study of the response potential of a sensory, motor or mixed nerve branch subjected to an electrical stimulus applied to the surface. The latter allows the direct and precise recording of the electrical activity of the muscle being studied, both in repose and in attempts at maximum contraction [41]. Another technique that determines the electrical activity of muscles is surface EMG. There are advantages and different application areas of sEMG in researches and in clinical practices [42,41]. In the study of muscle physiology, neural control of excitable muscle fibers is explained on the basis of the action potential mechanism. The electrical model for the motor action potential reveals how EMG signals provide us with a quantitative, reliable, and objective means of accessing muscular information [41,42,43]. When an alpha motoneuron cell is activated, the conduction of this excitation travels along the motor nerve's axon and neurotransmitters are released at the motor endplates. An endplate potential is formed at the muscle fibers and innervates the motor unit. Muscle fibres are composed of muscle cells that are in constant ionic equilibrium and also ionic flux. The semi-permeable membrane of each muscle cell forms a physical barrier between intracellular (typically negatively charged compared to external surface) and extracellular fluids, over which an ionic equilibrium is maintained [41,42,43]. These ionic equilibriums form a resting potential at the muscle fiber membrane (sarcolemma), typically -80 to -90mV (when not contracted). These potential differences are maintained by physiological processes found within the cell membrane and are called ion pumps. Ion pumps passively and actively regulate the flow of ions within the cell membrane [41,42,43]. When muscle fibers become innervated, the diffusion characteristics on the muscle fibre membrane are briefly modified, and Na^+ flows into muscle cell membranes resulting in depolarization. Active ion pumps in the muscle cells immediately restore the ionic equilibrium through the repolarization process which lasts typically 2-3ms [41,42,43]. When a certain threshold level is exceeded by the influx of Na^+ resulting in a depolarization of the cellular membrane, an action potential is developed and is characterized by a quick change from -80mV to +30mV. This monopolar electrical burst is restored in the repolarization phase and is followed by a hyperpolarization period. Beginning from the motor end plates, the action potential spreads across the muscle fibers in both directions at a propagation speed of 2-6m/s. The action potential leads to a release of calcium ions in the intracellular fluid and produces a chemical response resulting in a shortening of the contractile elements of muscle cells [41,42,43]. The depolarization-repolarization process described is a monopolar action potential that travels across the surface of the muscle fiber [41,42,43]. Electrodes in contact with this wave front present a bipolar signal to the EMG differential amplifiers because the electrodes are measuring the difference between two points along the direction of propagation of the wave front. EMG signals provide us with a viewing window into the electrical signals presented by multiple muscle fibres and are in fact a superposition of multiple action potentials [43].

3.1. Surface electromyography

Surface Electromyography is a non invasive technique for measuring muscle electrical activity that occurs during muscle contraction and relaxation cycles. EMG is unique in revealing what a muscle actually does at any moment during movement and postures. Moreover, it reveals objectively the fine interplay or coordination of muscles: this is patently impossible by any other means [40].

Surface EMG is widely used in many applications, such as:

Medical

- Orthopedic
- Surgery
- Functional Neurology
- Gait & Posture Analysis
- Urology (treatment of incontinence)
- Psychophysiology

Rehabilitation

- Post surgery/accident
- Neurological Rehabilitation
- Physical Therapy
- Physical Rehabilitation
- Active Training Therapy

Ergonomics

- Analysis of demand
- Risk Prevention

- Ergonomics Design
- Product Certification

Sports Science

- Biomechanics
- Movement Analysis
- Athletes Strength Training
- Sports Rehabilitation
- Motion analysis [41,42,43]

Although the noninvasive nature of surface EMG makes this technique ideal for clinical use and research, EMG data can be variable, which raises questions about the reliability of this technique [44]. Repeatability of EMG data is established for many isometric exercises but less is known about the reliability of this method of analysis during dynamic exercise, particularly ballistic movements [45,46,44]. Most studies assessing EMG reliability of data in dynamic movements have examined slow, controlled tasks, such as resistance training exercises or gait. Therefore, evaluation of the reliability of EMG during ballistic tasks is essential to determine the viability of this methodology for clinical and research applications [47,48-49-50,44]. Surface EMG, sometimes called kinesiological electromyography, is the electromyographic analysis that makes it possible to obtain an electrical signal from a muscle in a moving body [41]. It has to be added, by way of clarification, that according to this definition its use is limited to those actions that involve a dynamic movement. Nevertheless, it is also applicable to the study of static actions that require a muscular effort of a postural type [41].

The visual systems employed for motion analysis of cycling, even though scientific and accurate, can only indicate the apparent movements. It is often necessary to know how the movements are actually performed against a resistive load. For this reason electromyographic techniques are employed in conjunction with biomechanical analyses [51]. EMG is generally used to indicate which muscle groups are active during a given segment of the pedal revolution.

Surface electrodes are usually attached to the muscle groups to be studied. The action potentials generated are recorded during the pedaling action, thereby allowing the researcher to gain a more complete insight into the muscles employed and the extent of their involvement while pedaling [22]. Within EMG, a particular specialty has been developed wherein the aim is to use EMG for the study of muscular function and co-ordination. This area of research is usually called kinesiological EMG [52,47]. The general aims of kinesiological EMG are to analyze the function and co-ordination of muscles in different movements and postures, in healthy subjects as well as in the disabled, in skilled actions as well as during training, in humans as well as in animals, under laboratory conditions as well as during daily or vacational activities [52]. This is usually used by a combination of EMG, kinesiological and biomechanical measurement techniques [52,47]. Because there are over 600 skeletal muscles in the human body and both irregular and complex involvement of the muscles may occur in neuromuscular diseases and in voluntary occupational or sports movements [52,21,17]. The measurement of kinesiological EMG in sport and specific field circumstances, such as the track and/or soccer field, the alpine ski slope, the swimming pool and the ice rink, demands a specific technological and methodological approach, adaptable to both the field and the sport circumstances [52]. Sport movement techniques and skills, training approaches and methods, ergonomic verification of the human-machine interaction have, amongst others, a highly specialized muscular activity in common. The knowledge of such muscular action in all its aspects, its evaluation and its feedback should allow for the optimization of movement, of sports materials, of training possibilities and, in the end, of sports performance [52]. Drawing conclusions from a review of the EMG research of 32 sports, covering over 100 different complex skills, including methodological approaches, is an impossible task. EMG and sports is a vast area and a complete review is impossible, as information will be found scattered in many different journals, including those on the sports sciences, ergonomics, biomechanics, applied physiology, in different congress proceedings, and so on [52].

sEMG refers to surface electromyography and measures muscle activity in microvolts. This form of feedback allows us to determine if muscles not involved in a particular skill need to be relaxed and those muscles involved in a skill need to fire in the right sequence and with the right amplitude. In addition to using sEMG feedback for training purposes, the information can also provide insight into the athlete's strength and conditioning or the effects of an injury rehabilitation program [53].

EMG can also be used to examine the activation characteristics of specific muscle groups.

Amplitude and power spectrum of sEMG are commonly used to quantify neuromuscular activity and fatigue [54].

3.1.1. The limitations of sEMG

Because of the characteristics of electrodes used, sEMG enables us to study different muscles at the same time, without any inconvenience to the individual, with the advantage that the majority of sEMG equipment can accommodate different inputs simultaneously [55,41]. It also allows greater reproducibility of the traces obtained in different recordings. In addition, the recording obtained is more representative of the muscle as a whole rather than of a particular area. Nevertheless, as already discussed, obtaining traces that provide less information regarding the characteristics of the MUAPs is a limitation in those cases where this particular type of examination is of specific interest [41].

Another limitation is the fact that in some dynamic actions there can be displacement and modification of the volume of the muscle being analyzed. A change in the relative position of the muscle in relation to the electrode means that the same spatial relationship is not maintained between them, which affect the intensity of the signal that is recorded. Because of this, the best conditions for carrying out an sEMG, depending on the use and application required, are those that are similar to those needed for an isometric type of study [5,56,57,11].

The majority of activities in sport and occupational settings involve complex movement patterns often complicated by external forces, impacts and the equipment used during the movement. An electromyogram is the expression of the dynamic involvement of specific muscles within a determined range of that movement. The integrated EMG of that same pattern is the expression of its muscular intensity. However, intensity is not always related to force [12].

Mostly sEMG is used to investigate the activity of a series of muscles. The majority of scientists working in sports and occupational contexts measure EMG using surface electrodes [12,15]. Skeletal muscles do not always stay in the same place during complex dynamic movements and the entire muscle belly may not be fully under the skin, but covered by parts of other bellies or tendons and subcutaneous adipose tissue. It needs to be emphasized that the selection of muscles for EMG measurement requires careful consideration. Some of these choices can lead to erroneous registration, sometimes without being noticed by peer reviewers [12].

Many factors may affect the quality of EMG signals; they can be divided into physiological, physical, and electrical types. Some factors can be controlled by the investigator [58].

3.2. Origin of the EMG signal

Muscle tissue produce electrical potentials due to action potentials. With electrodes placed on surface or in muscle tissue, muscle action potentials can be determined. Several events must occur before contraction of muscle fibers. Central nervous system activity initiates a depolarization in the motoneuron [59,60]. The depolarization is conducted along the motoneuron to the muscle fiber's motor end plate. At the endplate, a chemical substance is released that diffuses across the synaptic gap and causes a depolarization of the synaptic membrane. This phenomenon is called muscle action potential. The depolarization of the membrane spreads along the muscle fibers producing a depolarization wave that can be detected by recording electrodes [60].

3.2.1. Skin preparation

Preparation of the skin is essential to avoid artifacts and receive an appropriate signal. Before placing the electrodes on skin, it must be ensured that the skin is clean and dry. The skin must be cleaned by using gel, cream or alcohol and then it should be dried [61,62,25]. If necessary, shave excess body hair. Cleansing of the skin is useful to provide EMG recordings with low noise levels. Appropriate preparation of the skin assures the removal of body hair, oils and flaky skin layers and, consequently, reduces the impedance in the electrode-gel-skin interface. Shaving, wetting and rubbing with alcohol, acetone or ether, are often considered for the cleansing of the skin [25].

Proper skin preparation and electrode positioning are essential elements in acquiring EMG measurements of high quality. Two key strategies govern electrode preparations (1) electrode contact must be stable (2) skin impedance must be minimized. While there are no general rules for skin preparations, the type of application and signal quality sought usually determines the extent of the skin preparation [43]. For example, given a targeted test condition if the movement is somewhat static or slow moving and only qualitative reading are desired, a simple alcohol swab around the area of interest is sufficient [43]. However, if dynamic conditions present risk of the introduction of movement artifacts like in walking, running or other planned accelerated movements, a thorough preparation is required. Some EMG systems have built in impedance checking circuit that sends an imperceptible burst of current through the electrodes and controlled measurements are correlated to a known impedance level to indicate the quality of the electrode contacts [43].

3.2.2. Electrode material, size, montage and positioning

Surface EMG is a helpful technique for the analysis of muscle activity. However, its efficacy is related to the correct electrode positioning, the adequate skin preparation and opportune recording instrumentation. In addition, it is mandatory to recognize artifacts which may alter EMG signals and choose a particular filtering procedure before any additional analysis [63].

Surface electrodes are usually made of silver/silver chloride (Ag/ AgCl), silver chloride (AgCl), silver (Ag) or gold (Au). Electrodes made of Ag/AgCl are often preferred over the others, as they are almost nonpolarizable electrodes, which mean that the electrode-skin impedance is a resistance and not a capacitance [25]. Therefore, the surface potential is less sensitive to relative movements between the electrode surface and the skin. Additionally, these electrodes provide a highly stable interface with the skin when electrolyte solution (for example gel) is interposed between the skin and the electrode [25]. Such a stable electrode-skin interface ensures high signal to noise ratios (for example the amplitude of EMGs exceeds fairly the noise amplitude), reduces the power line interference in bipolar derivations and attenuates the artifacts due to body movements [64,25]. The electrode should be placed between a motor point and the tendon insertion or between two motor points, and along the longitudinal midline of the muscle. The longitudinal axis of the electrode should be aligned parallel to the length of the muscle fibers. When an electrode is placed on the skin, the detection surface comes in contact with the electrolytes in the skin [65]. A chemical reaction takes place which requires some time to stabilize, typically in the order of a few seconds if the electrode is correctly designed. But, more importantly, the chemical reaction should remain stable during the recording session and should not change significantly if the electrical characteristics of the skin change from sweating or humidity changes. Given the high performance and small size of modern day electronics, it is possible to design active electrodes that satisfy the above requirements without requiring any abrasive skin preparation and removal of hair [65].

In localizing the site of detection of the electrode on the skin, a variety of approaches has been applied: (1) over the motor point; (2) equidistant from the motor point; (3) near the motor point; (4) on the mid-point of the muscle belly; (5) on the visual part of the muscle belly; (6) at standard distances of osteological reference points and (7) with no precision at all with respect to its placement [12].

4. Analysis of a movement

EMG enables us to record muscular activity, and it is often advisable to carry out a synchronized cinematic measurement at the same time. In this way, the two types of data can be contrasted and it is possible to establish:

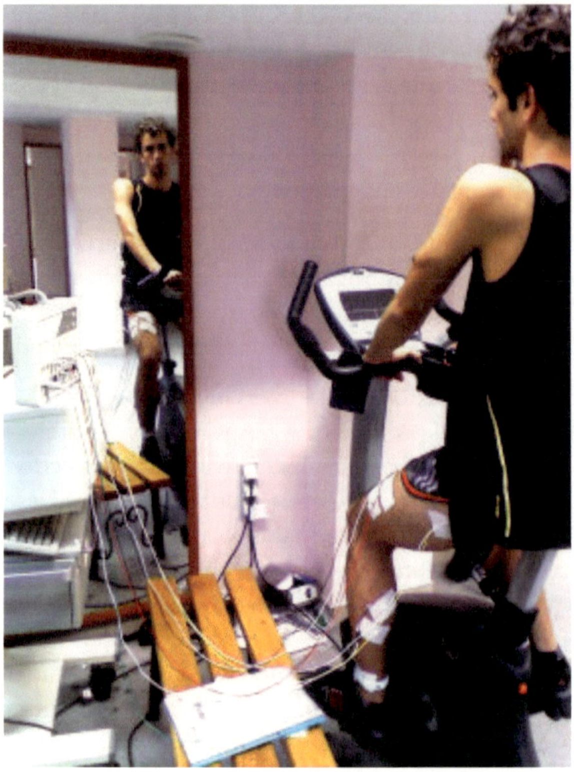

Figure 2. A research of lower extremity muscle groups [66] (Photograph shot during a study by Sozen H. et al.).

- How long the muscle is activated for, the start and end of the activation in relation to the articular position.
- The degree of muscular activity which itself reflects the level of muscular effort. However, this must not be confused with the level of muscular force, as the electrical signal detected is a function of the ionic concentration in the muscle [41].

The analysis of movement usually includes cinematic and kinetic study [52,47,41]. The cinematic study is responsible for determining the position, speed and acceleration parameters, both linear and angular. Different camera and marker systems are used for this purpose. A kinetic study determines the internal or external forces involved [41].

4.1. Evaluating sports performance

Surface EMG is commonly used to quantify the magnitude and timing of muscle activation during various physical tasks, that has broad application in sport science research [44]. The fact that sEMG can analyze dynamic situations makes it of special interest in the field of sports [11]. The improvement in the efficiency of a movement involves the correct use of the muscles, in terms of both economies of effort and effectiveness, as well as in the prevention of injury.

In a training process, improvements in these parameters can be sought, follow-up carried out and corrective measures or steps for improvement determined [5,13].

In particular, the performance of a task can be improved in terms of muscular activation and/or in terms of muscular fatigue, based on the analysis of the frequency of the electromyographic traces observed [9]. It has to be remembered that the EMG does not provide us with muscular force parameters, although it is an indicator of the muscular effort made in a particular action [67,12-57,11]. In relation to this, it is important to stress that the relationship between EMG activity and effort is only qualitative [5]. Recently, experiments have also been carried out in the sports area on applications for purposes such as the evaluation of the type of muscle fiber and the characterization of muscles [15,14].

4.2. Relationships between muscular force and EMG

Muscular force is the amount of force a muscle can produce with a single maximum effort. Enhanced muscular force can lead to improvements in the areas of performance, injury prevention, body composition, self-image, lifetime muscle and bone health, and chronic disease prevention [16]. There are many cases in which knowledge of the relationship between EMG and force is desired. If the relationship between force and EMG amplitude is simply linear, a direct regression equation yields a relatively simple technique to control prosthetic limb function [19].

Ergonomists could assess the load on various muscles by monitoring the EMG activity. The relationship between EMG and force also seems to depend on the nature of the muscle studied, since some investigators have reported a linear relationship for the adductor pollicis and first dorsal interosseous and soleus, and a nonlinear relationship for the biceps and deltoid [68]. There have been other, numerous examples of observations of nonlinear relationships between force and EMG amplitude [69,70].

It is clear that when considering the possible shape of the EMG force relationship, one needs to consider various features of the movement, such as the type of muscle contraction; the size and location of the active muscles; their role as agonists, synergists, or antagonists; air temperature [71,19] and the numerous other physiological and technical factors that affect the electromyogram [19].

4.3. Examples of current EMG studies in sciences of sports

EMG has been a subject of laboratory research for decades. Only with recent technological developments in electronics and computers has surface EMG emerged from the laboratory as a subject of intense research in particularly kinesiology, rehabilitation and occupational and sports medicine. Most of the applications of surface EMG are based on its use as a measure of activation timing of muscle, a measure of muscle contraction profile, a measure of muscle contraction strength, or as a measure of muscle fatigue [72]. Only a handful of research articles using EMG techniques were published in the early 1950s. Today, over 2500 research publications appear each year. The growth of the EMG literature and the availability of appropriate instrumentation and techniques might suggest that our understanding of the procedures used to record the EMG signal and the relevant analysis methods must be complete. Yet the interpretation of the signal remains controversial; and there are few sources available to help the novice electromyographer understand the physiological and biophysical basis of EMG, characteristics of the instrumentation, signal analysis techniques, and appropriate EMG applications [19].

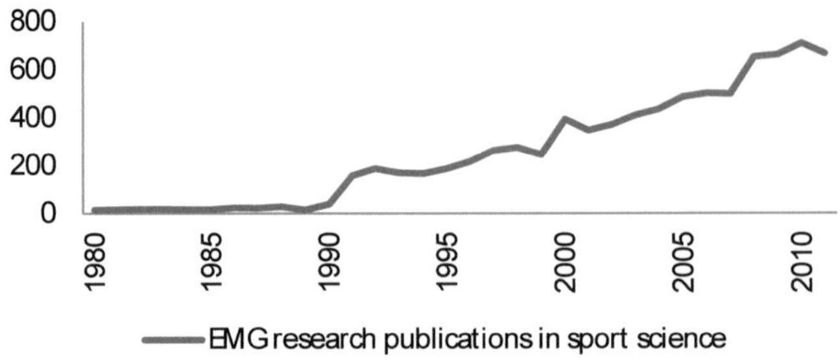

Figure 3. The growth in the number of EMG related publications in sport science since 1980s (drawn by Sözen H. based on data from Thomson ISI).

Sports science studies on exercise equipment often use electromyography. A study carried out by Sözen H. et al compared the muscle activation during the exercise on elliptical trainer, treadmill and bike equipment which are frequently used in the fields of rehabilitation and sport science. Determing the muscles used predominantly during the exercise on these three equipments may contribute to the regulation of available performance tests or the tests scheduled to be performed on these equipments. Besides, detemining in which muscle groups the equipments are used more efficiently for rehabilitation and treatment may help treatment be more successful. According to studies' results; it was found out that elliptical trainer equipment activated upper extremity muscles more when compared to treadmill and bicycle equipment. But, in the activation of lower extremity muscles, treadmill and elliptical trainer equipments are more advantageous compared to bike. As a result; elliptical trainer equipment is more advantageous to activate different muscle groups compared to treadmill and bicycle equipments. By more muscles groups' involving in action, more cardiorespiratory output, accordingly more energy consumption and production can be provided as a response to the exercise on elliptical trainer [1].

The studies that use surface EMG in sciences of sports are mostly related with determination of the mechanism of contraction and relexation of muscles while also dealing with evolution of injuries. The data obtained from these studies can be used in the following areas:

a. the evaluation of the technical development

b. the establishment of the suitable exercise programs

c. follow up of the development of the sportsmen

d. the choice of skills [34].

5. Conclusions

When the research in sciences of sports is thoroughly investigated, it is seen that usage of electromyography is rapidly increasing. Research and applications of such kind unite medical and sports sciences and thus help us understand the movement physiology of the human body.

Surface EMG, though often used for diseases of locomotion and movement disorders, may also be a tool for evaluation of performances of sportsmen. By this way the functional capacity of muscles which play the most active role in movement may be determined and this approach also yields designation of exercise programs and skill analysis that play an important role in success in various fields of sports.

Author details

Hande Türker[1] and Hasan Sözen[2]

1 Assoc. Prof. Dr. Faculty of Medicine, Department of Neurology, Ondokuz Mayıs University, Samsun, Turkey

2 Assist. Prof. Dr., Ordu University, School of Physical Education and Sports, Ordu, Turkey

References

[1] Sözen, H. Comparison of muscle activation during elliptical trainer, treadmill and bike exercise. Biology of Sport (2010). , 27, 203-206.

[2] Weiss, L, Silver, J. K, & Weiss, J. Easy EMG. Oxford, UK: Butterworth-Heinemann; (2004).

[3] Katirji, B. Electromyography In Clinical Practice A Case Study Approach. PA-USA: Mosby Elsevier; (2007).

[4] Soderberg, G. L, & Cook, T. M. Electromyography in biomechanics. Physical Therapy. (1984). , 64, 1813-1820.

[5] De Luca, C. J. The use of surface electromyography in biomechanics. Journal or Applied Biomechanics (1997). , 13-135.

[6] Monfort-panego, M, Vera-garcia, F. J, Sanchez-zuriaga, D, & Sarti-martinez, M. A. Electromyographic studies in abdominal exercises: a literature synthesis. Journal of Manipulative and Physiological Therapeutics (2009). , 32, 232-244.

[7] Marshall, P, & Murphy, B. The validity and reliability of surface EMG to assess the neuromuscular response of the abdominal muscle to rapid limb movement. Journal of Electromyography and Kinesiology (2003). , 13, 477-489.

[8] Potvin, J. R, & Bent, L. R. A validation of techniques using surface EMG signals from dynamic contractions to quantify muscle fatigue during repetitive tasks. Journal of Electromyography and Kinesiology (1997). , 7, 131-139.

[9] Balestra, G, Frassinelli, S, Knaflitz, M, & Molinari, F. Time-frequency analysis of surface myoelectric signals during athletic movement. IEEE Engineering Medicine and Biology Magazine (2001). , 20, 106-115.

[10] Maclsaac, D, Parker, P. A, & Scott, R. N. The short time Fourier transform and muscle fatigue assessment in dynamic contractions. Journal of Electromyography and Kinesiology (2001). , 11, 439-449.

[11] Farina, D. Interpretation of the surface electromyogram in dynamic contractions. Exercise and Sport Sciences Reviews (2006). , 34, 121-127.

[12] Clarys, J. P. Electromyography in sports and occupational settings: an update of its limits and possibilities. Ergonomics (2000). , 43, 1750-1762.

[13] Hendrix, C. R, Housh, T. J, Johnson, G. O, Mielke, M, Camic, C. L, Zuniga, J. M, & Schmidt, R. J. Comparison of critical force to EMG fatigue thresholds during isometric leg extension. Medicine and Science in Sports and Exercise (2009). , 41, 956-964.

[14] Beck, T. W, Housh, T, Fry, A. C, Cramer, J. T, Weir, J, Schilling, B, Falvo, M, & Moore, C. MMG-EMG cross spectrum and muscle fiber type. International Journal of Sports Medicine (2009). , 30, 538-544.

[15] Merletti, R, Rainoldi, A, & Farina, D. Surface electromyography for noninvasive characterization of muscle. Exercise and Sport Sciences Reviews (2001). , 29, 20-25.

[16] Fahey, T. D, Insel, P. M, & Roth, W. Fit & Well. NY, USA: McGraw-Hill; (2007).

[17] Draper, N, & Hodgson, C. Adventure Sport Physiology. UK: Wiley-Blackwell, A John Wiley & Sons Ltd; (2008).

[18] Castroflorio, T, Bracco, P, & Farina, D. Surface electromyography in the assessment of jaw elevator muscles. Journal of Oral Rehabilitation (2008). , 35(8), 638-645.

[19] Kamen, G, & Gabriel, D. A. Essentials of Electromyography. IL-USA: Human Kinetics; (2010).

[20] Russell, R, & Klebanoff, S. J. The smooth muscle cell. The Journal of Cell Biology (1971). , 50, 159-171.

[21] Guyton, A. C, & Hall, J. E. Textbook of Medical Physiology. PA, USA: Saunders Elsevier; (2011).

[22] Reilly, T, Secher, N, Snell, P, & Williams, C. Physiology of Sports. UK: Taylor & Francis; (1990).

[23] Hale, T. Exercise Physiology. UK: John Wiley & Sons Ltd; (2003).

[24] Kidd, G. L, & Oldham, J. A. Motor unit action potential (MUAP) sequence and electrotherapy. Clinical Rehabilitation (1988)., 2(1), 23-33.

[25] Garcia MACVieira TMM. Surface electromyography: Why, when and how to use it. Revista Andaluza Medicina Deporte (2011)., 4(1), 17-28.

[26] Merletti, R, & Parker, P. A. Electromyography. Canada: John Wiley & Sons; (2004).

[27] Lieber, R. L, & Friden, J. Morphologic and mechanical basis of delayed-onset muscle soreness. Journal of American Academy of Orthopaedic Surgeons (2002). , 10(1), 67-73.

[28] Mcardle, W. D, Katch, F. I, & Katch, V. L. Exercise Physiology. Energy, Nutrition and Human Performance. Baltimore: Williams & Wilkins; (1996).

[29] Stoppani, J. Encyclopedia of Muscle & Strength. IL, USA: Human Kinetics; (2006).

[30] Oh, S. J. Clinical Electromyography: Nerve Conduction Studies. USA: Lippincott Williams & Wilkins; (2003).

[31] Morgan, M. H. Nerve conduction studies. British Journal of Hospital Medicine Journal (1989).

[32] Clarys, J. P, Scafoglieri, A, Tresignie, J, Reilly, T, & Roy, P. V. Critical appraisal and hazards of surface electromyography data acquisition in sport and exercise. Asian Journal of Sports Medicine (2010)., 1(2), 69-80.

[33] Blumenstein, B, Bar-eli, M, & Tenenbaum, G. Brain and Body in Sport and Exercise Biofeedback Applications in Performance Enhancement. UK: John Wiley & Sons, Ltd; (2002).

[34] Cerrah, A. O, Ertan, H, & Soylu, A. R. Spor bilimlerinde elektromiyografi kullanımı. Spormetre Beden Eğitimi ve Spor Bilimleri Dergisi (2010). VIII(2): 43-49.

[35] Andersen, L. L, Andersen, C. H, Mortensen, O. S, & Poulsen, O. M. Bjornlund IBT., Zebis MK. Muscle activation and perceived loading during rehabilitation exercises: Comparison of dumbbells and elastic resistance. Physical Therapy (2010). , 90(4), 538-549.

[36] Hintermeister, R. A, Lange, G. W, Schultheis, J. M, Bey, M. J, & Hawkins, R. J. Electromyographic activity and applied load during shoulder rehabilitation exercises using elastic resistance. American Journal of Physical Medicine & Rehabilitation (1998)., 26, 210-220.

[37] Illyes, A, & Kiss, R. M. Shoulder muscle activity during pushing, pulling, elevation and overhead throw. Journal of Electromyography Kinesiology (2005). , 15(3), 282-289.

[38] Rivas, G. E, Jimenez, M. D, Pardo, J, & Romero, M. Manual de electromiografia clinica. Barcelona: Ergon; (2007).

[39] Ekstrom, R. A, Donatelli, R. A, & Carp, K. C. Electromyographic analysis of core trunk, hip, and thigh muscles during 9 rehabilitation exercises. Journal of Orthopaedic & Sports Physical Therapy (2007). , 37(12), 754-762.

[40] Basmajian, J. V, & De Luca, C. J. Muscle alive: their functions revealed by electromyography. Baltimore: Williams & Wilkins; (1985).

[41] Masso, N, Rey, F, Romero, D, Gual, G, Costa, L, & German, A. Surface electromyography applications in the sport. Apunts Medicine de Esport (2010). , 45(165), 121-130.

[42] Cram, J. R, Kasman, G. S, & Holtz, J. Introduction to Surface Electromyography. Gaithersburg, Md: Aspen Publishers; (1998).

[43] Quach, J. H. Surface electromyography: Use, design & technological overview. Project Report, Introduction to Biomedical Engineering. Canada: Concordia University; (2007).

[44] Fauth, M, Petushek, E. J, Feldmann, C. R, Hsu, B. E, Garceau, L. R, Lutsch, B. N, & Ebben, W. P. Realiability of surface electromyography during maximal voluntary isometric contractions, jump landings, and cutting. Journal of Strength and Conditioning Research (2010). , 24(4), 1131-1137.

[45] Bogey, R, Cerny, K, & Mohammed, O. Repeatability of wire and surface electrodes in gait. American Journal of Physical Medicine & Rehabilitation (2003). , 82, 338-344.

[46] Bolgla, L. A, & Uhl, T. L. Reability of electromyographic normalization methods for evaluating hip musculature. Journal of Electromyography Kinesiology (2007). , 17, 102-111.

[47] Sutherland, D. H. The evolution of clinical gait anysis part I: kinesiological EMG. Gait & Posture (2001). , 14(1), 61-70.

[48] Pitcher, M. J, & Behm, D. G. NacKinnon SN. Reliability of electromyographic and force measures during prone isometric back extension in subjects with and without low back pain. Journal of Applied Physiology Nutrition Metabolism (2008). , 33, 52-60.

[49] Kellis, E, & Katis, A. Reliability of EMG power-spectrum and amplitude of the semitendinosus and biceps femoris muscles during ramp isometric contractions. Journal of Electromyography Kinesiology (2008). , 18, 351-358.

[50] Mccarthy, C. J, Callaghan, M. J, & Oldham, J. A. The reliability of isometric strength and fatigue measures in patients with knee osteoarthritis. Journal of Manual & Manipulative Therapy (2008). , 18, 159-164.

[51] Hull, M. L, & Jorge, M. A method for biomechanical analysis of bicycle pedaling. Journal of Biomechanics (1985). , 18(9), 631-644.

[52] Clarys, J. P, & Cabri, J. Electromyography and the study of sports movements: a review. Journal of Sports Sciences (1993). , 11(5), 379-448.

[53] Micheli, L. J. Encyclopedia of Sports Medicine. CA, USA: SAGE Publication; (2011).

[54] Baars, H, Jöllenbeck, T, Humburg, H, & Schröder, J. Surface-electromyography: Skin and subcutaneous fat tissue attenuate amplitude and frequency parameters: proceedings of the XXIV ISBS Symposium, Salzburg, Austria; (2006).

[55] Vinjamuri, R, Mao, Z. H, Sclabassi, R, & Sun, M. limitation of surface EMG signals of extrinsic muscles in predicting postures of human hand: conference proceedings, Aug. Sept. 3 2006, 28th Annual International Conference of the IEEE; (2006). , 30-2006.

[56] Merletti, R. Lo Conte LR. Surface EMG signal processing during isometric contractions. Journal of Electromyography Kinesiology (1997). , 7, 241-250.

[57] Bishop, M. D, & Pathare, N. Considerations for the use of surface electromyography. KAUTPT (2004). , 11, 61-70.

[58] Puddu, G, Giombini, A, & Selvanetti, A. Rehabilitation of Sports Injuries. Germany: Springer; (2001).

[59] Tesch, P. A, Dudley, G. A, Duvoisin, M. R, Hather, B. M, & Harris, R. T. Force and EMG signal patterns repeated bouts of concentric or eccentric muscle actions. Acta Physiologica (1990). , 138(3), 263-271.

[60] Lamontagne, M. Application of electromyography in movement studies: proceeding of the 18th International Symposium on Biomechanics in Sports. Hong Kong, China; (2000).

[61] Zipp, P. Recommendations for the standardization of lead positions in surface electromyography. European Journal of Applied Physiology (1982). , 50, 41-54.

[62] Clancy, E. A, Morin, E. L, & Merletti, R. sampling, noise-reduction and amplitude estimation issues in surface electromyography. Journal of Electromyography and Kinesiology (2002). , 12(1), 1-16.

[63] Steele, C. Applications of EMG in Clinical and Sports Medicine. Rijeka: InTech; (2011).

[64] Geddes, L. A. Electrodes and the measurement of bioelectric events. New York, USA: Wiley, John & Sons; (1972).

[65] De Luca, C. J. Surface Electromyography: Detection and Recording. DelSys; (2002).

[66] Sözen, H. Eliptik bisiklet, koşu bandı ve bisiklet egzersizleri sırasında kas aktivasyonlarının karşılaştırılması. PhD thesis. Ondokuz Mayıs University, Samsun; (2009).

[67] Vilarroya, A, Marco, M. C, & Moros, T. Electromiografia cinesiologica. Rehabilitacion (1997). , 31, 230-236.

[68] Lawrence, J. H, & De Luca, C. J. Myoelectric signal versus force relationship in different human muscle. Journal of Applied Physiology (1983). , 54, 1653-1659.

[69] Woods, J. J, & Bigland-ritchie, B. Linear and non linear surface EMG force relationship in human muscle. American Journal of Physical Medicine & Rehabilitation. (1983). , 62, 287-299.

[70] Alkner, B. A, Tesch, P. A, & Berg, H. E. Quadriceps EMG force relationship in knee extension and leg press. Medicine and Science in Sports and Exercise (2000). , 32, 459-463.

[71] Bell, D. The influence of air temperature on the EMG force relationship of the quadriceps. European Journal of Applied Physiology (1993). , 67, 256-260.

[72] Hong, Y. International Research in Sports Biomechanics. NY, USA: Routledge; (2002).

Chapter 10

Evoked EMG Makes Measurement of Muscle Tone Possible by Analysis of the H/M Ratio

Satoru Kai and Koji Nakabayashi

Additional information is available at the end of the chapter

http://dx.doi.org/10.5772/55783

1. Introduction

1.1. Evoked EMG - Mechanism of evoked EMG

When we humans perform a physical activity, it is contraction of skeletal muscles that is responsible as its driving force. Active state of a skeletal muscle during motion can be viewed on an electromyogram (EMG). Because it is non-invasive and easy to handle, surface EMG has been widely used in the field of rehabilitation as in therapeutic exercise, training, motion analysis, and research.

When a peripheral nerve is subjected to percutaneous electrical stimulation, action potentials are induced in the innervated skeletal muscle. The induced action potential is recorded by evoked EMG, which includes the H-wave, the M-wave, and the F-wave (Fig. 1). The H-wave is a good indicator of the strength and distribution of the stimulus input from muscle spindle to the motor neuron pool, which lies at the site of the anterior horn of the spinal cord. The H-wave is commonly used, therefore, in the diagnosis of peripheral neuropathy (Kaeser 1973). The H-wave is also used to examine the state of muscle tone and spasticity, or other movement disorders of the central nervous system.

1.1.1. H-wave (H-reflex)

The name H-wave was derived from that of Johann Hoffmann, who found the response for the first time in 1918. Weak electrical stimulation can excite group Ia fibers from muscle spindle, and the antidromic impulse gets conducted to the spinal cord. Afferent fibers connect, via a synapse, with the alpha motor neuron in the spinal cord. Excitatory postsynaptic potential (EPSP) causes the excitement of the alpha motor neuron of the anterior horn cells in the spinal cord. The action potential that reaches from excitatory alpha motor neuron to skeletal muscle is called H-wave or H-response. With soleus or flexor carpi radialis muscle the H-wave is observed at rest, but in other muscles the H-wave can only be induced with mild voluntary contraction.

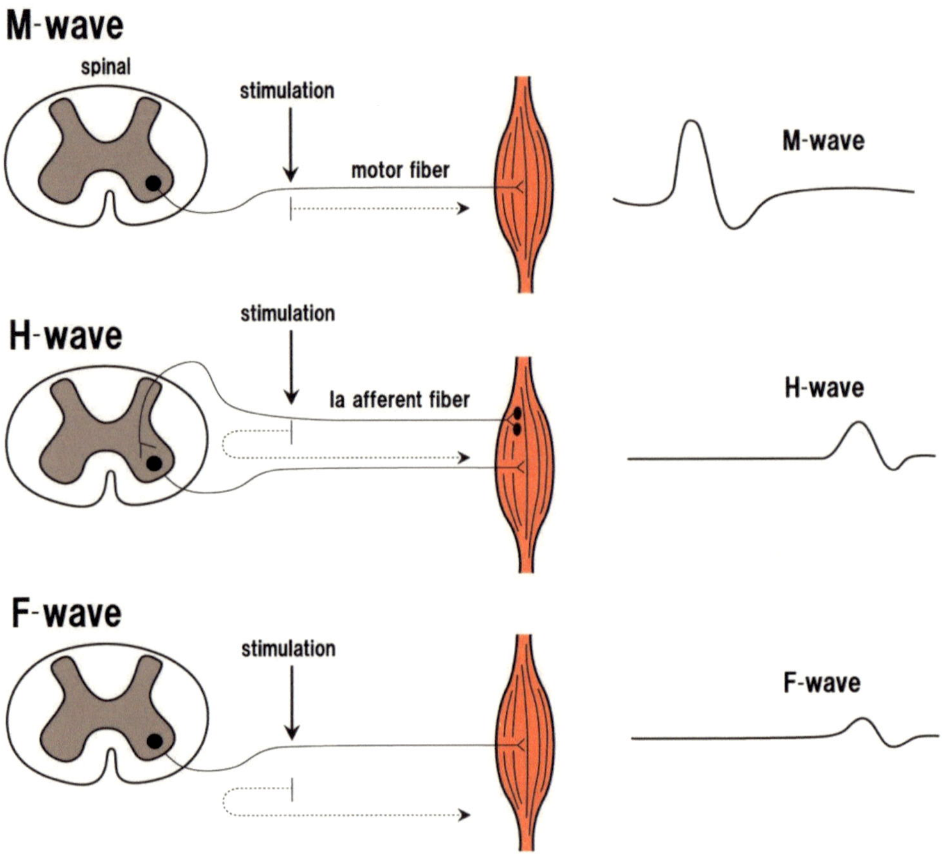

M-wave: Excitement is conducted to efferent. H-wave: Excitement is conducted via the monosynaptic reflex. F-wave: Excitement is conducted to antidromic.

Figure 1. Evoked EMG

1.1.2. M-wave (M-response)

Alpha motor neurons are activated directly by a gradual increase in the intensity of electrical stimulation, which occurs as the activity of Ia fiber is enhanced. The action potential of the skeletal muscle caused by this excitement is called M-wave or M-response.

1.1.3. F-wave (F-response)

If an alpha motor neuron receives a strong electrical stimulation, its antidromic impulse is conducted to axons of all motor neurons that have received the stimulus. The impulse is to

http://dx.doi.org/10.5772/55783

reach the innervated skeletal muscle after re-firing at part of the axon hillock of anterior horn cells in the spinal cord. The action potential in question is called F-wave or F-response. The F-wave is said to be evoked on any peripheral muscle.

1.2. Measurement of H- and M-wave

With evoked EMG, the action potential is derived from a skeletal muscle that is innervated by electrical stimulation conducted to peripheral nerves.

In this section, we briefly introduce the measurement method of H-wave in soleus muscle in accordance with the guidelines of clinical neurophysiology test as stipulated by International Federation of Clinical Neurophysiology. Kaeser advocated that the measurement of H-wave be standardized in the study of spinal reflex (Kaeser 1973). It is not always easy to apply his method in clinical situations, but we recommend that you should examine his method carefully because it is considered to be a correct way of recording the H-wave.

1.2.1. Postural position at measurement

Because H-wave is susceptible to the effects of posture, it is necessary to maintain the same posture during the measurement. A change in posture gives rise to changes in the length of muscles, which in turn bring on a change in the activity of muscle spindle receptors involved in the H-wave. That is how postural change can cause variability in H-wave.

When you try to evoke the H-wave of soleus muscle, it is important to prevent soleus muscle, and gastrocnemius muscle, from stretching. For the preventive purpose, you instruct the subject to mildly flex the knee joint (about 30 degrees). And because the H-wave of soleus muscle is inhibited by ankle dorsiflexion, the ankle joint is fixed at a mild plantar flexion position (about 20 degrees).

1.2.2. Stimulus conditions

The optimal duration of stimulation to elicit the H-wave is 0.5 ms or 1.0 ms; the choice is due to the difference in the strength-duration curves between axons of motor neurons and afferent group Ia fibers. Optimal conditions to excite group Ia fibers are 1) stimulation at a low enough intensity not to excite the axons of motor neurons, and 2) placement of the cathode of the stimulating electrode on the nerve, with the anode placed distal from the cathode on the run of the nerve. Because it is a reflex through a synapse, H-wave is easy to cause "habituation". That means that shorter stimulation intervals would tend to inhibit H-wave due to the decreased synaptic connection in the spinal cord. It is therefore important that the interval of stimulations be long enough, but you must also remember that the subjects would sometimes be poised when the stimulation interval is more than 5 seconds. For removal of the inhibitive influence of habituation, it is desirable to set the interval for stimuli at 10 seconds or more.

Clinically, it is often convenient, and optimal, to start with a rate of 1 Hz for H-wave measurement; the rate of stimulation is then decreased step by step (by 0.2-0.3 Hz) so that latency and amplitude can be measured.

1.2.3. Recording method (Fig. 2)

H-wave recording is often done with surface EMG. The skin surface is wiped clean before attaching an electrode to keep electrical resistance as low as possible. To record the H-wave from soleus muscle selectively, an electrode is firstly affixed between medial head and lateral head of gastrocnemius, and another is attached 3-5 cm distal from the first. It is important that electrodes be aligned along the long axis of the muscle for accurate measurement; values of the potential vary significantly if electrodes are placed across, at right angles or otherwise, in relation to the muscle's long axis.

Prevention of contamination from artifacts is also a major issue. Contamination of the potential induced by the latency of about 10 ms after the stimulus is highly likely specifically in terms of the inception and waveform of the H-wave. To remove artifact contamination, it is important that electrodes be securely earthed and the width and size of square wave of electrical stimulation be closely monitored.

As for H-wave amplitude, it increases as the motor neuron pool becomes more excitable due to weak voluntary muscle contraction, but H-wave latency hardly changes. Based on this characteristic, those muscle groups from which H-wave is hardly recorded at rest (e.g., tibialis anterior, extensor carpi radialis, and abductor pollicis brevis) can be induced to elicit recordable levels of H-wave.

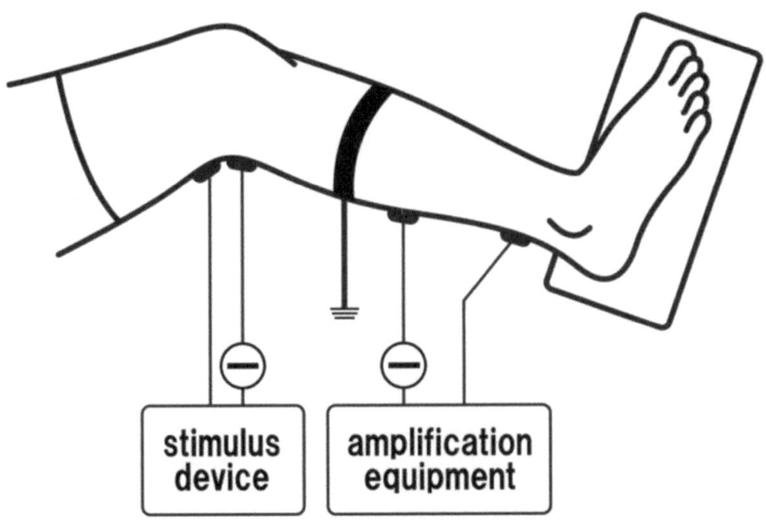

Figure 2. Recording method

1.2.4. Identification of waveforms

To elicit H-reflex from soleus muscle, a low-intensity electrical stimulation is applied on tibial nerve in the popliteal space, whereupon only those group Ia fibers with low threshold levels become selectively excited. The waveform which appears in the 20-30 ms latency is the H-wave

http://dx.doi.org/10.5772/55783

from soleus muscle. When the intensity of an electrical stimulus is gradually raised, group Ia fibers will be excited more. At the same time, alpha motor neuron which runs from the spinal cord to muscle fiber also becomes excited.

M-wave will appear at the 5-10 ms latency. If the stimulus intensity is raised, excitement of group Ia fibers will be lost and excitement of alpha motor neuron will become greater. H-wave amplitude decreases, whereas M-wave amplitude increases. H-wave is lost before M-wave reaches the maximum amplitude; only the M-wave may remain (Fig. 1).

H-wave latency is measured at the time when the value shows the first deflection from baseline. In the soleus H-wave, the first rising edge of the positive waveform is adopted as its latency because it is impossible to affix the recording electrode on the motor point. And its H-wave amplitude is defined by the difference in potential either from baseline to the top of negative waveform, or from the top of negative waveform to the top of next positive waveform.

It is important to ensure that the same measurement method is used for H-wave and M-wave amplitude. If these two amplitudes were measured differently, the H/M amplitude ratio would lose its reliability in the analysis of evoked EMG study.

1.3. To evaluate the muscle tone of skeletal muscle by analysis of the H/M ratio

Under uniform stimulus conditions, the amplitude size of an H-wave is determined by the strength of the stimulus and the excitability of the reflex arc. Thus, H-wave has been used as an indicator of the excitability of motor neurons in the anterior horn of the spinal cord.

In clinical practice, the ratio between the maximum amplitude of H-wave (Hmax) and that of M-wave (Mmax), or H/M ratio, is often adopted as a good index. The Hmax is taken to reflect the number of excited alpha motor neurons in the anterior horn of the spinal cord, when the condition is adjusted so as to maximize the input from group Ia fibers upon electrical stimulation. The Mmax, on the other hand, is thought to show the amplitude of complex muscle action potential when all the alpha motor neurons dominating the muscle (soleus muscle here) are excited synchronously. That is, of all the alpha motor neurons that dominate the targeted muscle (e.g., soleus muscle), the H/M ratio shows the percentage of excited alpha motor neurons upon electrical stimulation. In fact, correlation has been observed between the H/M ratio and the degree of spasticity. The H/M ratio shows marked increases in the elevated excitability of alpha motor neurons in the spinal cord, or in patients with spasticity.

Conversely, in cases of peripheral neuropathy, this H/M ratio is decreased. Because there is a great difference between individuals in the H/M ratio, it is more useful as a therapeutic tool in the same patient rather than as a general diagnostic tool. The H/M ratio would work when you tried to make an objective judgment of therapeutic effects on immediate change in the same patient, or when you tried to make a longitudinal change in a given condition also in the same patient.

It is surmised that if you observe changes in the H-wave at the time of intervention such as muscle contraction, vibration stimulation to the tendon, or muscle stretching, then those changes have in fact been brought on by the intervention, and not due to alterations in the physical condition such as electrode attachment and the like.

2. Vibration stimuli

2.1. Responses of skeletal muscle to vibration stimulation

Vibration stimulation has been used as one of the treatment modes for conditions of muscle tone of skeletal muscle, including spasticity. Its effects have in fact been reported. Unlike manual therapy, vibration stimulation is an excellent treatment method because it is expected to show a certain effect regardless of who uses it.

2.1.1. Physiological act on muscle cells

Though its detailed mechanism has not been elucidated, vibration stimulation acts directly on the contracted muscle cells to relax them (Vukas 1978, Ljung 1972, Ljung 1975).

2.1.2. Inhibitory act on muscle contraction

When skeletal muscle during a maximum contraction receives vibration stimulation, the muscle's action potential on EMG, nerve activity, and muscle output are reduced (Bongiovanni 1989, Kouzaki 2000, Stephen 2003, Konishi 2009). The inhibitory effect of muscle contraction is dependent on the conditions of vibration stimulation: the effect is greater if the frequency of the vibration stimulation is low, or if its amplitude is large (Desmedt 1978).

In recent reports, when stroke patients with a spastic upper limb received vibration stimulation on the limb, their upper limb function was shown to improve with a suppression of muscle tone (Noma 2012, Caliandro 2012).

In patients who underwent ACL reconstructive surgery or those with osteoarthritis, vibration stimulation to their quadriceps femoris muscle brought about neither an increase in neural activity as evaluated by integrated EMG nor a decrease in muscle output as evaluated by peak torque (Konishi 2002, Rice 2011). It is thought that this outcome was due to a failure in Ia afferent feedback, including dysfunction of the gamma-loop.

2.1.3. Neurophysiological mechanism

Muscle spindle senses a very small change in muscle length when a skeletal muscle receives vibration stimulation. And this information is transmitted to the fibers of group Ia or II, eventually to reach the spinal cord. In the spinal cord, the information serves as presynaptic inhibition through an interstitial cell and suppresses the alpha motor neuron (Gillies 1969, Shinohara 2005).

In addition, sustained vibration stimulation will selectively excite group Ia fibers. That will then bring about, in nerve endings, depletion of neurotransmitters and a rising threshold of group Ia fibers (Kouzaki 2000). It is believed that this is one of the reasons why a decrease is observed in the excitability of motor neurons in the spinal cord.

2.1.4. Conditions for vibration stimulation

The equipment that is used to apply vibration stimulation may vary from researcher to researcher, but the effect seems to be uniform as long as stimulation conditions are controlled in the same way. Stimulation conditions inevitably differ according to the research objective, but they are generally set at a frequency of 50-100 Hz and amplitude of 1-2 mm. The equipment is contacted at 20-30N on the body or tendon of the targeted skeletal muscle.

Effects that vibration stimulation has on the body depend on the duration of stimulation. The H/M ratio decreases immediately after the application of stimulation, and the inhibitory effect on spasticity has been confirmed in 5 minutes of stimulation (Noma 2012). Muscle output is reduced by a sustained stimulation of at least 20 minutes (Bongiovanni 1989, Kouzaki 2000, Stephen 2003, Konishi 2009).

2.2. Our previous study 1

Vibration stimulation on a skeletal muscle of healthy adults is known to bring on effects such as reflexivity contraction of an agonist muscle by muscle spindle Ia afferent nerve excitability, and inhibition of the antagonist muscle, called "tonic vibration reflex". Vibration stimulation also causes inhibition of monosynaptic reflexes such as the tendon reflex and stretch reflex while stimulation with vibration continues. These effects vary depending on stimulus conditions.

Clarified issue 1: Anterior horn cells in the spinal cord are suppressed by vibration stimulation from its onset to about 3 minutes into stimulation.

As a result of vibration stimulation on the triceps surae of healthy adults, the H/M ratio continues to decrease from 1 to 3 minutes after stimulus onset. After 4 minutes into stimulation, though the ratio continues to decrease somewhat, no significant difference was found between values at after 4 minutes and the value at 3 minutes of stimulation.

From these findings, it has been clarified that excitability of alpha motor neurons gets suppressed immediately after the intervention with vibration stimulation. Also clarified was that the decline of the H/M ratio reaches a steady state after 3 minutes of stimulation from its onset.

Clarified issue 2: It is recommended that vibration stimulation be applied on tendon.

If vibration stimulation is to be adopted in clinical settings, it is essential that an appropriate set of stimulus conditions should be considered for each of the clinically different cases. A site of stimulation is certainly one of the factors for the treating therapist to take into account.

Based on the results of our study, the H/M ratio was significantly lower after the onset of vibration stimulation on both muscle belly and the tendon ($p<0.01$). In addition, when stimulus to the belly was compared with stimulus to the tendon, the H/M ratio was significantly lower in the latter ($p<0.05$). In other words, to suppress muscle tone using a vibration stimulus, it is recommended that a stimulus be applied on the tendon.

2.3. Our previous study 2

When vibration stimulation is applied on skeletal muscle, the amount of output and muscle activity of the stimulated skeletal muscle is decreased. This finding should help to bring on a change in the pattern of muscle activity during action (Table 1).

It may be possible to facilitate the activity of the muscle that is important to knee joint extension, namely vastus lateralis muscle, when vibration stimulation decreases its activity. In fact, we have confirmed that, when vastus lateralis muscle was stimulated by vibration, the reduction in the amount of muscle activity was observed in only vastus lateralis muscle among quadriceps femoris muscles (Table 2).

There may be a possibility of enhancing the activity of inner muscles, which were long assumed to be unsusceptible to strengthening, provided that you can selectively suppress just those muscles you want to suppress. It is hoped that our future studies will clarify this issue as well.

Pre-vibration	Post-vibration
250.0 ± 25.4	220.5 ± 16.2

Mean±standard deviation

Table 1. Muscle force of quadriceps femoris muscle before and after vibration stimulation (%BW).

	Pre-vibration	Post-vibration
Rectus femoris muscle	174.5 ± 29.2	121.2 ± 52.3
Vastus medialis muscle	143.8 ± 34.2	102.1 ± 68.5
Vastus lateralis muscle	113.6 ± 49.1	95.5 ± 37.8 *

*p<0.05: pre-vibration vs post-vibration

Mean±standard deviation

Table 2. Muscle activity of quadriceps femoris muscle before and after vibration stimulation (%iEMG).

2.4. Previous studies by other authors

2.4.1. Spasticity of upper limb in stroke patients is suppressed by 5 to 10 minutes of vibration stimulation

If vibration stimulation of about 5 to 10 minutes is applied on the spastic muscle of a stroke patient's upper limb, the following will be observed: a decrease in the H/M ratio indicative of the excitability level of anterior horn cells in the spinal cord; improvement of motor function and of Modified Ashworth Scale indicative of the degree of spasticity; and improvement of Functional Ability Scale using Wolf Motor Function Test. In some treatment cases, an immediate effect was recorded after the intervention.

The nervous system of a spastic stroke patient may be restructured and/or strengthened by adjusting the level of CNS excitability using a vibration stimulus in combination with training on the nervous system. It is anticipated that further effects that vibration stimulation has on spastic muscle in stroke patients will be revealed in the near future.

2.4.2. Muscle activity and the amount of skeletal muscle output are reduced by more than 20 minutes of vibration stimulation

Vibration stimulation on a sustained maximum muscle contraction case can reduce the firing frequency of the nerve cells involved in the maximum contraction, and subsequently the muscle output will decrease. In addition, more than 20 minutes of vibration stimulation on quadriceps femoris muscle can bring on a reduction in the peak torque and integrated EMG.

If you apply these findings clinically, it is possible to suppress the excessive and abnormal muscle activity that occurs as a compensatory motion during action, and subsequently to let the patient have efficient training.

However, in patients with osteoarthritis of the knee and also in patients who have undergone ACL reconstruction and therefore need onerous training, no decrease of the peak torque and integrated EMG occurs after the vibration stimulation. Abnormal gamma motor neurons are believed to be involved, and the abnormality results from reduced afferent nerve activity of the joints.

All in all, clinical application of vibration stimulation on patients with musculoskeletal disorders awaits further trials because there remain some unsettled issues.

3. Inhibitory and facilitative effects of muscle tone in normal healthy subjects

This section provides an overview of the effects of inhibition and facilitation by physical stimuli on skeletal muscle of healthy subjects. We shall then consider the current state surrounding the physical stimulus in the field.

3.1. Pressure stimulation

A decreased H/M ratio was observed by air pressure in the splint on triceps surae muscle of the lower limb (Robichaud et al., 1992) and radiocarpal flexor muscle of the upper limb (Agostinucci et al., 2006) both in healthy subjects.

Pressure stimulation causes a decrease in blood flow, leads to the state of lack of oxygen, and adversely affects the site of compression of the cell, tissue, or organ. What then would be an appropriate duration and compression strength to apply without bringing on undesirable effects? In a study of healthy Japanese youths, the condition of 5 minutes at 50 mmHg was recommended as appropriate (Miura et al., 2011). A pressure of up to 50 mmHg did not result in any statistically significant differences in blood flow compared with no-addition pressure stimuli. But at this time the excitability of soleus muscle motor neurons was inhibited in the spinal cord.

3.2. Whole Body Vibration (WBV)

Studies using WBV include the examination of its longitudinal and acute effects. Indices that are adopted to verify or refute those effects are as follows: muscle activity, muscle strength, power, height by counter jump, body balance, and mechanical competence of bones.

3.2.1. Acute effects

Neuromuscular stimulation derived from WBV is the likely source of previously observed changes in athletic performance. The tonic vibration reflex is a response elicited from vibration directly applied to a muscle belly or tendon. This reflex is characterized by activation of muscle spindles primarily though Ia afferents and activation of extrafusal muscle fibers through alpha motor neurons (Cormie et al., 2006).

Vibration has been shown to stimulate transient increases in certain hormones, such as growth hormone and IGF-I (Cormie et al., 2006).

A study exists in which the flexibility of hamstring muscle of the lower limb was examined by varying the frequency of vibration stimulation. It showed that there was a 10% increase in flexibility at 20 Hz and no change at 40 Hz (Cardinale et al., 2003).

Vibration is detected not only by spindle, but also by the skin, the joint and secondary endings. All those structures contribute to the facilitatory input to the gamma-system which in turn affects sensitivity of the primary endings. Modulation of neuromuscular response to vibration is then to be referred not just to spindle activation, but to all the sensory systems in the body. Various parameters can affect the synergies in the sensory system and determine specific responses. Vibration is thought mainly to inhibit the contraction on antagonist muscles via Ia inhibitory neurons. However there is some evidence as well that vibrations can also produce co-activation (Cardinale et al., 2003).

A previous study investigated the acute effects of WBV on back and abdominal muscle activity. Muscle activity with vibration showed a low to moderate increase in trunk muscle activation (Wirth et al., 2011).

3.2.2. Long-term effects

A 4-month WBV-loading induced a significant 8.5% mean increase in jump height of young healthy adults. This improvement was already seen after 2 months of the vibration. Lower limb extension strength was also enhanced by the 2-month vibration period. Intervention with a 4-month WBV enhanced jumping power in young adults, suggesting neuromuscular adaptation to the vibration stimulation. On the other hand, the vibration-intervention showed no effect on dynamic or static balance of the subjects (Torvinen et al., 2002).

3.2.3. The difference between athletes and normal healthy subjects

There are many reports in which knee extensor strength and jump performance improved after stimulation with WBV in healthy subjects. In contrast, no improvement was observed in sprint-trained athletes and elite female field hockey players. This means either that the effect of daily training was greater than the stimulatory effect with WBV or that its cumulative activity and inhibitory effects were retained in the body system. It is suggested that the stimulating effect of WBV is probably greater in subjects that do not exercise every day.

4. Inhibitory and facilitative effects of muscle tone in patients with pathological disorder

Section 4 presents an overview of the effects of inhibition and facilitation provided by the physical stimulus on skeletal muscles in people with pathological disorder. We shall then consider the existing state surrounding the equipment used in rehabilitation.

In the field of rehabilitation, people with muscle hypo-tone are induced to undergo activities that facilitate muscle activity, and those with muscle hyper-tone are given activities that inhibit muscle activity. In general, when standing position is sustained there will be increases in muscle tone from that posture. Therapists often suppress the excessive muscle activity in such cases. Muscle hypo-tone from paralysis or hemiplegia is usually treated with a facilitative method using electrical stimulation or proprioceptive neuromuscular stimulation. At the present time, it is not clear to what extent these physical means are effective; it needs continued investigation. Physical therapy stands for intervention with physical means in people with physical disturbance so that their physical disorder is alleviated. For that purpose, application of clinical and kinesiologic EMG is one of the most effective methods.

4.1. In people with cerebrovascular accident

Cerebrovascular Accident (CVA) is a general term for diseases such as subarachnoid hemorrhage, rupture of a cerebral aneurysm, and cerebral infarction. Disturbances after a CVA are various in severities. What was the onset of a CVA like, was there early treatment, or was the site known at the time of its onset? These are the questions that help determine how severe CVAs turn out to be. Sequelae such as motor paralysis, sensory disturbances, and language disorder occur in about one-third of the patients who suffered CVA.

4.1.1. Electrical stimulation

When the antagonist muscle of spastic paralysis undergoes electrical stimulation, its muscle spasticity is suppressed. This suppression is brought on by reciprocity through the Ia inhibition in the spinal cord, which in turn results from an adjustment of the reflective circuit. If the spastic muscle itself is subjected to electrical stimulation in such a case, a decrease in muscle tone occurs through the antagonist inhibition. Upon application of electrical stimulation to rectus femoris muscle of the lower limb, facilitation of the flexion of the hip joint and the extension of the knee joint occurs through suppression of the muscle tone of hip flexor muscle and knee extensor muscle, respectively. Thus, gait itself turns out to show improvement.

If a muscle receives electrical stimulation, what will be the reaction of the muscle? Electrical stimulation to a paralyzed muscle, for instance, will cause the amount of muscle activity to increase. This is referred to as the carry over effect.

4.1.2. Pressure stimulation

Pressure stimulation on spastic muscle of people with CVA brings about an effect that is similar to the effect it has on healthy people. Air pressure in a splint to triceps surae muscle of the lower limb in people with spastic paralysis caused a decrease in the H/M ratio (Robichaud et al., 1992). And the same was seen in spastic muscle of the upper limb: radiocarpal flexor muscle in people with neurological diseases, when stimulated by air pressure in the splint, registered a lowered H/M ratio (Agostinucci et al., 2006).

4.2. In people with spinal cord injury

Spinal cord injury (SCI) is a disorder caused by damage to the spinal nerve running through the spinal canal. SCI often brings on motor paralysis or sensory disturbances caused by their proprioceptive CNS diseases, leading eventually to impaired autonomic nervous system. Hypertensive tendon reflexes are often seen in the patient.

4.2.1. Pressure stimulation

When air pressure in a splint is applied to soleus muscle of the lower limb in people with SCI, alpha motor neuron reflex excitability is suppressed (Robichaud et al., 1992).

4.2.2. Therapeutic massage

When people with SCI were given massage treatment for 3 minutes, there was a decrease in the amplitude of H-reflex when compared with what it was before the massage (Goldberg et al., 1994).

4.2.3. Whole Body Vibration (WBV)

When WBV is applied on a person with SCI, residual effects of medication for muscle spasticity will sometimes be recognized. And because the duration of stimulation differs among researchers, a simple comparison is difficult (Ness et al., 2009).

There is a report in which the adopted cycle of WBV treatment consists of the following: 4 bouts of 45 seconds with one minute of seated rest between bouts, done on 3 days a week lasting for 4 weeks.

4.3. In people with Parkinson's disease

Parkinson's disease (PD), often caused by depletion of dopamine in the substantia nigra of the midbrain, is a disease that indicates a variety of movement disorders. Rigidity, tremor, akinesia, amimia, and pill-rolling phenomenon are the characteristic symptoms. By taking L-dopa, people with PD can alleviate these symptoms.

4.3.1. Whole Body Vibration (WBV)

4.3.1.1. Acute effects

With WBV, scores of Unified Parkinson's Disease Rating Scale (UPDRS) tremor and rigidity improved compared with no intervention. There is no evidence, however, that WBV is effective in improving knee proprioception and other clinical measures of sensorimotor performance, such as balance and mobility (Lau et al., 2011).

4.3.1.2. Long-term effects

WBV had no significant effects, or was only slightly effective, on UPDRS motor scores (Lau et al., 2011).

4.4. In people with multiple sclerosis

Multiple sclerosis (MS) is a chronic inflammatory, demyelinating disease of the central nervous system. The most prevalent symptoms of this disease include sensory changes, visual disturbances, fatigue, and micturition disorders (Jackson et al., 2008).

4.4.1. Whole Body Vibration (WBV)

4.4.1.1. Acute effects

There is no evidence that WBV is effective in improving peak torque values for both quadriceps and hamstring muscles (Jackson et al., 2008).

4.4.1.2. Long-term effects

Under the duration of 5 training sessions per 2-week cycle for 20 weeks, WBV did not improve leg muscle performance or functional capacity in mildly to moderately impaired people with MS (Broekmans et al., 2010). Also 8-week exercise is effective in improving standing balance and timed up-and-go test (Mason et al., 2012). But there are differences in stimulation frequency and duration between the two reports. That makes it difficult to determine whether WBV is or is not effective in the long run.

4.5. In people with knee osteoarthritis

4.5.1. Whole Body Vibration (WBV)

Previous research investigated WBV as an alternative strengthening regimen in the rehabilitation of people with total knee arthroplasty (TKA) compared with traditional progressive resistance exercise (TPRE). Post-TKA subjects received physical therapy with WBV or with TPRE for 4 weeks. There was a significant increase in knee extensor strength and improvements in mobility both with WBV and with TPRE.

With an addition of WBV to squat training, elderly people with knee osteoarthritis (OA) were evaluated on functional performance and self-report of disease. A total of 23 elderly subjects participated. There was no statistically significant difference in functional performance and self-report of disease status between groups of squat training with or without WBV.

4.6. Summary

We therapists realize after all that, at the present time, WBV effectiveness against SCI, PD, MS, and knee OA has not been established. There are reasons for that: disease mechanisms have not been clarified, and optimum conditions such as stimulation frequency are not definitely set yet. And in intervention studies, one cannot completely eliminate the influence of other factors. It is unfortunate that not enough high-level evidence-based research has been done or published.

Though rather limited in scope, we therapists can help people with disabilities, or even people without disabilities, by suppressing the muscle tone of a given muscle through the spinal cord loop.

5. Health science research with EMG

In research using EMG, there are two groups of studies: clinical and kinesiologic. Kinesiologic EMG is to record the response during motion of the body.

Clinical EMG

1. EMG as a diagnostic aid in cases in which causes of muscle weakness and muscle atrophy are neurogenic or myogenic
2. EMG as a means to confirm the lesion site and properties of peripheral nerve injury
3. EMG as a means to confirm abnormal muscle activity
4. EMG in cases that are not classifiable as 1, 2, or 3 above

Likely target diseases are amyotrophic lateral sclerosis, polymyositis, carpal tunnel syndrome, and Bell's palsy.

Cases of kinesiologic EMG are as in the following:

1. EMG to check presence or absence of muscle activity
2. EMG to measure timing and duration of muscle activity
3. EMG to measure amount of muscle activity

4. EMG as basis of biofeedback to patients
5. EMG to determine matters relative to muscle fatigue
6. EMG to measure reaction time on external stimuli
7. EMG to evaluate motor control
8. EMG to assess gait
9. EMG to evaluate motor learning
10. EMG for purposes not classifiable as 1 to 9 above.

In recent years, the study of human-machine interfaces became fairly popular. For example, equipment is used to amplify muscle activities of a person with disabilities, which will then be relayed to a robot so it can put them into effect for the disabled person. Or EMG is made use of as a vital part of technique to convey information from a robot to a human subject through the human senses. We shall introduce some of these studies.

In the field of rehabilitation, the type of equipment has been developed that controls movements of a joint by the muscle discharge in people with disabilities. The equipment sends a command from electrodes attached to the forearm of the robot to its artificially created fingers to control. The number of sensors attached on the disabled person increased gradually, so it became possible to control the intensity of such delicate movements as tapping or lifting. Numerous researches have also been done on motion control by an exoskeleton. The target joints now include forearm, elbow joint, shoulder joint, upper limb, cervix, hip joint, knee joint and lower limb, as well as a wide variety of fingers and hands. In upper limb research, starting from motions of three degrees of freedom (3-DOF), it has now reached the level of 7-DOF motions. Research on reaction time has also shown improvement; in the line of research on hand reactions, delays of only 100 ms have been attained. Research has also been done on robot-assisted therapy on upper limb recovery after stroke, but not much that is revolutionary has come out of it so far. Perhaps we can expect to see this line of research grow in the future.

We consider it possible that robot-assisted therapy may eventually help an individual patient become free from environmental and personal factors. Introduction of the so-called ICF (International Classification of Functioning, Disability and Health) model may be something that is revolutionary.

6. Conclusion

Verification of inhibitory effects of muscle tone by vibration stimulation as we did above, though it is only the beginning, seems to point to further development in the future. Significance may be found in the fact that healthy people can be checked using simple equipment. In the literature, a certain level of effectiveness of vibration stimulation is found in people with disabilities; determination of the optimum stimulation conditions will certainly be researchers' next point of interest. In studies using other physical means, it seems necessary to set conditions for measuring the effectiveness of the given means. Overall, studies of equipment-aided therapies tell us that aided-therapies seem to be superior to non-aided therapies because you can minimize the individual difference between techniques of intervention. This may be true in day-to-day therapeutic sessions as well as in the examination of the effect of physical therapy.

Acknowledgements

The authors are grateful to Mr. Kensuke Tokaichi for refining the English of the manuscript.

Author details

Satoru Kai[1] and Koji Nakabayashi[2]

1 Faculty of Allied Health Sciences, Kansai University of Welfare Sciences, Japan

2 Department of Physical Therapy, Takeo Nursing and Rehabilitation School, Japan

References

[1] Agostinucci, J, Holmberg, A, Mushen, M, Plisko, J, & Gofman, M. (2006). The effects of circumferential air-splint pressure on flexor carpi radialis H-reflex in subjects without neurological deficits, *Percept. Mot. Skills*, , 103, 565-579.

[2] Bongiovanni, L. G, Hagbarth, K. E, & Stjernberg, L. (1989). Prolonged muscle vibration reducing motor output in maximal voluntary contractions in man, *J. Physiol* , 423, 15-26.

[3] Broekmans, T, Roelants, M, Alders, G, Feys, P, Thijs, F, & Eijnde, B. O. (2010). Exploring the effects of a 20-week whole-body vibration training programme on leg muscle performance and function in persons with multiple sclerosis, *J. Rehabil. Med* , 42, 866-872.

[4] Caliandro, P, Celletti, C, Padua, L, Minciotti, I, Russo, G, Granata, G, La Torre, G, Granieri, E, & Camerota, F. (2012). Focal muscle vibration in the treatment of upper limb spasticity: A pilot randomized controlled trial in patients with chronic stroke, *Arch. Phys. Med. Rehabil,* Apr 13.

[5] Cardinale, M, & Lim, J. (2003). The acute effects of two different whole body vibration frequencies on vertical jump performance, *Med. Sport* , 56, 287-292.

[6] Cormie, P, Deane, R. S, Triplett, N. T, & Mcbride, J. M. (2006). Acute effects of whole-body vibration on muscle activity, strength, and power, *J. Strength Cond. Res* , 20, 257-261.

[7] Desmedt, J. E, & Godaux, E. (1978). Mechanism of the vibration paradox: excitatory and inhibitory effects of tendon vibration on single soleus muscle motor units in man, *J. Physiol* , 285, 197-207.

[8] Gillies, J. D, Lance, J. W, Neilson, P. D, & Tassinari, C. A. (1969). Presynaptic inhibition of the monosynaptic reflex by vibration, *J. Physiol* , 205, 329-339.

[9] Goldberg, J, Seaborne, D. E, Sullivan, S. J, & Leduc, B. E. (1994). The effect of therapeutic massage on H-reflex amplitude in persons with a spinal cord injury, *Phys. Ther* , 74, 728-737.

[10] Jackson, S. W, & Turner, D. L. (2003). Prolonged muscle vibration reduces maximal voluntary knee extension performance in both the ipsilateral and the contralateral limb in man, *Eur. J. Appl. Physiol* , 88, 380-386.

[11] Jackson, K. J, Merriman, H. L, Vanderburgh, P. M, & Brahler, C. J. (2008). Acute effects of whole-body vibration on lower extremity muscle performance in persons with multiple sclerosis, *JNPT*, , 32, 171-176.

[12] Kaeser, H. E. (1973). Evoked muscle and sensory nerve action potentials in polyneuropathies. In: *Handbook of Electroencephalography and Clinical Neurophysiology*, Elsevier, Amsterdam, , 16A, 36-44.

[13] Konishi, Y, Fukubayashi, T, & Takeshita, D. (2002). Possible mechanism of quadriceps femoris weakness in patients with ruptured anterior cruciate ligament, *Med. Sci. Sports Exerc* , 34, 1414-1418.

[14] Konishi, Y, Kubo, J, & Fukudome, A. (2009). Effects of prolonged tendon vibration stimulation on eccentric and concentric maximal torque and EMGs of the knee extensors, *Journal of Sports Science and Medicine*, , 8, 548-552.

[15] Kouzaki, M, Shinohara, M, & Fukunaga, T. (2000). Decrease in maximal voluntary contraction by tonic vibration applied to a single synergist muscle in humans, *J. Appl. Physiol* , 89, 1420-1424.

[16] Lau, R. W. K, Teo, T, Yu, F, Chung, R. C. K, & Pang, M. Y. C. (2011). Effects of whole-body vibration on sensorimotor performance in people with Parkinson disease: A systematic review, *Phys. Ther*, 91, 198-209.

[17] Ljung, B, & Sivertsson, R. (1972). The inhibitory effect of vibrations on tension development in vascular smooth muscle, *Acta. Physiol. Scand* , 85, 428-430.

[18] Ljung, B, & Hallgren, P. (1975). On the mechanism of inhibitory action vibrations as studied in a molluscan catch muscle and in vertebrate vascular smooth muscle, *Acta. Physiol. Scand* , 95, 424-430.

[19] Mason, R. R, Cochrane, D. J, Denny, G. J, Firth, E. C, & Stannard, S. R. (2012). Is 8 weeks of side-alternating whole-body vibration a safe and acceptable modality to improve functional performance in multiple sclerosis?, *Disabil. Rehabil* , 34, 647-654.

[20] Miura, N, Kurosawa, K, Hirose, M, & Suzuki, T. (2011). Inhibitory effects of pressure on soleus muscle motor neuron excitability and flow volume in healthy adults, *Rigakuryoho Kagaku*, , 26, 773-776.

[21] Nakabayashi, K, Kodama, T, Mizuno, K, Ikeda, T, Kai, N, Fukura, T, & Kai, S. (2011). The inhibitory effect of vibration stimulus on muscle tone of the triceps surae: Analysis of the H/M ratio, *Rigakuryoho Kagaku*, , 26, 393-396.

[22] Nakabayashi, K, Kodama, T, Matsumoto, N, Yamamoto, H, Nomiyama, M, Fukura, T, & Kai, S. (2012). Muscle tone inhibitory effects of vibration applied to the tendon and muscle belly of the triceps surae, *Rigakuryoho Kagaku*, , 27, 151-154.

[23] Ness, L. L, & Field-fote, E. C. (2009). Effect of whole-body vibration on quadriceps spasticity in individuals with spastic hypertonia due to spinal cord injury, *Restor. Neurol. Neurosci* , 27, 623-633.

[24] Noma, T, Matsumoto, S, Shimodozono, M, Etoh, S, & Kawahira, K. (2012). Anti-spastic effects of the direct application of vibratory stimuli to the spastic muscles of hemiplegic limbs in post-stroke patients: a proof-of-principle study, *J. Rehabil. Med,* 44, 325-330.

[25] Rice, D. A, Mcnair, P. J, & Lewis, G. N. (2011). Mechanisms of quadriceps muscle weakness in knee joint osteoarthritis: the effects of prolonged vibration on torque and muscle activation in osteoarthritic and healthy control subjects, *Arthritis Res. Ther* R151, 13

[26] Robichaud, J. A, Agostinucci, J, & Linden, D. W. V. (1992). Effect of air-splint application on soleus muscle motoneuron reflex excitability in nondisabled subjects and subjects with cerebrovascular accidents, *Phys. Ther*, 72, 176-183.

[27] Shinohara, M, Moritz, C. T, Pascoe, M. A, & Enoka, R. M. (2005). Prolonged muscle vibration increases stretch reflex amplitude, motor unit discharge rate, and force fluctuations in a hand muscle, *J. Appl. Physiol* , 99, 1835-1842.

[28] Torvinen, S, Kannus, P, Sievanen, H, Jarvinen, T. A. H, Pasanen, M, Kontulainen, S, Jarvinen, T. L. N, Jarvinen, M, Oja, P, & Vuori, I. (2002). Effect of four-month vertical whole body vibration on performance and balance, *Med. Sci. Sports Exerc,* 34, 1523-1528.

[29] Vukas, M, Sivertsson, R, & Ljung, B. (1978). Inhibitory effects of vibrations on contractility of isolated rabbit papillary muscle, *Scand. J. Clin. Lab. Invest* , 38, 415-419.

[30] Wirth, B, Zurfluh, S, & Muller, R. (2011). Acute effects of whole-body vibration on trunk muscles in young healthy adults, *J. Electromyogr. Kinesiol* , 21, 450-457.

Chapter 11

Underwater Electromyogram for Human Health Exercise

Koichi Kaneda, Yuji Ohgi, Mark Mckean and
Brendan Burkett

Additional information is available at the end of the chapter

http://dx.doi.org/10.5772/55115

1. Introduction

1.1. Why exercise in water has become popular?

The physical qualities of water are well established and include buoyancy, water drag force, hydrostatic pressure and thermal conductivity [1]. The large difference in these physical qualities, compared to land-based activities, affect the human body in both physiologic and biomechanical aspects. An example of this is buoyancy, which acts vertically against gravity on the immersed object thus decreasing weight of the human body. The buoyancy level is equal to the mass of water displaced by the immersed object and is based on the accepted Archimedean principle. When a human is immersed in water up to the level of pubis around 40% of weight is accounted for, 50% at umbilical, 60% at xiphoid, and almost 80% at the level of axillary [1, 2]. When immersed to their lower limb joint and waist in a water environment, humans can easily move, without gravitational overload, due to the buoyancy effect.

Water drag force is composed of three types of drag; surface drag, form drag and wave drag [3]. Surface drag is affected by viscosity of water and the surface quality of the immersed object. For example, the roughness of the surfaces of the object might increase surface drag, however, this depends on the speed of movement of the object as seen in the decreased drag on a golf ball due to the dimples [3]. Form drag depends on the shape and size of the immersed object, whilst wave drag directly opposes the object's movement through water. Water drag force increases proportionally by the frontal projected area and square of moving velocity [4]. Therefore, humans need to exert a much greater force to overcome water drag force when moving in water due to a greater frontal surface area [3].

Hydrostatic pressure is related to water density and depth. Water density is about 800 times greater than air. When at a water depth of 1 meter, hydrostatic pressure increases about

73.5mmHg [1], which is similar to normal diastolic blood pressure. Hydrostatic pressure causes blood to shift from the lower extremities to the thoracic region [5], and also affects lung, renal and other endocrine functions [6]. Thermal conductivity, which is about 25 times faster than air, also affects the human circulatory system [1]. When a human is immersed in water with a lower than thermo-neutral temperature, peripheral vasoconstriction occurs and increases the blood shift to the thoracic region [7]. This thermoregulation effect has been used for a range of therapeutic practices [1].

As briefly described above, the water physical qualities can be very beneficial for the human body. In addition to those effects, exercising in a water environment is a safe environment and may reduce the incidence of falling [8]. A wide range of people including those who have difficulty moving on land due to obesity, a lower-limb disorder, through to those who are healthy or want to improve their fitness may benefit from utilizing the water environment [8, 9].

1.2. Why knowledge of muscle activity during exercise in a water environment is important?

When exercising in water, the benefits of buoyancy and water resistance mainly occur because these qualities act directly on the exercise motion. For example, weight reduction, due to buoyancy, may contribute to the upward or downward motion, and additional loading by water resistance would strongly affect the motion in any direction. Therefore, the instructors of water exercise need to consider the effect of water specific qualities can play on the human body.

As a method of understanding the loading or offloading effect of water specific qualities on human body, investigation of muscle activity is considered an important tool. This provides information regarding the degree of muscle loading during exercise in water, and also provides a basis to apply health and rehabilitation exercise in a water environment more effectively. It is easily hypothesized that the muscle activity would be changed during exercise in water, compared with the same exercise on land. However, there is a challenge in measuring muscle activity in a water environment.

In consideration of these points, firstly, this chapter focuses on the methodology and its validity of collecting muscle activity data in a water environment, with special mention regarding a waterproofing method. Following this, the muscle activity modality for walking, running and many other exercise forms in water are also featured. Walking and running exercise in water are the most popular and basic exercise forms of water exercise [9]. This chapter focuses on walking, running and other water exercise forms which is based on gait, for example, walking with long step, walking with twisting, walking with kicking and so on. Finally, this chapter provides an informative suggestion for exercise participants and instructors.

2. How to collect underwater electromyogram (EMG)?

2.1. The methodology for the collection of muscle activity in underwater environment

Measuring muscle activity by EMG method is challenging because most EMG devices are not waterproofed. As with all electronic devices, water immersion can be dangerous. Because of this risk, most research has used silver-silver-chloride surface EMG electrodes as passive surface electrodes [10, 11]. Some researchers who have investigated muscle activity using EMG devices developed their own waterproofing methods [10, 11] of which there are two types. The first type attached a waterproof seal onto the electrodes placed on the local muscle of interest [10, 11], and the second wears a dry suit on the whole body created for EMG collection [10, 12].

Waterproofing the seal onto the electrodes usually involves attaching transparent film and/or a foam pad (Foam Pad, 75A: Nihon Kohden, Tokyo, Japan) and this method has been used successfully in previous research [10, 11]. For even better waterproofing, transparent film and/ or foam pad are attached in combination [10, 11]. This is achieved by sealing a small piece of transparent film over the electrodes which are attached on the muscle belly to be studied. Then, fill up the slight gap between electrodes leads and transparent film with putty. Finally, use a large piece of transparent film to cover over the small size film and putty (Figure 1).

A

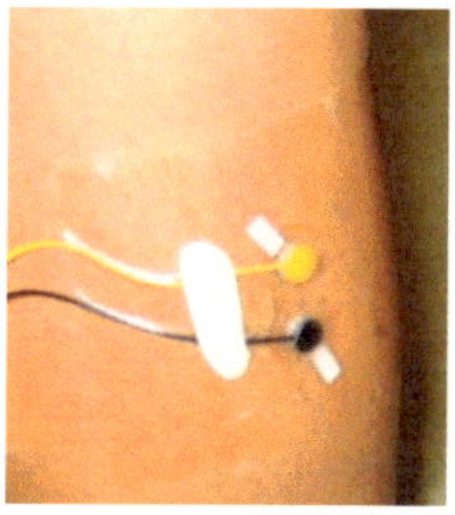

B

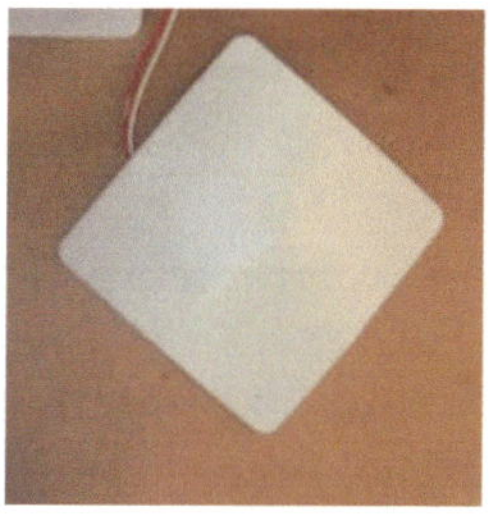

A: doubled by transparent films with putty. B: covered by foam pad.

Figure 1. Waterproofing of surface electrodes. [Pictures were taken by the authors]

Even when this strict waterproofing is applied the water can sometimes immerse under the films cause interference with the electrodes. Therefore, when using this method, the EMG signal has to be monitored continuously throughout the experiment to ensure the data is not affected by water intrusion. When water intrusion under the films or electrodes occurs, a high frequency noise and/or baseline fluctuation on the wave data would be observed. If an abnormal data reading is confirmed due to water intrusion, the electrodes attachment has to be removed and re-applied and the experiment procedure should be started over again. In addition to the waterproofing to the electrodes, the code of each electrode should be taped along with body segment to avoid unexpected tension by water resistance and swinging by exercise motion in water which may prevent or interfere with the normal motion (Figure 2). Due to the series of extensive electrode attachments, waterproofing procedures and establishing the settings for collecting data of underwater EMG, the procedure for underwater EMG takes considerably longer to perform compared with testing in the land environment.

A whole body dry suit has been developed for the collection of underwater EMG, specifically for water sports activities to allow full range of motion [10, 12]. This suit consists of waterproof material with the arm, leg and neck openings tightly sealed. Once the electrodes are attached on the subject, the electrodes and its leads are well covered from the water due to the fully enclosed suit. The advantages of this suit include less set up time than waterproofing and

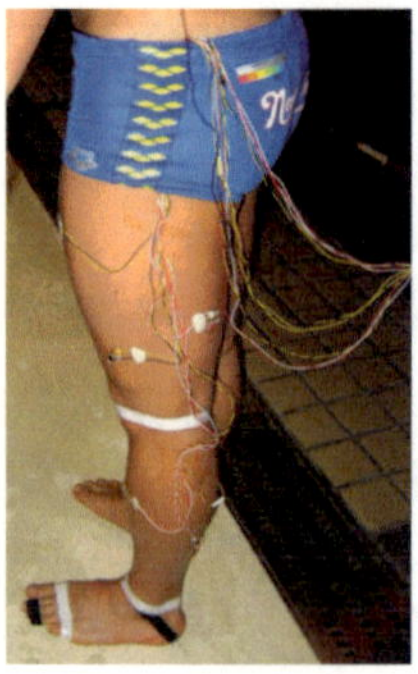

Figure 2. Electrodes and its codes attachment for underwater EMG experiment. [Picture was taken by the authors]

enable longer EMG data collection periods due to increased comfort the suit provides in the water environment. However, the suit would disadvantage subjects who do not fit the standard size of the suit, and this waterproof method still requires further refinement to limit water intrusion at the openings [10, 12].

2.2. The effect of human water immersion on EMG data

The other issue for EMG recording in a water environment is whether the EMG data is affected by water immersion, even if the electrodes are waterproofed. However the EMG data seems to have little attenuation from water immersion if the waterproofing is completely implemented [10, 13-16]. There are numerous studies regarding the influence of water immersion for EMG data collection using waterproofed and non-waterproofed electrodes attached on human muscles [10, 13-16]. Rainoldi et al. [13] investigated the effect of EMG recording by using surface electrodes attached on Biceps Brachii in conditions of dry land, in water with waterproofed or not. The subjects conducted 50% of isometric maximal voluntary contraction (MVC) as determined by a load cell. The results showed that there was no attenuation on EMG recordings in averaged rectified value (ARV) and root mean square (RMS) value with waterproofed condition, whilst the non-waterproofed condition showed significant reduction of the EMG data. In addition to that, the same circumstances were seen in the signal spectrum analysis. The authors concluded that waterproofing was required for EMG recording in water environment to avoid large signal artifacts, to ensure constant recording conditions for the whole experimental session duration, and to avoid time consuming alternative correction technique to remove low frequency artifacts. Pinto et al. [14] investigated the effect on surface EMG recording of isometric MVC between on land and in water. The EMG was recorded from Biceps Brachii, Triceps Brachii, Rectus Femoris and Biceps Femoris. The results showed that the EMG data of each muscle was not affected by water immersion, however the force production of the hip extension decreased significantly in water. This study also reported a significant intra-class correlation coefficient from moderate to high (0.69-0.92) for the EMG recording and the authors concluded that the environment did not influence the EMG data in MVC. With respect to a reduction of EMG data without waterproofing in water environment, Carvalho et al. [15] reported that the reduction was around 37.1-55.8% in the water condition without waterproofing compared with the land or the water with waterproofing in both MVC and 50% of MVC trials. Recently, Silvers et al. [16] reported the validity and reliability of EMG recording by waterproofing in water exercise suggesting future EMG studies should conduct MVC testing in water for data normalization and confirm the post-exercise verification of EMG recording. It can be then assumed due to the body of previous research that the collection of EMG data during water environment is not influenced by water immersion if the electrodes were waterproofed, however, it might be more reliable to verify post-experiment EMG recordings and/or normalization in water MVC.

3. The characteristics of muscle activity during walking in water

3.1. Muscle activity in lower limb muscles

One of the most basic forms of exercise in water is walking gait. Walking in water provides significant changes on your body. A number of investigations have been conducted on the physiological aspects of water walking [17, 18, 19], and more recently, biomechanics and kinesiology research has been published [11, 20-25]. Research into muscle activity has focused mainly on lower limb muscles due to the fact that walking exercise in water is generally conducted at the waist depth or deeper [8, 9, 18, 19]. Research of the lower limb muscles activity during walking in water has been reported by the authors at subject's self-selected slow, moderate and fast speed in comparison to those same selected speeds for land walking [11, 20]. Subjects included nine young men and they walked along the swimming pool deck for the land trial and in a 1.1m deep swimming pool. The EMG data was collected from Tibialis Anterior (TA), Soleus (SOL), Medial Gastrocnemius (GAS), Rectus Femoris (RF), VastusLateralis (VL), and Long Head of Biceps Femoris (BF) on subject's left side with 2000Hz sampling rate. The EMG data was normalized by MVC on land in each muscle. Data processing involved the raw EMG data being filtered using 4th-order low-pass and high-pass filters with cut-off frequencies of 500 Hz and 10 Hz, respectively. And then, the filtered EMG data was transferred to digital data, and the root mean square (RMS) of each phase calculated on a 100-ms window of data (i.e. 50 ms both before and after the data point of interest), and expressed as percentages of MVC (%MVC). This study evaluated the muscle activity in each cycle phase as to a stance phase from a heel contact to a toe-off, and a swing phase from the toe-off to the next heel contact. A paired Student's-t-test was applied for a statistical comparison between two conditions. Figure 3 and Figure 4 showed the result of the study.

As a result of the stance phase (Figure 3), significantly lower %MVC were observed during water-walking compared to land-walking in the SOL and GAS muscles at all speeds ($P < 0.05$). On the other hand, the TA and BF were significantly higher during water-walking than land-walking at normal and fast speeds ($P < 0.05$). In the swing phase, RF was significantly higher during water-walking than land-walking at all speeds, but the other muscles tended to be lower during water-walking than land-walking at all speeds especially in the TA (slow), SOL (moderate), VL (moderate and fast) and BF (slow and moderate) as significance (Figure 4).

Muscle activity during walking is not dramatically large if it is expressed in %MVC regardless of the condition. Basically, TA seems to activate during stance phase to stabilize the ankle joint against the water resistance added to whole body during water walking [21]. This may explain why the TA activity was significantly higher during water-walking in moderate and fast speeds (Figure 3). There was no phase where the TA had to stabilize the ankle joint during swing phase, resulting in lower TA activity during water-walking than land-walking. However, Nakazawa et al. [22] concluded that the inter-subject and intra-subject variability were higher in the TA response during water-walking. Therefore, more precise investigation of TA during water-walking is required. The muscle activity of SOL and GAS dramatically decreased during water-walking due to a reduction of weight bearing by buoyancy. Further investigation of these muscles by Miyoshi et al. [23] reported a different role of SOL and GAS muscles during water-walking. They concluded that the SOL was affected by walking speed and gravity stress, while the GAS was affected by only walking speed. In BF, more activation is needed to generate propulsive force against water resistance force by extending hip joint during stance phase. A larger hip joint extension moment during water-walking throughout the stance phase than that during land-walking was confirmed by Miyoshi et al. [24]. In the swing phase, the RF muscle activates more during water-walking than land-walking to overcome water resistance force for forwarding lower limb [21]. Interestingly, the %MVC of the other muscles decreased during water-walking compared to land-walking. It is presumed that this is due to a lack of or smaller impact force in water than that on land, reducing the need for VL and BF muscles to prepare for shock absorption at heel contact. As described above, lower limb muscle activity shows different modalities depending on walking style.

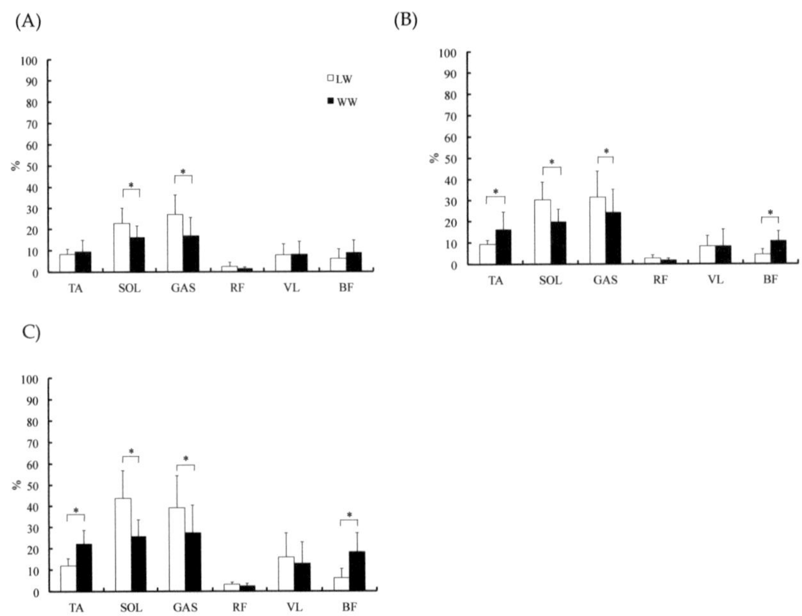

A: slow, B: moderate, C: fast.
LW: land-walking, WW: water-walking.
*: significant difference between water-walking and land-walking (P < 0.05).

Figure 3. The mean ± standard deviation (SD) of %MVC value in each lower limb muscle at each speed during stance phase. [Modified from reference 11]

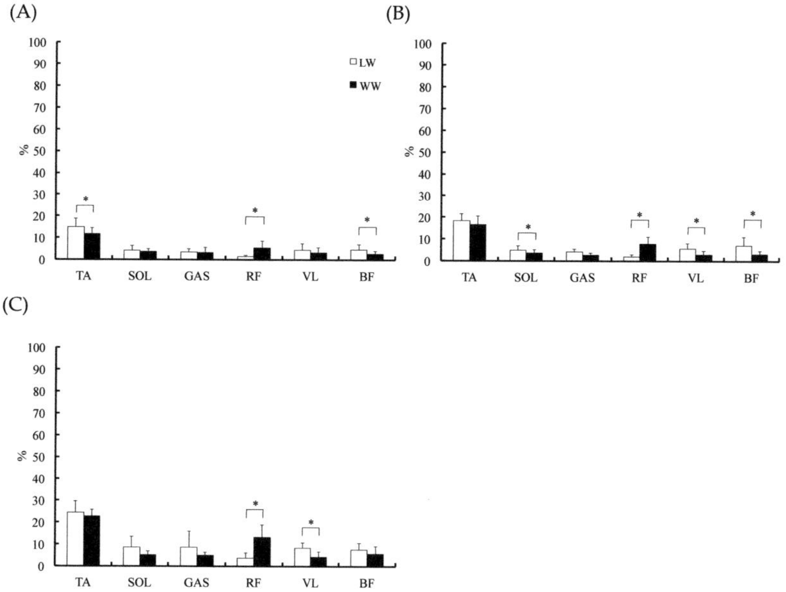

A: slow, B: moderate, C: fast.
LW: land-walking, WW: water-walking.
*: significant difference between water-walking and land-walking (P < 0.05).

Figure 4. The mean ± standard deviation (SD) of %MVC value in each lower limb muscle at each speed during swing phase. [Modified from reference 11]

3.2. Muscle activity in hip and trunk muscles

There are a limited number of studies investigating hip and trunk muscle activity during water-walking, and the EMG data around hip and trunk muscles during water and land based walking [25, 26]. In the author's investigation [25], the surface electrodes were attached to the subject's left side and the muscles studied included Adductor Longus (AL), Gluteus Maximus (GMa), Gluteus Medius (GMe), Rectus Abdominis (RA), Obliquus Externus Abdominis (OEA), and Erector Spinae (ES, the position of L2). The data reduction methods were also applied with the same method as mentioned in lower limb analyzes. The EMG data collected by 2000Hz sampling rate was normalized by MVC (%MVC) on land in each muscle with 4th-order 500Hz low-pass and 10Hz high-pass filters, and the root mean square (RMS) on a 100-ms window of data applied. Figure 5 and 6 showed the results of the Student-t's-t-test.

In the stance phase (Figure 5), the OEA was significantly lower %MVC during water-walking than that during land-walking in all speeds ($P < 0.05$). The RA showed significantly lower %MVC during water-walking than land-walking only in slow speed. A significantly higher %MVC was seen during water-walking than land-walking in the GMe and ES at fast speed. In the swing phase, the AL and ES showed significantly higher muscle activity during water-walking than that during land-walking at all speeds, however, all other muscles activity were lower during water-walking than land-walking in the OEA at all speeds, the GMa and GMe at moderate, and the GMa and RA at fast with significant level ($P < 0.05$), respectively.

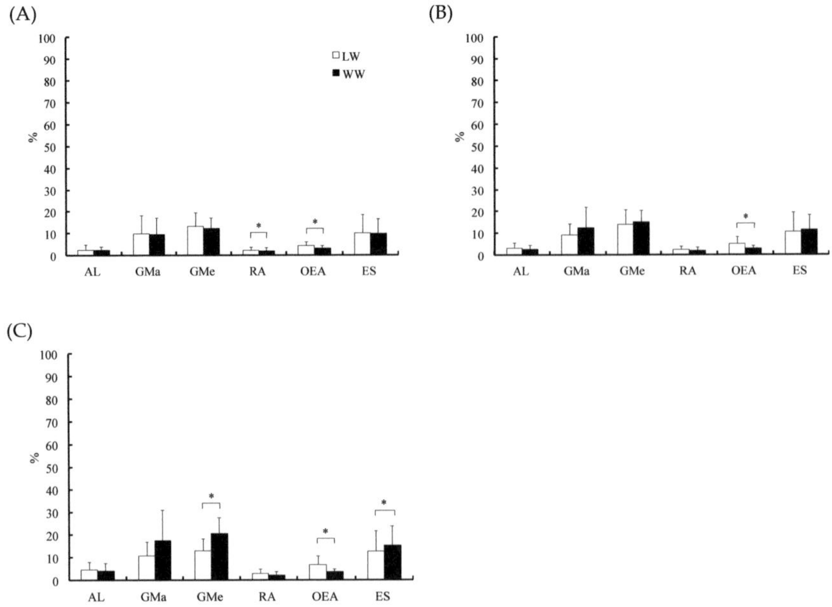

A: slow, B: moderate, C: fast.
LW: land-walking, WW: water-walking.
*: significant difference between water-walking and land-walking (P < 0.05).

Figure 5. The mean ± standard deviation (SD) of %MVC value in each hip and trunk muscle at each speed during stance phase. [Modified from reference 25]

Similar to the %MVC of lower limb muscle, the %MVC of hip and trunk muscles were also not as large during each walking style. The highest level of the %MVC in the hip and trunk muscles is around 20%. In addition to that, the mean differences in some muscles were very small, for example, the RA in both phase, the GMa and GMe in the swing phase. This should be taken into account for a more precise interpretation when applied to an actual exercise situation. Regardless of the fact, there are many noticeable changes when walking in water, compared with walking on land. Adductor Longus muscle appears to activate to stabilize pelvis and thigh segment [27, 28] during swing phase and does not fluctuate by water resistance force. Moreover, one of the important functions of AL is hip joint flexion matched to swing phase, during which relatively larger water resistance force added to lower limb. In respect to the stability during walking, GMe would act to increase stability of pelvis on the femur [28] against large water resistance force especially in the fast speed. Obliquus Externus Abdominis acts in body twisting yet the activity of OEA seems to decrease throughout walking in water compared with walking on land. Considering the results of the muscle activity, trunk twisting during water-walking might be less than that during land-walking. However, there is no evidence about movement in the transverse plane, and further research is needed to clarify this. Despite the fact that ES also acts in body twisting as well as OEA, the results showed higher activity in the ES during water-walking than that during land-walking. It is suggested that ES is compelled to activate against increased water resistance force on trunk during

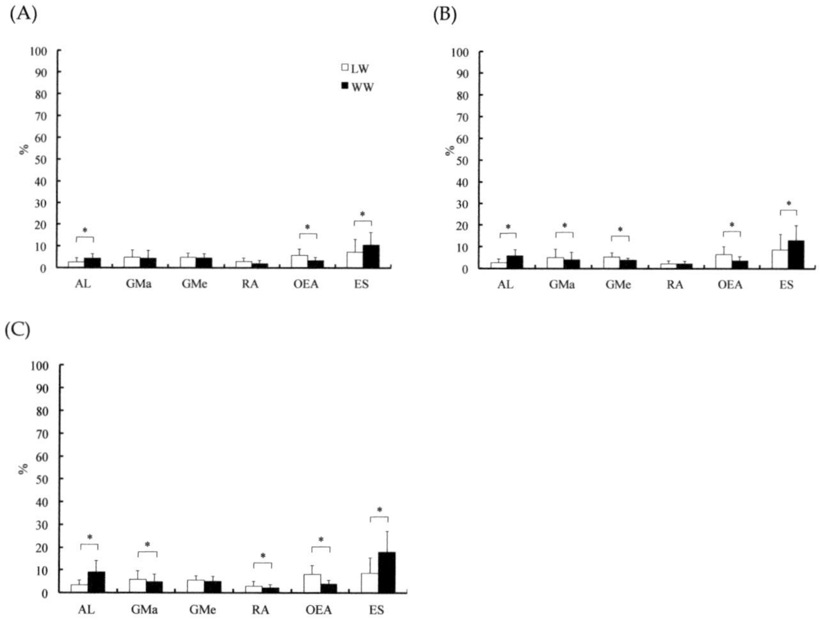

A: slow, B: moderate, C: fast.
LW: land-walking, WW: water-walking.
*: significant difference between water-walking and land-walking (P < 0.05).

Figure 6. The mean ± standard deviation (SD) of %MVC value in each hip and trunk muscle at each speed during swing phase. [Modified from reference 25]

propulsion of the body. As evidence for this, the trunk forward inclination angle is larger during water-walking than land-walking (Figure 7), which is a counteractive reaction to deal with increased frontal water resistance force.

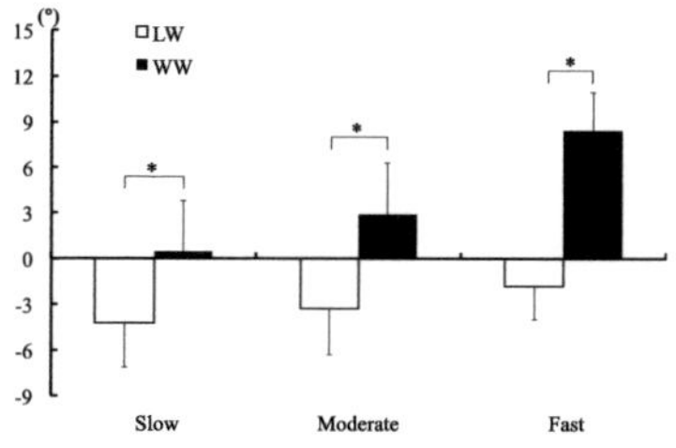

LW: land-walking, WW: water-walking
*: significant difference between water-walking and land-walking (P < 0.05)
Positive: forward inclination
Negative: backward inclination

Figure 7. Trunk inclination angle during walking. [Modified from reference 25]

Trunk muscles show different muscle activity between water and land based walking, as well as lower limb. However, when humans walk on a treadmill apparatus, most muscle activity decreased during water compared with land in both lower limb and trunk area [29]. In this case, the walking speed was set as one-half to one-third of the land walking in reference to the oxygen consumption [17]. Furthermore, muscle activity during treadmill water-walking without water flow further decreased muscle activity than with flow set to the same speed to the walking speed [29]. The differences between with or without treadmill may be due to the treadmill function moving the leg backward automatically without force generation during stance phase. Further, it would be possible that the displacement of the lower limb moves through less distance on treadmill walking than without treadmill in swing phase since human would be at the same position during treadmill walking. Although no previous research has clarified the biomechanical difference between walking with and without treadmill in water, researchers, exercise instructors and participants should pay attention to the differences of the muscle activity modality to determine more appropriate exercise and specific prescription according to water-walking style selected.

4. The characteristics of muscle activity during deep-water running

4.1. Muscle activity in lower limb and trunk

Deep-Water Running (DWR) is one of the unique exercise forms in water environment. Using a floatation device around the waist (Figure 8), people move their feet as if running without touching the bottom of the swimming pool.

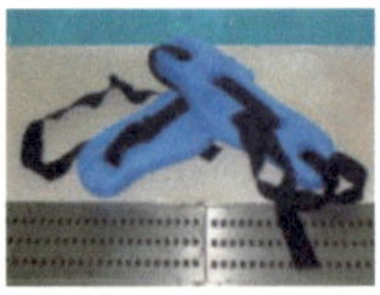

Figure 8. Aqua Jogger (Excel Sports Science Inc., Japan) used for DWR exercise. [Picture was taken by the authors]

This exercise form has been widely used for aerobic training and cross training for performance enhancement in athletes [30], and rehabilitation training [31]. Previous studies have investigated muscle activity during DWR by the authors and compared this with water-walking and land-walking [11, 20, 25]. The results of %MVC level in lower limb muscles and hip and trunk muscles during those exercises are presented in Figure 9, 10 and 11. The measurement procedure, environment settings and the analysis methods were the same as the previous investigation comparing water-walking and land-walking by the authors [11, 20, 25]. In the DWR, the data was collected for one cycle from a maximal knee flexion to a maximal knee extension during the backward swing phase, and from the maximal knee extension to the next maximal knee flexion during the forward swing phase. These phases represent the stance and swing phase in walking exercise, respectively. One-way repeated measures analysis of variance (ANOVA) with Tukey's post-hoc test was applied for the statistic comparison.

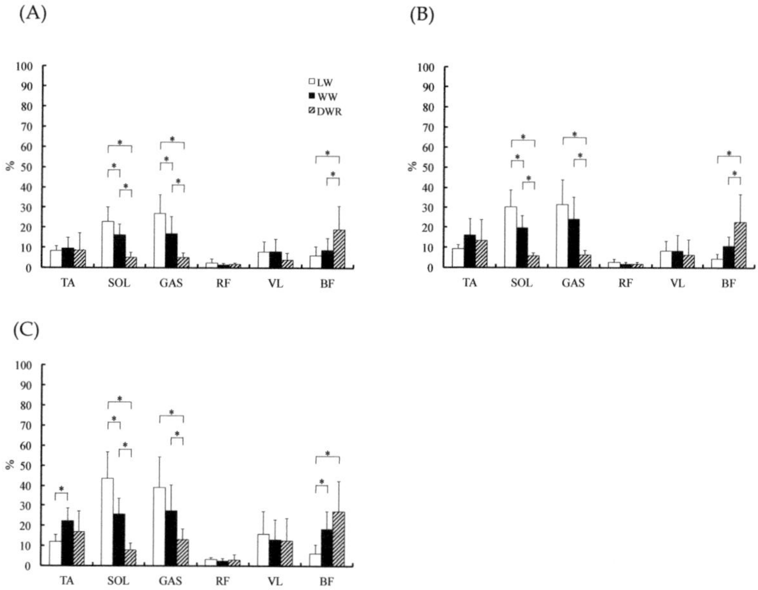

A: slow, B: moderate, C: fast.
LW: land-walking, WW: water-walking, DWR: Deep-Water Running
*: significant difference (P < 0.05).

Figure 9. The mean ± SD of %MVC value in each lower limb muscle at each speed during backward swing phase. [Modified from reference [11]

As seen in Figure 9 and 10, the characteristics of the DWR, %MVC of the SOL, GAS in the backward swing phase, and the VL in the forward swing phase were dramatically decreased compared with water- and land-walking (P<0.05). This is likely a result of the non-contact phase during DWR compared to land walking. On the other hand, %MVC of the BF in both swing phases, and the RF in forward swing phase were much higher than land- and sometimes water-walking (P<0.05). The knee and hip joint range of motion (ROM) was increased during DWR when comparedto both land- and water-walking (Figure 12), which would cause the higher %MVC in the RF and BF. Similarly this increased ROM of the hip would also result in higher %MVC of the GMa, AL and GMe during the DWR than during water- and land-walking. Increased ROM directly indicates that thigh and knee extension and flexion muscles receive greater water resistance force. Further, it is likely that the AL and GMe activated to stabilize the pelvis against femur during an unstable floating situation as in DWR [25].

Interestingly, the %MVC of the RA, OEA and ES were higher during DWR than water- and land-walking throughout one-cycle (P<0.05, Figure 11). The authors speculated that maintaining forward inclination during DWR would increase the RA and OEA muscles activation

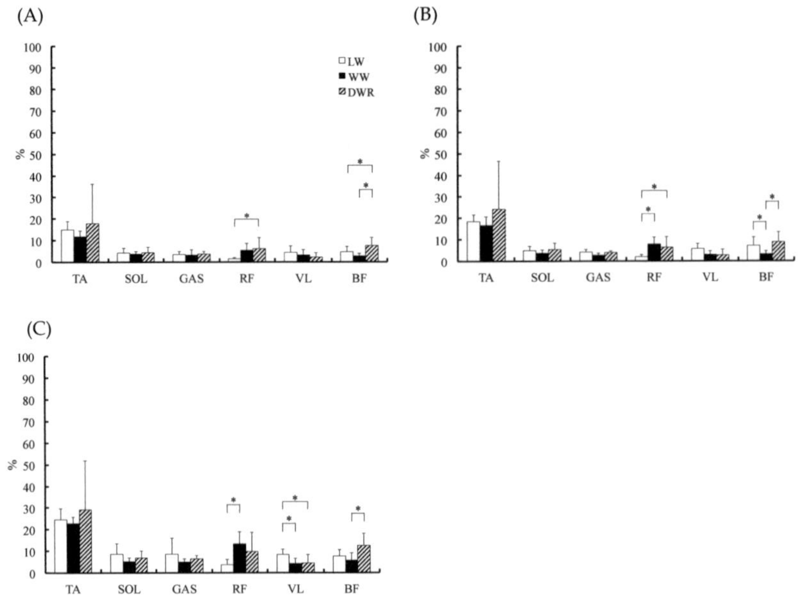

A: slow, B: moderate, C: fast.
LW: land-walking, WW: water-walking, DWR: deep-water running
*: significant difference (P < 0.05).

Figure 10. The mean ± SD of %MVC value in each lower limb muscle at each speed during forward swing phase. [Modified from reference 11]

(Figure 13). However, it is important not to lean forward excessively which would explain the ES muscle activity needed to maintain forward inclination posture.

The DWR seems to use muscles of the hip and trunk more than water- and land-walking. Muscle activity comparing running on land and DWR was studied by Masumoto et al. [32]. This study reported the EMG data of the DWR in comparison with running on land treadmill for TA, GAS, RF and BF muscles. Masumoto et al. [32] revealed that TA and GAS muscle activity; when calculated as the average EMG; was clearly lower in DWR than land treadmill running for the same rating of perceived exertion (RPE). Similarly, RF and BF muscles tended to be lower in DWR than land treadmill running. Further investigation comparing running and DWR is necessary for more detailed understanding of muscle activity behavior during DWR.

4.2. Muscle activity difference between two types of deep-water running

There are various styles of DWR depending on the type of floatation device and its usage. Previous research has investigated muscle activity during DWR using aqua pole (Pole Running: PR, Figure 14), and compared this with the DWR using an aqua belt (Belt Running: BR, Figure 8). Subjects sat on the aqua pole with one leg either side instead of using upper body (Figure 15). The results showed the mean ± SD value of the EMG data as %MVC during one cycle in the TA, SOL, GAS, RF, VL, BF, AL, GMa, GMe, RA, OEA and ES muscles (Figure 16 and 17).

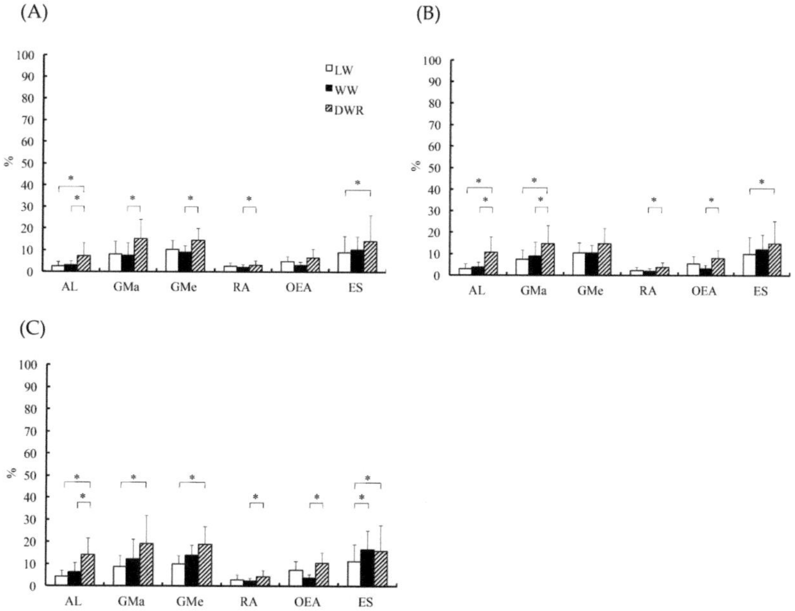

A: slow, B: moderate, C: fast.
LW: land-walking, WW: water-walking, DWR: deep-water running
*: significant difference (P < 0.05).

Figure 11. The mean ± SD of %MVC value in each hip and trunk muscle at each speed during one cycle. [Modified from reference 25]

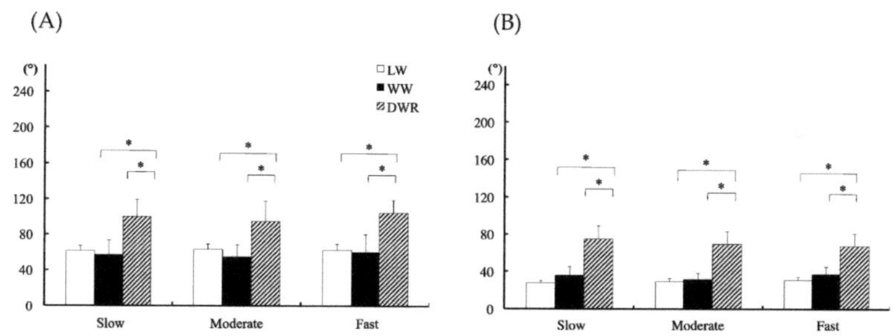

LW: land-walking, WW: water-walking, DWR: deep-water running
A: knee joint, B: hip joint
*: significant difference (P < 0.05)

Figure 12. The mean ± SD of the knee and hip joints ROM during each exercise. [Modified from reference 25]

In summary, the muscle activity during both Belt Running and Pole Running reported similar values. However, the SOL tended to be higher activity during Pole Running than Belt Running, whilst the VL tented to be higher activity during Belt Running than Pole Running. The reasons for the difference in the SOL activity is difficult to determine, however, the different activity level in the VL which acts on knee extension motion, was considered to be due to the different

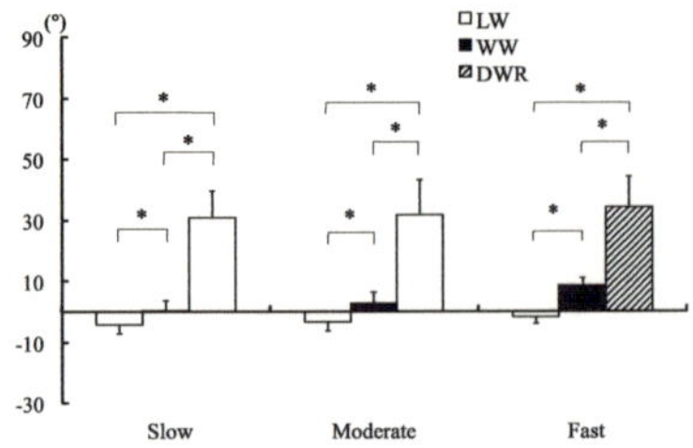

LW: land-walking, WW: water-walking, DWR: deep-water running
*: significant difference (P < 0.05)
Positive: forward inclination
Negative: backward inclination

Figure 13. The mean ± SD of the trunk inclination angle during each exercise. [Modified from reference 25]

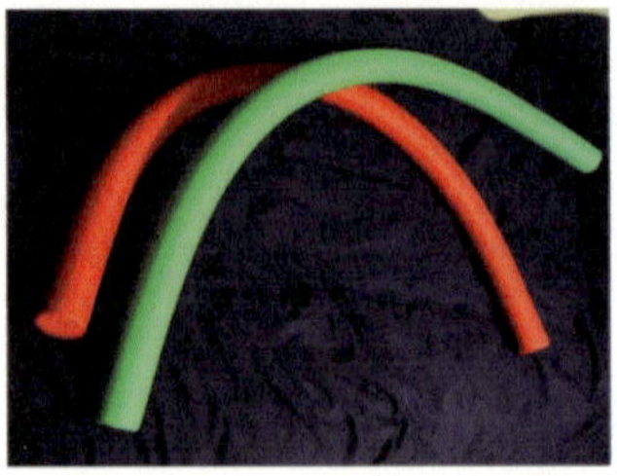

Figure 14. Aqua Pole (Footmark Corp., Japan) used for DWR exercise. [Picture was taken by the authors]

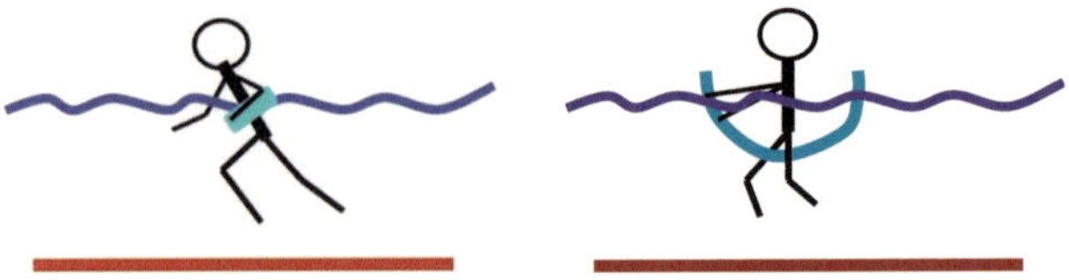

Figure 15. Belt Running (BR) and Pole Running (PR). [Pictures were created by the authors]

knee joint ROM during exercise, where the ROM of Belt Running was greater than that of Pole Running (Figure 18).

In hip and trunk muscles, the AL, RA and OEA muscles tended to have higher activation during Belt Running than Pole Running. The reason for this result is that the exercise style where subjects place aqua pole between their legs in Pole Running may require AL muscle to be less involved in the movement as the subject legs are wider apart during Pole Running than Belt Running. The higher muscle activity of RA and OEA muscles during Belt Running may be due to the trunk inclination angle being larger than that used in Pole Running (Figure 19). Thus, Pole Running is comparably a more upright position compared to Belt Running, which may explain the slight differences of muscle activity during the two forms of exercise. Researchers, instructors and participants can design a variety of exercise styles by simply varying the type of floatation device used in the activity.

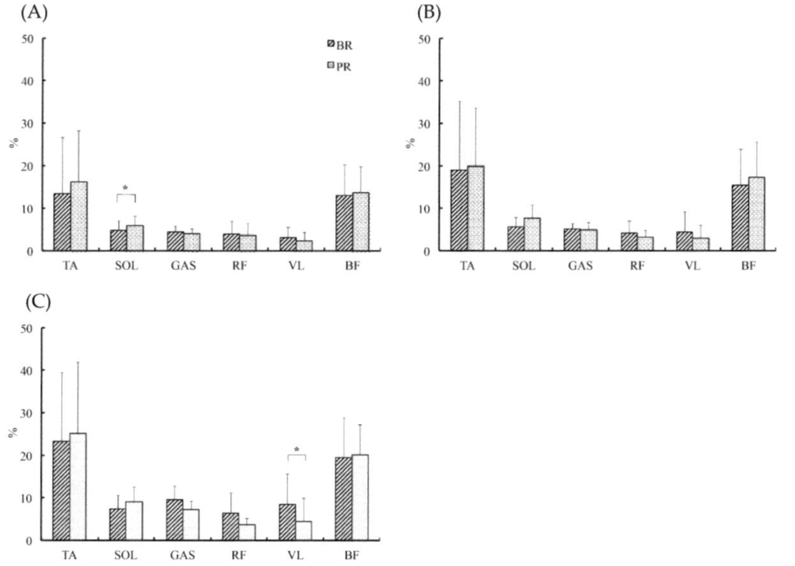

A: slow, B: moderate, C: fast.
BR: Belt Running, PR: Pole Running.
*: significant difference ($P < 0.05$).

Figure 16. The mean ± SD of %MVC value in each lower limb muscle at each speed during Belt Running and Pole Running. [Unpublished data]

There is still a limited amount of research published on muscle activity during DWR as well as running in water. When determining the most suitable style or type of activity in DWR for rehabilitation and cross training, further insight into muscle activity during the running would be a very useful regardless of running style.

5. Insight into muscle activity during various exercises in water

There are many types of exercise in the water environment and walking and running in water are representative of the common forms. The authors reported the effect of buoyancy and water resistance during exercise in water and categorized exercises by its movement direction [33]. The exercise category was reported as follows: forward walking and backward walking as a horizontal movement, squat and calf raise as a vertical movement, and leg range and leg pendulum motion as a both horizontal and vertical included movement. Nine male subjects were involved in this study, where muscle activity of TA, SOL, GAS, RF and BF was measured. Each exercise was conducted both in water and on land conditions at the same pace. The data was collected at 1000Hz, and calculated integrated EMG (IEMG). Time constant was 0.03sec that is equal to 5.3Hz high pass filter. Results showed IEMG values during each exercise were dramatically decreased in the water condition compared with the land condition. Predominantly the agonist muscles were active in the vertical movement and both horizontal and

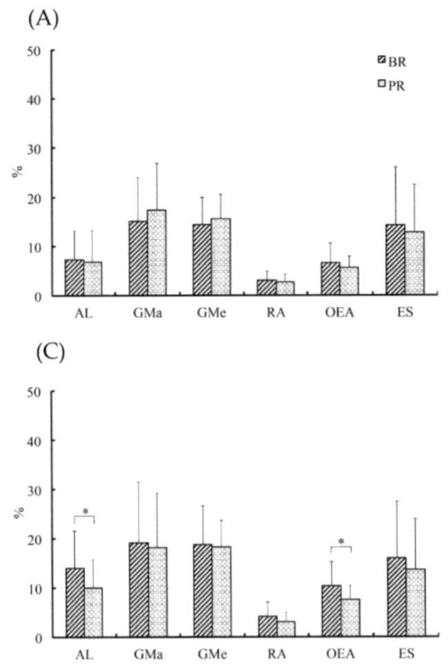

A: slow, B: moderate, C: fast.
BR: Belt Running, PR: Pole Running.
*: significant difference (P < 0.05).

Figure 17. The mean ± SD of %MVC value in each hip and trunk muscle at each speed during Belt Running and Pole Running. [Unpublished data]

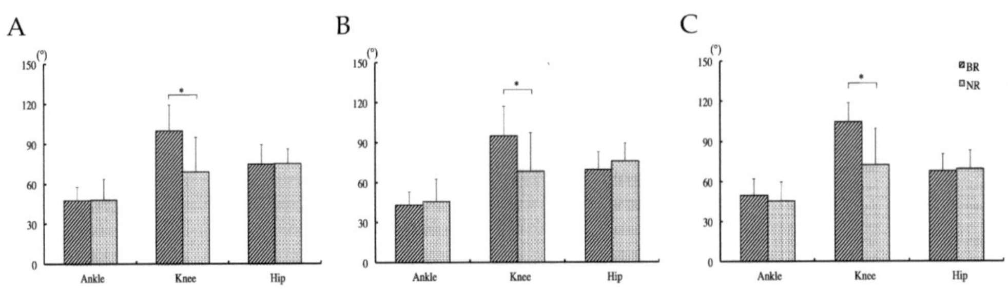

BR: Belt Running, PR: Pole Running
A: slow, B: moderate, C: fast.
*: significant difference (P < 0.05)

Figure 18. The mean ± SD of the lower limb joint ROM during each exercise. [Unpublished data]

vertical included movement, for example, RF in the squat, GAS in the calf raise, RF in the leg range, and RF and BF in the leg pendulum motion (Figure 20). In contrast, the EMG values were more increased in the water condition than the land condition in the horizontal movement especially for the thigh muscles (Figure 20). It can be said that the only horizontal movement in water environment gives higher muscle stimulus than the same exercise on land.

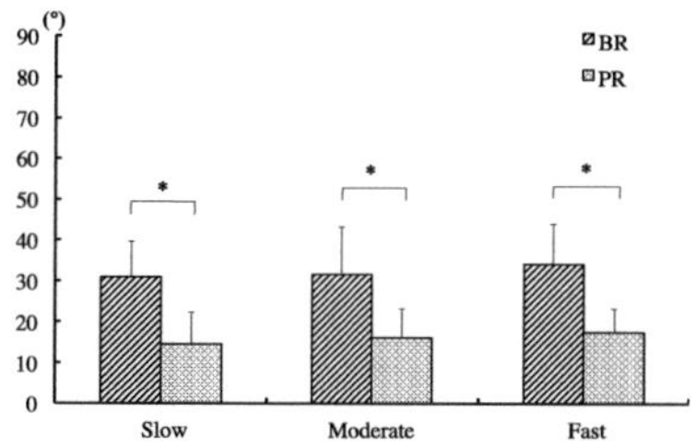

BR: Belt Running, PR: Pole Running
*: significant difference (P < 0.05)
Positive: forward inclination

Figure 19. The mean ± SD of the trunk inclination angle during Belt Running and Pole Running.

Therefore, it was suggested that vertical and both horizontal and vertical included movement in water environment are useful for rehabilitation training from injury or disability due to the lower levels of stress in water activity than on land.

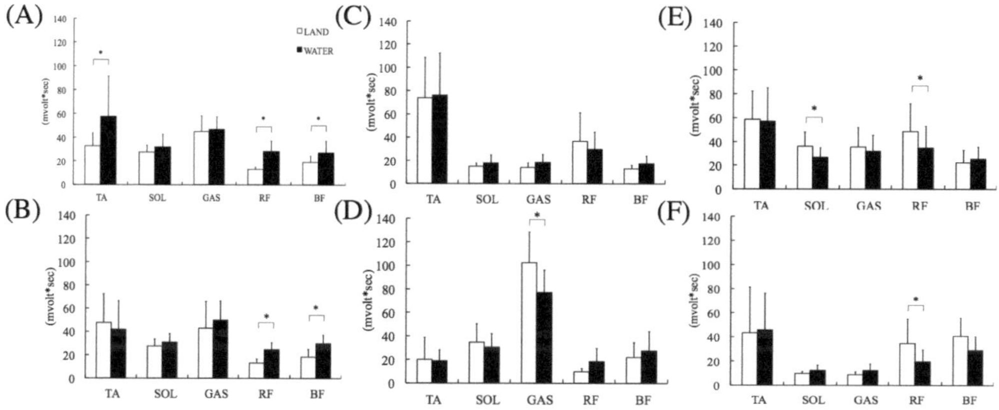

A: forward walking, B: backward walking, C: squat, D: calf raise, E: leg range, F: leg pendulum motion. [Modified from reference 33]
*: significant difference (P < 0.05)

Figure 20. The mean ± SD of the lower limb muscle activity during water and land exercise.

Further research by the authors has investigated lower limb and trunk muscle activity in ten kinds of water exercise [Unpublished data]. The mean EMG values of each muscle were shown in Figure 21. The data was collected at 1000Hz, and the mean EMG values were calculated from %MVC of RMS values with 100ms window of the data applied during one cycle of each exercise form. The exercises performed in this study were: forward walking, backward walking, DWR, normal running, side walking, walking with long step, walking with trunk twisting, walking with kicking, walking with knee-up, walking with elbow-knee alternative touching. These exercises are considered basic variations of walking exercise in water which are often implemented in practical exercise sessions.

As seen in the figure 21, normal running in water stimulated every muscle except the RA and the OEA muscles compared to the other exercise forms. This indicates normal running provides a high intensity activity for these muscles. The DWR was apparently an effective exercise for the BF, AL, RA and OEA muscles, especially abdominal muscles as seen in the comparison with water- and land-walking in the former section. The walking with kicking exercise clearly activated the VL and RF because those muscles were the agonist muscle for the walking with kicking motion, and this exercise stimulated abdominal muscles slightly more when compared to the other exercises. The VL muscle activity was comparably higher in the normal running, side walking, walking with long step, walking with trunk twisting and walking with kicking than the other exercises which may be due to those exercises requiring the body to be immersed deeply or require stronger extension of the knee joint during this motion. The walking with knee up exercise could be said to be of a low intensity exercise as it showed lesser EMG values than the others in every muscle. The walking with elbow-knee alternative touching exercise tended to show a high muscle activity especially in the hip and trunk muscles. It was speculated that the muscle activity for this exercise happened during standing phase in measured muscles resulting from the attempt to stabilize against upper body motion moving dynamically. As just described, the figure showed the features of the muscle activity modality during several exercises in water, but further video analysis investigation would be needed for understanding the cause of the muscle activity more precisely.

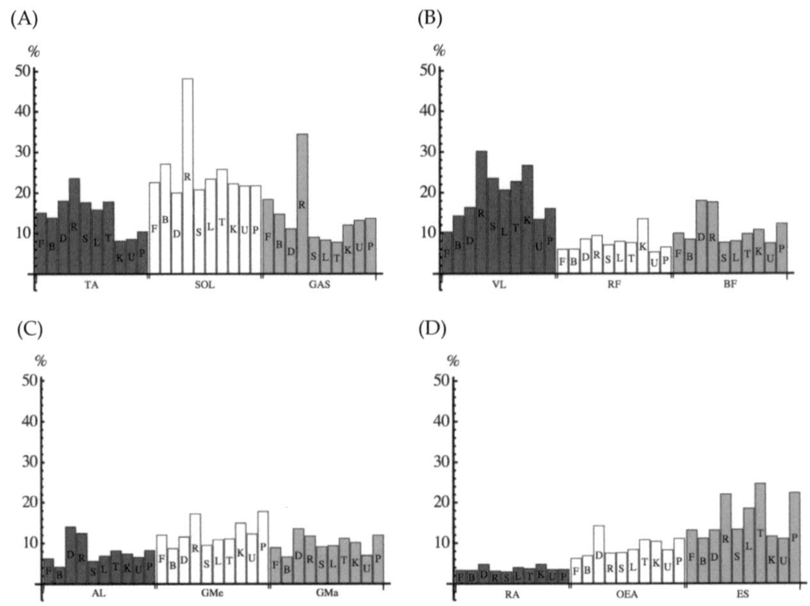

A: shank muscles, B: thigh muscles, C: hip muscles, D: trunk muscles
F: forward walking, B: backward walking, D: DWR, R: normal running, S: side walking, L: walking with long-step, T: walking with trunk-twisting, K: walking with kicking, U: walking with knee-up, P: walking with elbow-knee alternative touching

Figure 21. The mean %MVC value of the lower limb, hip and trunk muscle during exercise in water. [Unpublished data]

6. Rehabilitation training in water for regaining normal walking, is it truly effective?

The EMG characteristics introduced in this chapter are used in the comparison of the EMG data such as mean value or quantity. However, it is important to evaluate the quality of EMG signal to identify where the stimulus happened as the mean value is nothing more than the representative mean of the data for the targeted period. The quality analysis for EMG signal of exercise in water is a comparison of the wave forms that accompany exercise movement. Normalization from 0 to 100% of one cycle was applied so as to compare the muscle activity time course pattern [26, 34]. However, there was no statistical comparison made to the time course pattern. Instead the authors compared the time course pattern of walking exercise in water and on land by applying a cross correlation function. This correlation was then used in discussing the similarity of muscle activity patterns between water- and land-walking, as well as the usability of walking in water as a form of rehabilitation training. The hypothesis being that a water environment may have the benefit of less gravity stress and greater safety in preventing falling accidents. In addition, training of the targeted movement may be more effective and movement function specific [35] in water than on land. Thus, further investigation of the similarity of muscle activity between water- and land-walking would provide increased understanding regarding the use of water activity and exercise prescription for rehabilitation.

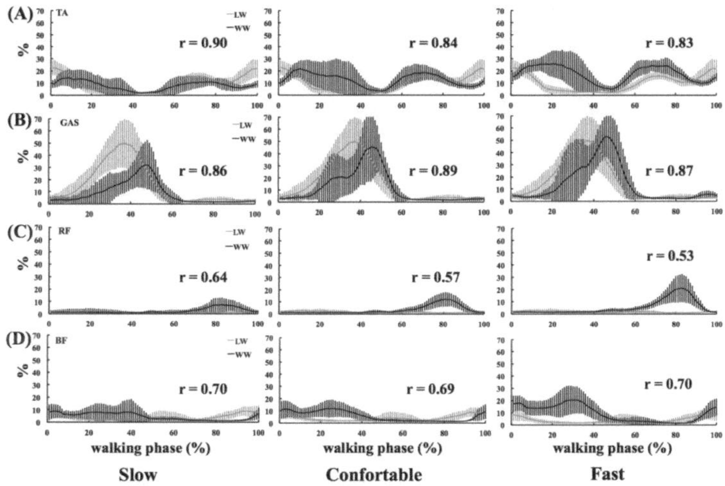

Values are mean ± SD of the subjects
A: TA, B: GAS, C: RF, D: BF
LW: land-walking, WW: water-walking
r: cross correlation coefficient

Figure 22. The normalized time course pattern of %MVC during walking in water and on land. [Modified from reference [36]

In the study by the authors [36], nine male subjects walked in water and on land condition at self-selected slow, comfortable, and fast speed in water as well as comfortable speed on land.

During each effort, the muscle activity of TA, GAS, RF and BF were collected at 2000Hz with a time constant of 0.03sec equal to 5.3Hz high-pass filter. After the collection, the data was filtered with low and high pass filter of 500Hz and 10Hz, respectively. Then, the data was full-wave rectified and low-pass filtered with moving average at 5 Hz to obtain the linear envelope. Following this, the data was normalized from heel contact (0%) to next heel contact (100%), and expressed as %MVC. The comparison was then made between each water-walking speed and confortable speed of the land-walking.

A normalized time course pattern and results of the cross correlation analysis are shown in Figure 22. The cross correlation coefficients were moderate in the RF and BF (r = 0.53 - 0.70), and were high in the TA and GAS (r = 0.83 - 0.90). This showed the muscle activity pattern of the water-walking were similar to that of the land-walking even in the slow and fast speed. Moreover, as seen in the figure 22, the muscle activation was higher during the water-walking than land-walking during most part of one full stride for all muscles except the GAS. This suggests the water-walking would be able to simulate the land-walking very closely regardless of the speed of the water-walking, and stimulate the thigh muscles and TA sufficiently even in the slow speed. The authors also suggest that even during slow speed, water-waking is an effective exercise modality for muscle training in a similar way to normal walking on land.

A possible limitation can be seen when applying normalization method to time course pattern in that the normalization process resulted in apparent cancelations in time length changes which may alter the sequencing and timing of events especially in exercise in water due to the buoyancy and water resistance affect on the movement duration. In addition, changing the time length may also distort the time course pattern, where the exact timing may not be comparable between the same timing of two wave forms (i.e. does the 50% of land-walking truly match to the 50% of water-walking in normalized data?). This should be considered in studying outputs from EMG modality of water-walking.

7. Conclusion

This chapter focused on muscle activity during exercises in water especially variations of gait (walking and running) and other activities of daily living. Descriptions on how to waterproof electrodes, placing the electrodes on the muscle of interest, and the verification of EMG collection in the water environment was then discussed. The authors also suggest that when the electrodes are waterproofed appropriately, EMG recording is not affected by water immersion. Namely, we can measure muscle activity correctly even in underwater condition without any artifact.

In summary of the reported characteristics of muscles activity during walking in water, TA and thigh muscles and ES tended to show higher activity than land-walking with self-selected pace. There was a lower activity than land-walking with Triceps Surae muscle, VL and abdominal muscle. Further, most muscles tended to decrease their activity when walking on treadmill apparatus, compared to land treadmill walking. During DWR the characteristics of muscle activity for the thigh, hip and trunk muscles show higher activity than walking in water and/or on land, whilst the muscle activity of Triceps Surae muscle decrease dramatically. From these

http://dx.doi.org/10.5772/55115

results the authors concluded that muscle activity would probably decrease in DWR, when compared to land treadmill running. In addition, the muscle activity modality can be changed significantly by using different flotation devices. In the results of the comparison between water exercise and land exercise, the muscle activity modality was affected by the physical qualities of water (buoyancy and water resistance). For example, horizontal movement in water tended to increase agonist muscle activity, hence vertical movement and horizontal- and vertical-included-movement decreased agonist muscle activity. The water physical qualities would affect the posture during exercise and result in changes to muscle activity modality. The muscle activity characteristics in fundamental variations of water-walking vary its pattern resulting in unique movements, and the characteristics basically conform with exercise direction. Running in water, with feet touching the bottom of the swimming pool, generated the highest muscle activity. Walking in water with knee up has the lowest intensity among variations of water exercise when exercising in self-selected moderate pace.

This chapter introduced research comparing the EMG of water-walking to land-walking. The results concluded that the shank and thigh muscle activity during water-walking was similar to that of land-walking. Identifying the water environment can simulate land-walking in respect to muscle activity even at slow speed. This reinforces the concept in water environment as a legitimate and effective exercise. In addition, the water environment provides increased safety with respect to falls. In summary, the water environment would be very beneficial especially not only for the physically fit but also for people wishing to regain the normal motion which may be difficult to achieve on normal land environment.

Acknowledgements

The authors thank PhD Hitoshi Wakabayashi in Chiba Institute of Technology, PhD Daisuke Sato in Niigata University of Health and Welfare, and Professor Takeo Nomura in NPO Tsukuba Aqua Life Research Institute for your contributing to the data collection related in this chapter.

Author details

Koichi Kaneda[1,2,3*], Yuji Ohgi[1], Mark Mckean[4] and Brendan Burkett[4]

*Address all correspondence to: koichi@sfc.keio.ac.jp koichikaneda.japan@gmail.com

*Address all correspondence to: kkaneda@sea.it-chiba.ac.jp

1 Graduate School of Media and Governance, Keio University, Fujisawa City, Kanagawa, Japan

2 Education Center of Chiba Institute of Technology, Japan

3 Japan Society for the Promotion of Science, Graduate School of Media and Governance, Keio University, Fujisawa City, Kanagawa, Japan

4 Faculty of Science, Health, Education and Engineering, University of the Sunshine Coast, Sippy Downs, Queensland, Australia

References

[1] Becker BE. Aquatic therapy: scientific foundations and clinical rehabilitation applications. Physical Medicine and Rehabilitation 2009;1(9) 859-872.

[2] Miyoshi T, Shirota T, Yamamoto S, Nakazawa K, Akai M. Functional roles of lower-limb joint moments while walking in water. ClinBiomech 2005;20(2) 194-201.

[3] Burkett BJ. Sports Mechanics for Coaches (3rd ed.). Human Kinetics; 2010.

[4] Naemi R, Easson WJ, Sanders RH. Hydrodynamic glide efficiency in swimming. Journal of Science and Medicine in Sport 2011;13(4) 444-451.

[5] Arborelius M Jr, Ballidin UI, Lilja B, Lundgren CE. Hemodynamic changes in man during immersion with the head above water. Aerospace Medicine 1972;43(6) 592-598.

[6] Reilly T, Dowzer C, Cable NT. The physiology of deep-water running. Journal of Sports Sciences 2003;21 959-972.

[7] Bonde-Petersen F, Schultz-Petersen L, Dragsted N. Peripheral and central blood flow in man during cold, thermoneutral, and hot water immersion. Aviation Space and Environmental Medicine 1992;63(5) 346-350.

[8] Sato D, Kaneda K, Wakabayashi H, Nomura T. The water exercise improves health-related quality of life of frail elderly people at day service facility. Quality of Life Research 2007; 16(10) 1577-1585.

[9] Kaneda K, Sato D, Wakabayashi H, Hanai A, Nomura T. A comparison of the effects of different water exercise programs on balance ability in elderly people. Journal of Aging and Physical Activity 2008a;16(4) 381-392.

[10] Masumoto K, Mercer JA. Biomechanics of human locomotion in water: an electomyographic analysis. Exercise and Sports Science Review 2008;36(3) 160-169.

[11] Kaneda K, Wakabayashi H, Sato D, Uekusa T, Nomura T. Lower extremity muscle activity during deep-water running on self-determined pace. Journal of Electromyography and Kinesiology 2008b;18(6), 965-972.

[12] Mercer, J.A., Groh, D., Black, D., Gruenenfelder, A. (2005). Technical note: Quantifying muscle activity during running in the water. Aquatic Fitness Research Journal 2005;2(1) 9-15.

[13] Rainoldi A, Cescon C, Bottin A, Casale R, Caruso I. Surface EMG alterations induced by underwater recording. Journal of Electromyography and Kinesiology 2004;14(3) 325-331.

[14] Pinto SS, Liedtke GV, Alberton CL, da Silva EM, Cadore EL, Kruel LF. Electromyographic signal and force comparisons during maximal voluntary isometric contractionin water and on dry land. European Journal of Applied Physiology 2010;110(5) 1075-1082.

[15] Carvalho RG, Amorim CF, Perácio LH, Coelho HF, Vieira AC, Karl-Menzel HJ, Szmuchrowski LA. Analysis of various conditions in order to measure electromyography of isometric contractions in water and on air. Journal of Electromyography and Kinesiology 2010;20(5) 988-993.

[16] Silvers WM, Dolny DG. Comparison and reproducibility of sEMG during manual muscle testing on land and in water. Journal of Electromyography and Kinesiology 2011;21(1) 95-101.

[17] Evans BW, Cureton KL, Purvis JW. Metabolic and circulatory responses to walking and jogging in water. Research Quarterly 1978;49(4) 442-449.

[18] Gleim GW, Nicholas JA. Metabolic costs and heart rate responses to treadmill walking in water at different depths and temperatures. American Journal of Sports Medicine 1989;17(2) 248-252.

[19] Kaneda K, Ohgi Y, Tanaka C. Gender differences in metabolic responses during water walking. International Journal of Aquatic Research and Education 2010;5(4) 421-431.

[20] Kaneda K, Wakabayashi H, Sato D, Nomura T. Lower extremity muscle activity during different types and speeds of underwater movement. Journal of Physiological Anthropology 2007;26(2) 197-200.

[21] Kato T, Sugagima Y, Koeda M, Fukuzawa S, Kitagawa K. Electromyogram activity of leg muscles during different types of underwater walking. Advances in Exercise and Sports Physiology 2002;8(2) 39-44.

[22] Nakazawa K, Yamamoto S, Yano H. Muscle activation patterns during walking in water. In: Taguchi K, Igarashi M, Mori S. (ed.) Vestibular and Neural Front. Amsterdam: Elsevier Science; 1994. p255-258.

[23] Miyoshi T, Nakazawa K, Tanizaki M, Sato T, Akai M. Altered activation pattern in synergistic ankle plantarflexor muscles in a reduced-gravity environment. Gait and Posture 2006;24(1) 94-99.

[24] Miyoshi T, Shirota T, Yamamoto S, Nakazawa K, Akai M. Lower limb joint moment during walking in water. Disability and Rehabilitation 2003;25(21) 1219-1223.

[25] Kaneda K, Sato D, Wakabayashi H, Nomura T. EMG activity of hip and trunk muscles during deep-water running. Journal of Electromyography and Kinesiology 2009;19(6) 1064-1070.

[26] Barela AM, Stolf SF, Duarte M. Biomechanical characteristics of adults walking in shallow water and on land. Journal of Electromyography and Kinesiology 2006;16(3) 250-256.

[27] Adelaar RS. The practical biomechanics of running. American Journal of Sports Medicine 1986;14(6) 497-500.

[28] Cavanagh PR. Biomechanics of distance running. Champagne, IL: Human Kinetics Books; 1990.

[29] Masumoto K, Takasugi S, Hotta N, Fujishima K, Iwamoto Y. Electromyographic analysis of walking in water in healthy humans. Journal of Physiological Anthropology Applied Human Science 2004;23(4) 119-127.

[30] Reilly T, Dowzer C, Cable NT. The physiology of deep-water running. Journal of Sports Sciences 2003;21(12) 959-972.

[31] Assis MR, Silva LE, Alves AM, Pessanha AP, Valim V, Feldman D, Neto TL, Natour J. A randomized controlled trial of deep water running: Clinical effectiveness of aquatic exercise to treat fibromyalgia. Arthritis and Rheumatism 2006;55(1) 57-65.

[32] Masumoto K, Delion D, Mercer JA. Insight into Muscle Activity during Deep Water Running. Medicine and Science in Sports and Exercise 2009;41(10), 1958-1964.

[33] Kaneda K, Kimura F, Akimoto T, Kono I. Differences in underwater and land-based leg muscle activity. Japanese Journal of Physical Fitness and Sports Medicine 2004;53(1) 141-148. In Japanese.

[34] Barela AM, Duarte M. Biomechanical characteristics of elderly individuals walking on land and in water. Journal of Electromyography and Kinesiology 2008;18(3) 446-454.

[35] Bernstein NA. On dexterity and its development. 2nd ed. Mahwah, NJ: Lawrence Erlbaum: 204-44, 2003.

[36] Kaneda K, Sato D, Wakabayashi H, Ohgi Y, Nomura T. Quantitative analysis on the muscular activity of lower extremity during water walking. Scientific Proceedings of the 27th International Conference on Biomechanics in Sports, p807-810, 17-21 August, 2009, Limerick, Ireland.

Chapter 12

Recent Trends in EMG-Based Control Methods for Assistive Robots

R. A. R. C. Gopura, D. S. V. Bandara,
J. M. P. Gunasekara and T. S. S. Jayawardane

Additional information is available at the end of the chapter

http://dx.doi.org/10.5772/56174

1. Introduction

Any person would like to spend his or her entire life time as an individual without becoming a dependant person by any means. Nonetheless, there are several instances where a human being would fail to achieve this due to physical problems which preventing him/her from acting as an individual. In most cases, after a stroke, brain or orthopedic trauma, brain damage due to an accident or a cognitive disease the victim will definitely have to undergo physical or cognitive rehabilitation in order to get him used to changed body conditions. In modern society, a considerable percentage of population is physically weak due to aging, congenital diseases, physical diseases and occupational hazards [1, 2]. Such people need a dexterous assistive methodology to regain the normal activities of daily living (ADL). Not only they, those with a missing limb (e.g. due to an amputation), should also be furnished with necessary aids which would enable them to regain the individuality. The development of proper devices for the purpose of rehabilitation, human power assistance and as replacements to body parts has a long history [3, 4] which has reached a high point due to recent developments in technology, such as robotics, biomedical signal processing, soft computing and advances in sensors and actuators over the past few decades. With many advances, capabilities and potential, still biological signal based control has a long way to go before reaching the realm of professional and commercial applications [5].

Most of the studies [5-7] that considered the integration of biomedical signal processing with robotics have achieved tremendous development in the area of assistive robotics. Assistive robots can mainly be classified into three areas: orthoses, prostheses and other types. An orthosis is worn as an external device to the existing body part, while a prosthesis is used as a replacement for the lost body part [5, 8]. The meal assistive robot [9], assistive wheel chair [10] and assistive humanoid robot [10] are some examples of the other types of assistive robots. Both orthoses and prostheses directly interact physically and cognitively with the wearer. Therefore, they are expected to provide physiological and mental comfort to the user, without letting the user feel a difference while functioning/assisting correctly to perform the required motion. However, the controlling of the robot according to human motion intention is not an easy task [11, 12]. Therefore, in the integration of the human with a robot, the selection of a proper control input signal to reflect the correct motion intention would be very important. So far research is being carried out considering different biological signals such as Electromyography (EMG), Mechnanomyogram (MMG), Electroencephalography (EEG) Electrooculography (EOG) and Electrocorticogram (EcoG) [13, 14, 15] as the main input signal to the robot controller. Among them, the EMG signal, which is the measurement of the electrical activity of muscles at rest and during contraction, has obtained promising results in the case of controlling robotic prostheses and orthoses by correctly interpreting the human motion intention [16, 17]. Basically, EMG based control is a sophisticated technique concerned with detection, processing, classification and application of EMG to control assistive robots. EMG can be applied to control assistive robots in various manners by considering data acquisition, feature extraction and classification [18]. Some of the available exoskeleton robots controlled based on EMG are the orthotic exoskeleton hand [19], exoskeleton robot for tremor suppression [20], SUEFUL-7 [6] etc. In addition, DEKA Arm [21], Saga Prosthetic Arm [22], and Manus Hand [23] are some of the available prosthetic devices with EMG based controlling. Many researchers from different institutions have been working on EMG based control methods over several decades and their contribution has greatly influenced a new era of EMG based control of assistive robots [5, 24, 25].

This chapter presents a comprehensive review of EMG based control methods of recent upper-limb orthoses and prostheses. Initially, it explains the detection and processing of EMG and available EMG extraction systems. Next, ways of categorization of EMG based control methods are explained. Here EMG based control methods are categorized in detail, based on the structure of the controller algorithm, as pattern recognition based controls and non-pattern recognition based controls. Most of available control methodologies used with assistive robots are pattern recognition based controls [18, 19, 24, 26, 27]. The control methods belonging to non-pattern recognition based controls [28-30] are rare. Further, comparison of EMG based control methods of upper-limb exoskeleton robots and upper-limb prostheses are presented considering the features of the control method. In addition, the conclusion and future directions of EMG based control methods of assistive robots are described.

The next section focuses on the procedure of EMG detection and processing. Section 3 describes the categorization of EMG based control methods. The review of EMG based control methods of upper-limb exoskeleton robots and upper-limb prostheses together with a comparison of control methods are presented in section 4. The final section briefly outlines the conclusion and future directions.

2. Procedure of EMG detection

Detection of EMG signals can be done mainly in two ways, namely non-invasive and invasive [5]. Surface EMG (sEMG) electrodes are used for the former, while intramuscular EMG (iEMG) electrodes are used for the latter. Placement of surface EMG electrodes is comparatively easier than intramuscular EMG electrodes. However noise and other disturbances are inherent in surface EMG detection [5]. Intramuscular EMG electrodes are placed close to the Motor Unit Action Potentials (MUAP), and as a result the influence of other disturbances is not dominant. It provides a better accuracy and repeatability of the EMG signal [25]. As shown in Fig. 1, the EMG extraction process includes several steps. The initial step is the selection of the most significant muscle of the human body relevant to the required motion. After the muscle is selected, the next important step is the placement of electrodes. In the case of sEMG, the electrodes should be placed in the belly area of the muscle for maximum signal extraction.

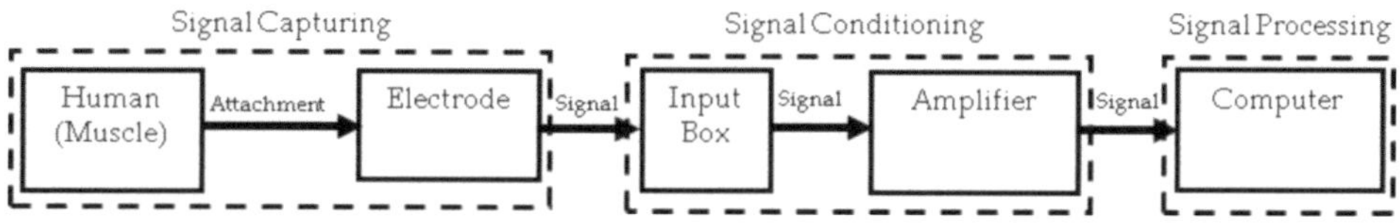

Figure 1. EMG signal extraction process

The electrode should be placed onto the relevant muscle after cleaning the skin surface. There are a few types of surface electrodes, some of which need a gel [31] to be applied between the skin and the electrode and some [32] which instead use an adhesive tape to ensure proper contact between the muscle and the electrode. Signals from several electrodes are then fed into the input box and subsequently passed to the amplifier. The output of the amplifier can be fed into a computer via data cards or any other data communication interface and can be recorded or manipulated in the required way. In most EMG based control methods a raw EMG signal is processed to extract the features of the signal. Several feature extraction methods are available for this purpose [5]: mean absolute value, mean absolute value slope, waveform length, zero crossings, root mean square value, *etc*. The features of the raw EMG signal have to be extracted in real time to use EMG as input signals to the controller of the assistive robots. Most robots use Root Mean Square (RMS) as the feature extraction method of raw EMG mainly due to ease of analyzing real time information of EMG signal.

There are a number of commercially developed EMG acquisition systems available [31-34] (see Fig. 2). They could be used for both medical and research purposes. Some of the leading EMG acquisition system manufacturers are Nihon Kohden Co. [31], Delsys [32], BioSemi [33], and Cambridge Electronic Design [34]. The Delsys EMG system shown in Fig. 2(a) is widely used in research, whilst the Nihon Kohden EMG system shown in Fig. 2(b) is widely used for medical applications. Nevertheless, there are other models in Nihon Kohden which also support for research [31]. The BioSemi EMG system shown in Fig. 2(c) could also be used in research applications. The next section will explain the classification of EMG based control methods

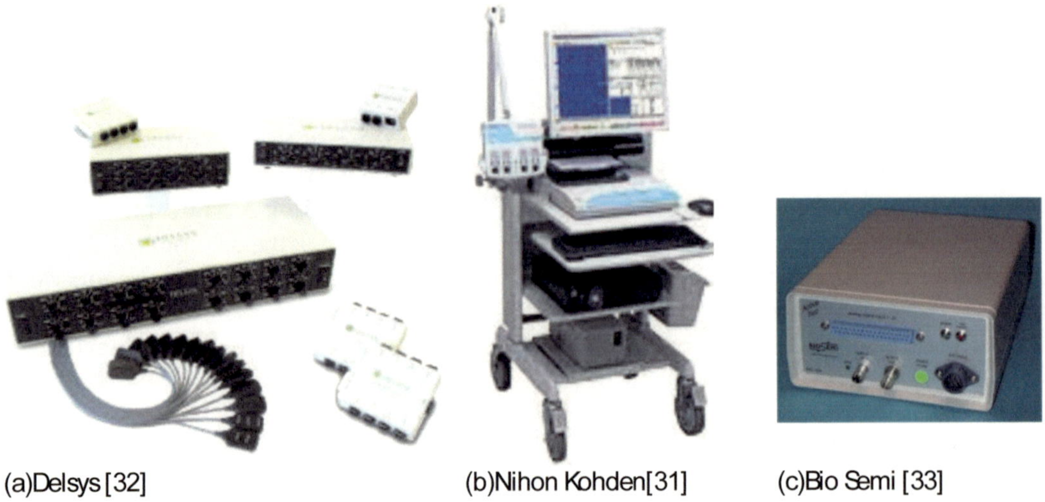

Figure 2. Available EMG acquiring systems

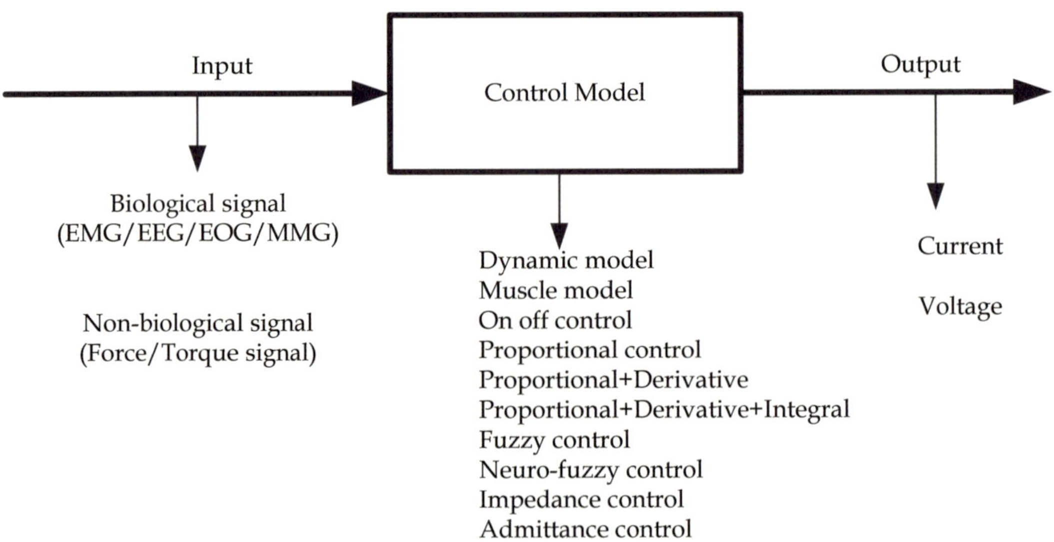

Figure 3. Control method classification for assistive robots

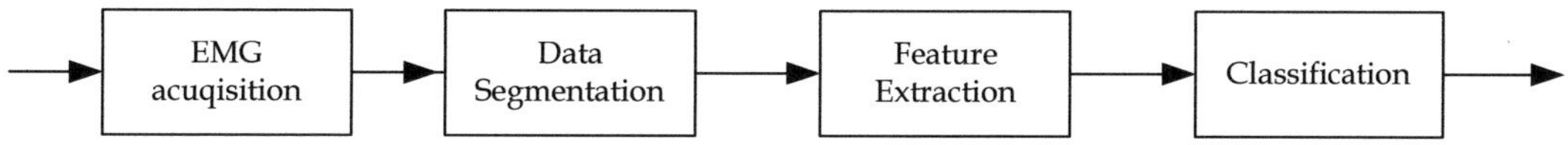

Figure 4. EMG processing sequence in pattern recognition based control

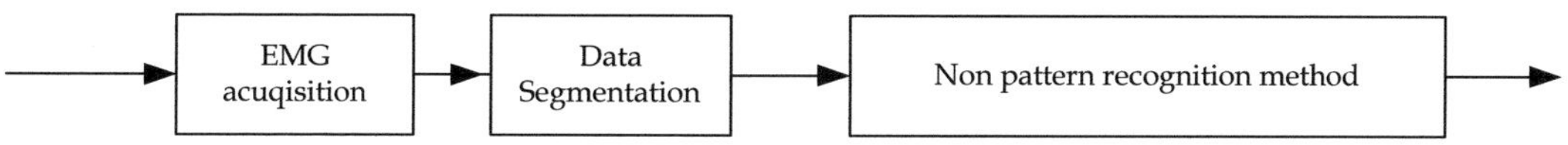

Figure 5. EMG processing sequence in non-pattern recognition based control

3. Categorization of EMG based control methods

Control methods of assistive robots based on EMG can be categorized mainly according to the input information to the controller, architecture of the control algorithm, output of the controller and other ways. Figure 3 shows the ways of categorization of EMG based control methods. In this chapter, the EMG based control methods of assistive robots are categorized based on the architecture of the control method. Considering the EMG signal processing method in the architecture of the controller the EMG based control methods can be categorized mainly as pattern recognition based and non-pattern recognition based [5, 25]. Control methods of many assistive robots are designed with pattern recognition based control methods and it provides an accurate control action compared to non-pattern recognition based EMG based control [5]. However, several intermediate steps (see Fig.4) are applied with a pattern recognition method such as data segmentation, feature extraction, and classification [5, 25]. The accuracy of pattern recognition based control is greatly improved by methods of feature extraction and classification [5, 25]. Robots such as, SUEFUL-7 [6], NEUROExos [27], W-EXOS [11], DEKA Arm [21], Saga Prosthetic Arm [22], Manus Hand [23] are on pattern recognition based control. The non-pattern recognition based control method involves only a few steps (see Fig.5).

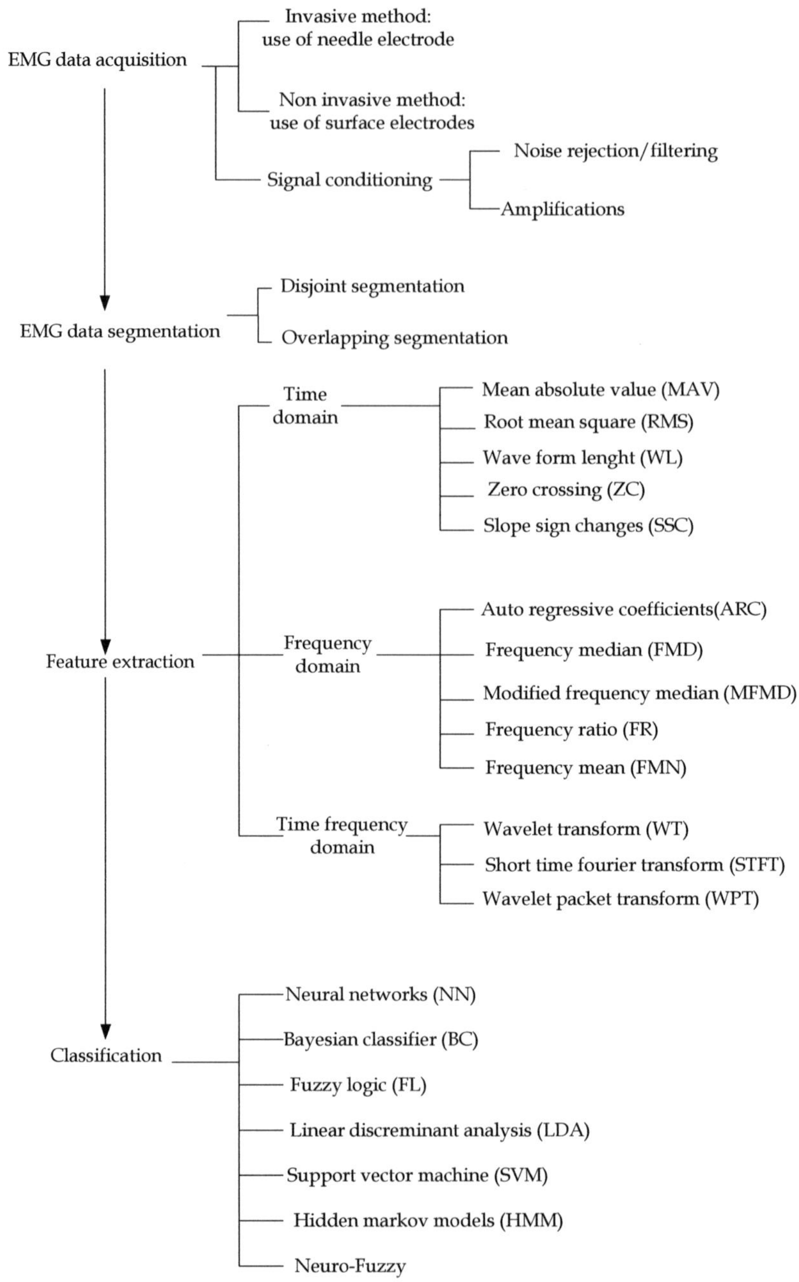

Figure 6. Steps of pattern recognition based EMG processing

EMG processing in pattern recognition based control [5] and non-pattern recognition based control are further illustrated in the next subsections.

3.1. Pattern recognition technique

The different steps coming under pattern recognition such as data acquisition, data segmentation, feature extraction and classification can be further broken down into sub areas considering available options as shown in Fig. 6. Next subsections present further categorization of data segmentation, feature selection and classification respectively coming under the pattern recognition based EMG based control method.

Data segmentation: The EMG signal has two states: transient and steady. In the transient state, the muscle goes from rest to a voluntary contraction level [5]. Constant contraction of the muscle can be seen under the steady state. In addition the EMG signal in the transient state shows a large deviation of error compared to the steady state level. Therefore, in many cases, the steady state signal is used for the analysis of EMG. For the better result of data segmentation, the selected time slot should be equal to or less than 300ms. This includes segment length and processing time to generate the control command. In addition bias and variance of features can be minimized by selecting adequately a large time slot and it contributes to better classification performance [5, 12, 19]. Data segmentation is carried out with two major techniques: overlapping segmentation [5, 25], and disjoint segmentation which uses segments with predetermine length for feature extraction. Also processing time is a small portion of segment length and thus processor is idle for remaining time of the segment. The new segment slides over the current segment and has small incremental time for overlapping segmentation technique. According to [25], overlapping segment method increases processing time and hence better for the data segmentation [5].

Feature selection: Due to the large number of inputs and randomness of the signal, it is impractical to feed the EMG signal directly to the classifier [6, 18]. Therefore, it is necessary to create the feature vector, where sequence is mapped into a smaller dimension vector. Success of any pattern recognition problem depends almost entirely on the selection and extraction of features. According to the literature, features fall into one of three categories: time domain, frequency domain and time scale domain [25]. Many assistive robots use time domain analysis for feature extraction and in most cases, RMS calculation is adapted for feature extraction [6, 35]. Assistive robots based on frequency domain and time frequency domain were scarce.

Classification: Extracted features need to be classified into distinctive classes for the recognition of the desired motion pattern [5]. Several external factors, such as fatigue, electrode position, perspiration and posture of the limb may causes changes in the EMG pattern over time. Therefore, this leads to large variations in the value of a particular feature. The important feature of the classifier is the ability to identify the unique feature throughout the varying pattern due to other influences. The speed of the classifier is an important aspect for generating required output from the controller. Further, training of the classifier is another way to improve the response of the control system of the assistive robot. Depending on the performance of the subject, practice required for rehabilitation etc can be customized through a training of the classifier and it produces the expected rehabilitation training for the patient too. According to the literature, several methods are used for EMG classifications. Some of them are Neural network [5, 35], Fuzzy logic [25], Neuro-fuzzy logic [5, 25], Probabilistic approach etc.

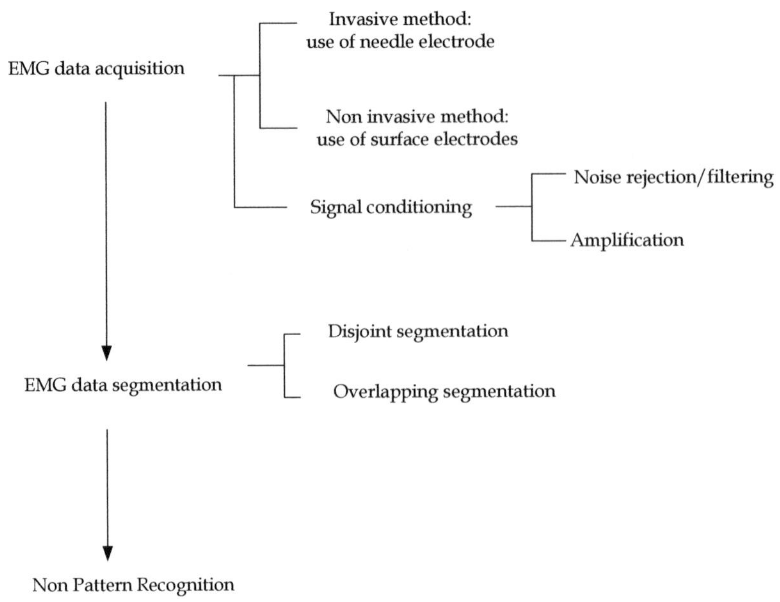

Figure 7. Steps of non-pattern recognition based EMG processing

3.2. Non Pattern recognition technique

In the non-pattern recognition based method accuracy is not as high as the pattern recognition based method. The two main steps coming under non-pattern recognition based method can further be broken down into sub areas considering available options as shown in the Fig. 7. Typically, non-pattern recognition based method includes proportional control, threshold control etc. This is a simple structure and in most cases it uses ON/OFF control [5]. During the review, control methods of assistive robots based on non-pattern recognition based control were hardly found. This may be due to poor accuracy, low level of response, etc.

4. Review of EMG based control method of assistive robots

This section presents a review of EMG based control methods of upper-limb exoskeleton robots and prostheses. For this review, several databases including IEEE explorer, Science direct and Google scholar were used. In total, more than forty five numbers of conferences and journal papers are included and reviewed. Further, EMG based control methods of upper-limb exoskeleton robots and prostheses are compared considering their country of origin, input signals, structure of the controller and special features. Table 1 shows the comparison of EMG based control method of assistive robots.

Reference	Country of origin	Input signal	Structure of controller	Special features
Hand exoskeleton [27]	Germany	EMG	Uses blind source separation to recover the original EMG signal	Developed for hand rehabilitation. Adding force sensors will increase the complexity of blind source separation. increased when combined force sensors
Neuro-fuzzy exoskeleton robot [18]	Japan	EMG and force signal	Multiple neuro-fuzzy controllers are used to take the effect of posture changes during motion	Mean absolute value (MAV) of EMG signal used to controller. Force sensor signals are used to control robot at low muscle activity
Exoskeleton hand [19]	USA	EMG	Uses binary, variable and reaching control algorithms	Suitable control algorithm is needed to provide accepted level of rehabilitation
Hand rehabilitation robot [24]	Italy	EMG	Input signals are fed to the microcontroller via serial connection	Motor speed varies according to joint angle variation of fingers
SUEFUL-7 Upper limb exoskeleton [6]	Japan	EMG and force sensor signal	Neuro-fuzzy controller with muscle model oriented control method. Impedance controller is applied to change the impedance parameters	Joint torques and weights of muscle-model matrix are changed according to posture changes.
Proportional EMG control upper limb exoskeleton [27]	Italy	EMG	EMG based proportional controller. Proportional control gains, K_{bic} and K_{tric} are used to determine the output	Exoskeleton provides extra torque when it works at high proportional gains. This provides better assistance according to level of EMG activity
W-EXOS [35]	Japan	EMG and force signal	EMG based fuzzy-neuro controller. Fuzzy rules are used to determine torque required according to motion intention	Allows flexible and natural motion to user according to motion intention.
Saga Arm [22]	Japan	EMG and Kinematic signal	EMG based fuzzy controller and a kinematic based controller	Transhumeral Prosthetic Arm developed for predefined daily activities
Manus Hand [23]	Spain	EMG	Based on EMG signal of three levels	A command language was developed for the 3-bit input signal of EMG
Finger Prosthesis [46]	AUS	EMG	Post-processing Classification using LIBSVM and kNN	An improved control algorithm has being proposed
EMG based Robotic Hand [36]	Japan	EMG	Based on ANN classification	Together with motion capturing data, joint angles can be calculated for controlling purposes
DEKA arm [21]	USA	EMG/ pressure signals	Uses TMR controlling with pressure signals from the foot	Modular based controlling could be realized

Table 1. Comparison of EMG based control method of assistive robots

A considerable numbers of literature of EMG based control methods show the usage of different methods for EMG processing. This may give a number of options to researchers to conduct experiments for EMG processing in different angles. Most of EMG based assistive robots use surface EMG electrodes for EMG signal detection and few robots use needle electrodes [8, 13]. It was found that all methods of EMG processing belong to one of three main categories: time domain, frequency domain and time-frequency domain [5]. Another important aspect of an EMG based control method is signal classification. Generally, accuracy of EMG based control method highly depends on method of classification and which helps to identify muscles to generate the required output from the EMG based control method [18]. Different robots use different techniques for signal classification and many of them are based on neuro-fuzzy, fuzzy logic and neural network. All assistive robots considered for this review used an EMG signal as its main input signal and the architecture of the controller varies from one type to other. Some of them are based on proportional control and others use advanced control methods such as PID control. In another way, controllers can be classified based on its model as dynamic model [25], muscle model or other method. EMG based control methods of upper-limb exoskeleton robots and prostheses are respectively presented and reviewed in the next subsections. The authors make every possible effort to include all recent EMG based control methods of assistive robots in the next section. The logic for selecting particular control method is its key features and novelty.

4.1. EMG based control methods of upper-limb exoskeleton robots

Different approaches have been proposed by various researchers in the past in order to estimate the muscle torque starting from EMG activation. These methods include neural networks, neuro-fuzzy classifier, hill model *etc* [27]. In the next subsections, several EMG based control methods of upper-limb exoskeleton robots are reviewed.

4.1.1. EMG based control of hand exoskeleton

The hand exoskeleton robot with EMG control has been developed by researchers from the University of Berlin, Germany [26]. This mainly focuses to use by patients who have limited hand mobility. Figure 8 shows the EMG control method for a hand exoskeleton with blind source separation. The construction of the design allows controlling the motion of finger joints. Researchers have presented the difficulties in the application of EMG algorithms. One such drawback is the identification of the correct muscle responsible for a particular motion. In other words, only a subset of muscles responsible for hand movement is sampled by the surface electrodes [26]. Another difficulty is the EMG signal separation for relevant motion. This needs a suitable process to recover the underlying original signals. Armin *et. al.*, have proposed a blind source separation method to recover the underlying original signals developed by a particular motion of muscle [26]. Initially signals are filtered by a weighted low pass differential filter. Then an inverse demixing matrix which, results from an iterative algorithm [4] approximates the separation about 1.5dB for close proximity sensors. Subsequent to the separation, the signals are used for control purposes. However, integration of additional sensors and additional DoF complicates the separation and further, the position of electrodes increases the complexity. Therefore, blind source separation has practical limitations in working with EMG sensors with force sensors.

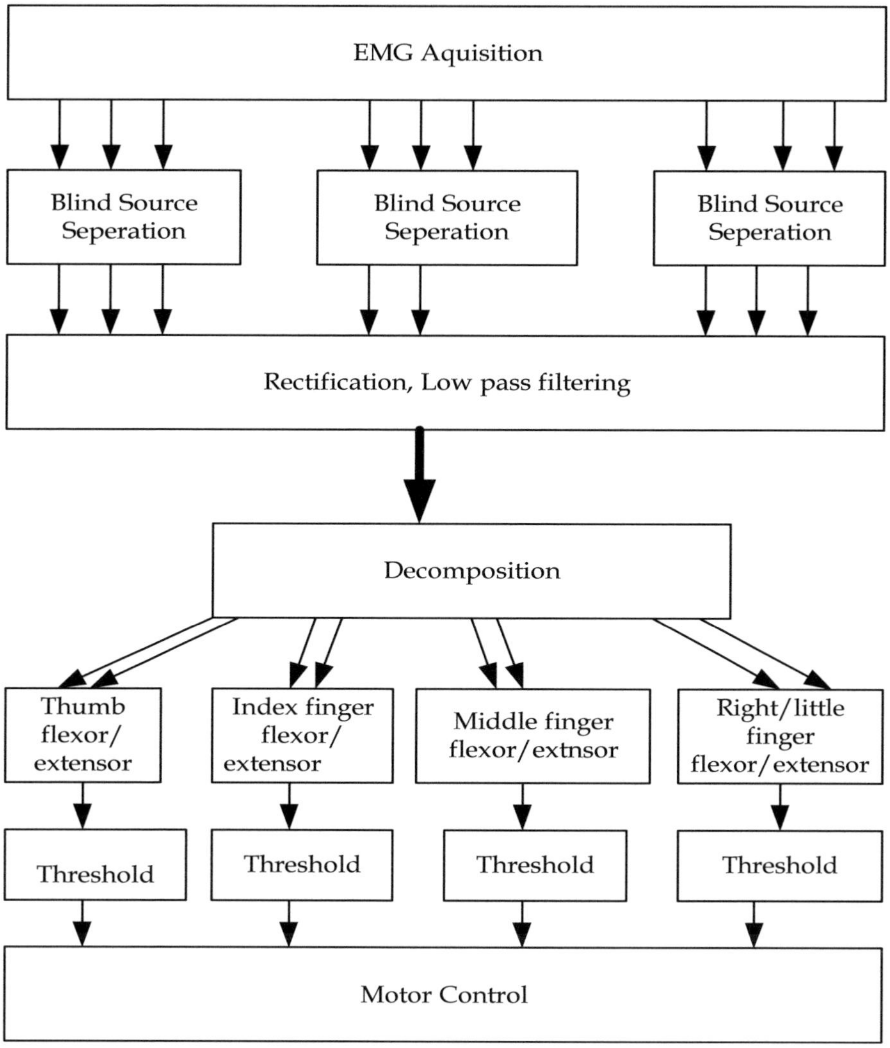

Figure 8. Structure of the control method with blind source separation [26]

4.1.2. EMG based neuro-fuzzy control method

Kiguchi *et al.* [18] have developed an exoskeleton robot and it is controlled based on EMG signals. The robot is used to assist the motion of physically weak persons such as elderly, disabled and injured [37-39]. Although EMG signals directly reflect the human motion intention, it is difficult to control the robotic exoskeleton since the strength of EMG varies with factors like physical and physiological conditions, placement of electrodes, shift of electrodes and high nonlinearity of muscle activity for a certain motion. Therefore, Kiguchi *et al* proposed a neuro-fuzzy controller with EMG signals which provides flexible and adaptive nonlinear control for the exoskeleton robot in real time. The architecture of the controller is shown in the Fig. 9. Mean absolute value (MAV) is used to extract the features of the EMG signal due to its

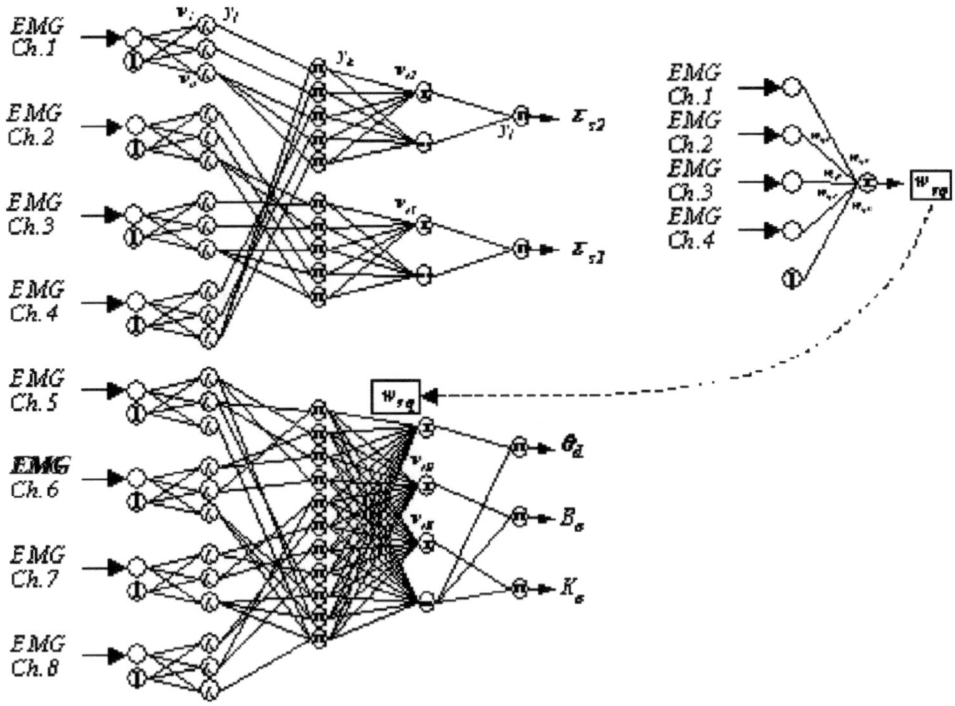

Figure 9. Architecture of neuro-fuzzy controller [18]

effectiveness in real time control compared with other methods such as mean absolute value slope, zero crossing, slope sign changes or wave form length [16, 18]. The hierarchical controller consists mainly of three stages: input signal selection stage, posture selection region stage and neuro-fuzzy control stage. The first stage consists of EMG based control according to the muscle activity levels of the robot and the second stage consists of neuro-fuzzy control according to the motion of the human and finally the controller determines desired torque command for each joint via neuro-fuzzy controller. This helps to realize the effective motion assistance for the robot user. In the first stage, input information to the controller is selected in accordance with the user's muscle activity levels. The control is carried out based on EMG, however, when muscle activity is low, the control signal is generated by force sensors. The second stage of the controller basically works in accordance with the user's arm posture. Different postures may cause different control rules and this leads to complexity of controller. In this situation, multiple neuro-fuzzy controllers have been proposed. The desired torque commands are finally generated by the neuro-fuzzy controller in their last stage.

This EMG based control method employed controller adaptation to realize the desired motion assistance for any subject. Further, the controller is capable of adapt itself to physical and physiological condition of any user of robot. However, this adaptation of the controller imposes training prior to use the assistive robot and it may take a considerable time resulting in a lack of motivation.

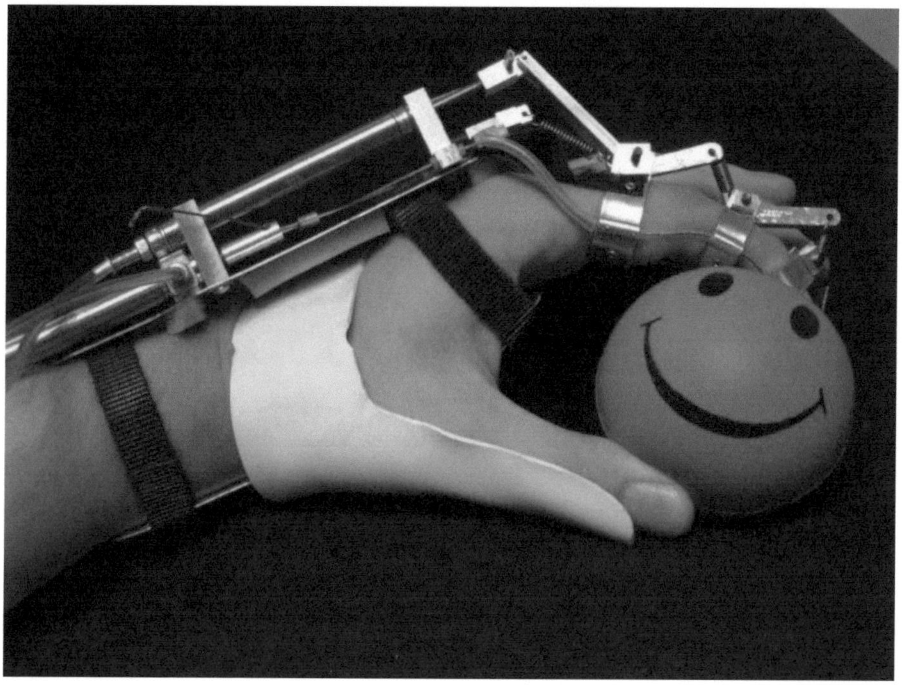

Figure 10. Orthotic exoskeleton hand control by EMG [19]

4.1.3. *EMG controlled orthotic exoskeleton hand*

Researchers from Carnegie Mellon University, USA have developed a light weight, low profile orthotic exoskeleton (see Fig. 10) which is controlled by using EMG signals [19]. Matsuoka *et al.* further extended their research on discovering the best control methodology for EMG based control of exoskeleton robots. Their observations are presented through conducting experiments under three control scenarios [19]. According to [19], they have conducted EMG based control through Binary control algorithm [40], Variable control algorithm [19] and Natural reaching algorithm [19].

The binary control algorithm provides either 'ON' or 'OFF' states to the outputs or actuators based on EMG activity. This is a more primitive type of control method and it does not cover any intermediate state of function. This problem is overcome when adopting a variable control algorithm which defines the intermediate state and guarantees the smooth function of robotic actuators via an EMG signal. The natural reaching algorithm is suitable for subjects who are paralyzed completely in one of the arms. Authors concluded that the suitable control algorithm is one of the important aspects for better control of the exoskeleton robot with an EMG signal. This determines the type of object being carried by user and the type of interaction needed for it. Therefore, identification of the control algorithm enhances the effective use of the EMG signal for exoskeleton robot control. However, the experiments have not been carried out to determine the effectiveness of the natural reaching algorithm.

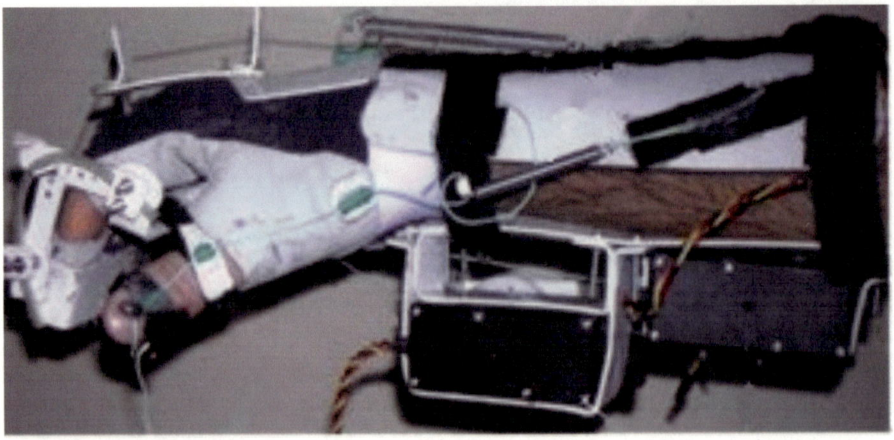

Figure 11. Hand exoskeleton [24]

4.1.4. EMG based controlled exoskeleton for hand rehabilitation

Giuseppina *et al* from Italy have worked on developing a hand exoskeleton system (see Fig. 11) which is also controlled by EMG signals [24]. This is mainly developed for hand rehabilitation where people have partially lost the ability to correctly control their hand movements. Figure 12 shows the control flow chart of the hand rehabilitation robot. During the research they have selected the relevant muscle to capture the finger motion and EMG electrodes are placed in order to minimize the noise due to the movements. This is one of the important factors to be considered when placing dry electrodes on the skin. The control system of the robot consists of microcontroller and EMG acquisition systems. Processed EMG signals are communicated with the microcontroller via serial connection. Finally the microcontroller generates the command signal required to drive the actuator and control real positions by means of sensory inputs. Threshold is defined in order to distinguish the real electric activity of the muscle from other interferences. According to [24], the relationship between motor speed, $v(t)$ and joint angle position, $\theta(t)$ is obtained as in equation (1).

$$v(t) = A\{1 - \theta(t)\} \tag{1}$$

where A is defined as an opportunely chosen factor.

According to (1), they are able to control the motor speed which is proportional to the hand opening and progressively it reaches zero when the fingers are flexing. This control method is more suitable for advanced rehabilitation processes. At the same time it takes the effect of natural variability of the EMG signal into account.

4.1.5. Muscle-model-oriented EMG based control of an exoskeleton robot

The SUEFUL -7 is an upper-limb exoskeleton robot mainly developed to assist motion of physically weak individuals. In the robot EMG signals are used as the main input signal to the

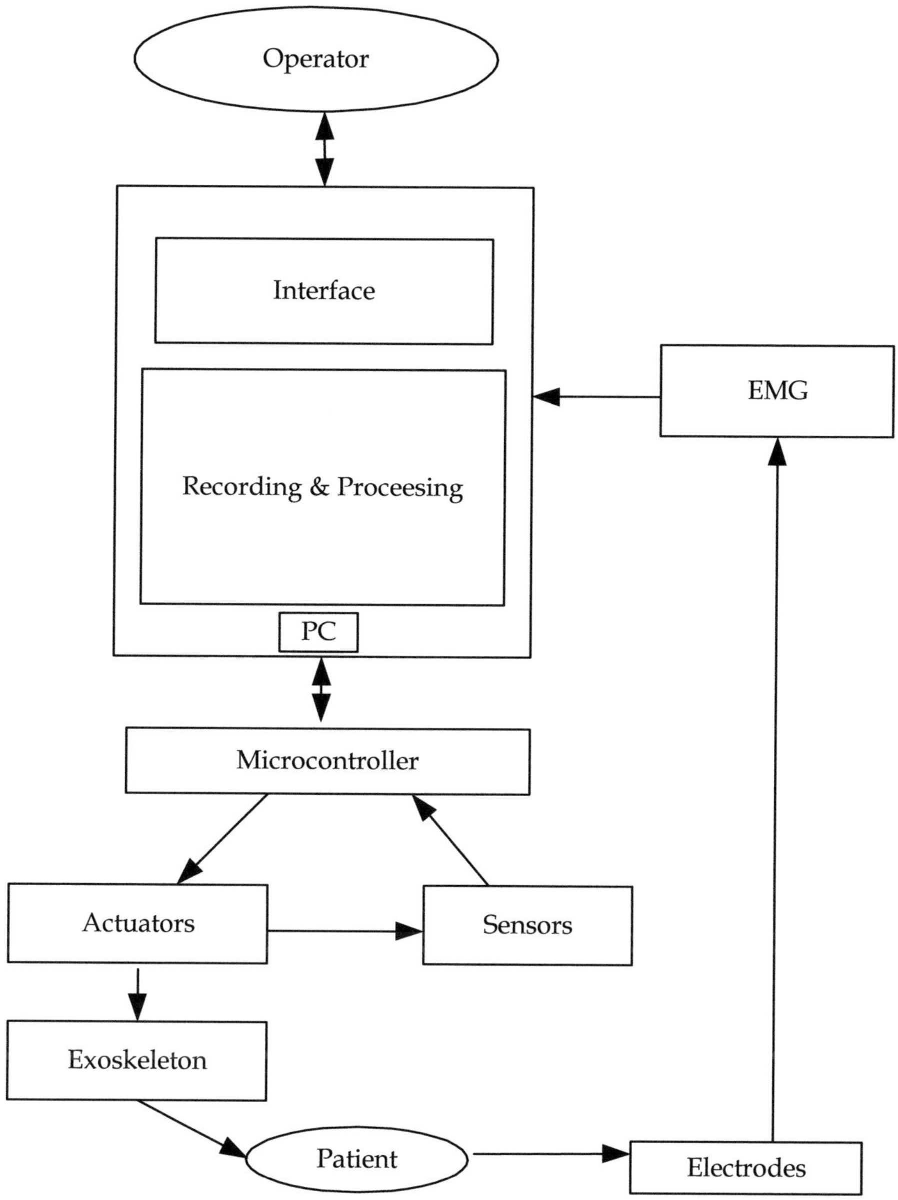

Figure 12. Control flow chart of hand rehabilitation robot [24]

controller (see Fig. 13). In order to obtain the real time control, a muscle-model-oriented control method has been proposed for the robot. This control method is more suitable compared to the fuzzy-neuro control method, where it needs a higher number of fuzzy rules in case of higher DoF. An impedance controller is applied with a muscle-model-oriented control method and impedance parameters are then adjusted in real time as a function of upper-limb posture and EMG activity level [6].

The controller of the SUEFUL-7 [6] uses EMG signals of the user as the primary input information. Also, forearm force, hand force and forearm torque are used as subordinate input information for the controller [6]. This hybrid nature of the control method is a guarantee to activate the SUEFUL-7 even with low EMG signal level. On the other hand, when EMG signals are high, the robot is controlled mainly by the EMG signal generated by user motion. The features of the raw EMG signal are extracted through RMS calculation. This RMS of EMG is fed to the controller. In order to identify the 7DoF motions the EMG signals of sixteen locations are measured with surface electrodes.

The correct joint torque is affected by the posture of the upper limb and it changes the relationship between EMG signals and generated joint torques. Further, this posture variation is nonlinear and stochastic [6]. Fuzzy reasoning is therefore applied to estimate the effect of posture change. Neuro-fuzzy modifier is then applied to modify the muscle model matrix by means of adjusting weights in order to take the effect of changes of posture of the upper limb effectively. Online adaptation of the neuro-fuzzy modifier is important if the robot is expected to be used for different uses. Therefore, the neuro-fuzzy modifier is trained for each user using relevant information. The overall structure of the controller (see Fig. 13) consists of two stages.

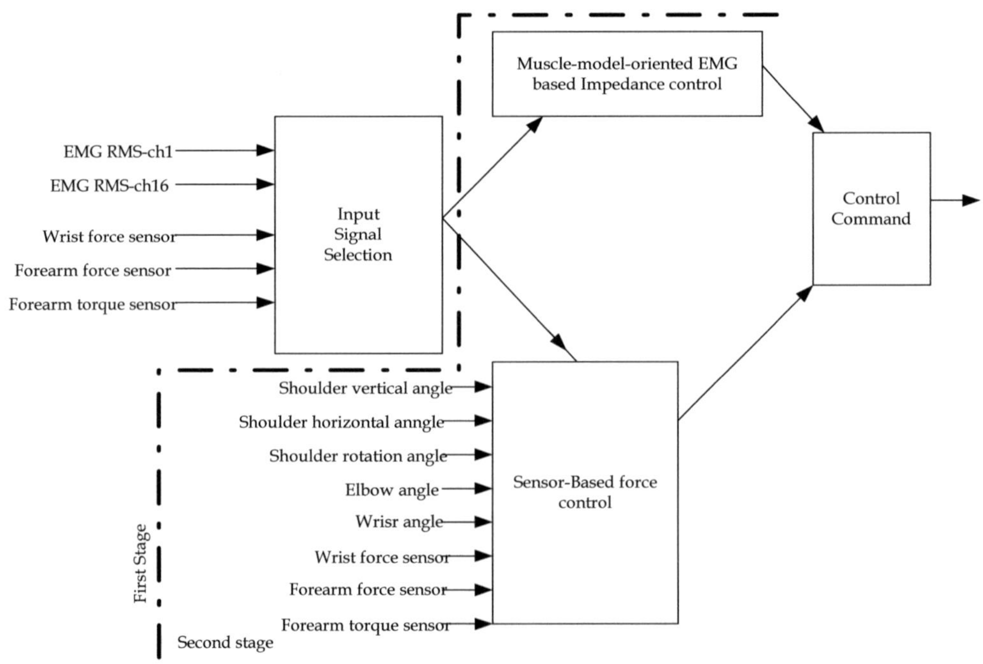

Figure 13. Structure of SUEFUL-7 controller [6]

The first stage is the input signal selection and the second stage is muscle model oriented EMG based impedance control. Proper input information is selected to the controller according to muscle activity levels in the first stage. Depending on the RMS of the EMG signal, muscle model oriented EMG based control or sensor based force control is selected under the second stage and it is fed as a control command to the robot.

4.1.6. Use of EMG to tremor suppression control

Tremor is defined as the involuntary motion that may occur in various parts of the body, such as the leg or arm. An essential tremor is the most common tremor disorder of the arm and it may occur during a voluntary motion such as writing, painting, etc. If the essential tremor occurs in the arm, the person may not be able to achieve sensitive tasks properly with certain tools [20].

Saga University, Japan has developed an EMG based control method to suppress the tremor of the hand [20]. The features of the EMG signals are extracted from the RMS and fed to the controller. Sixteen EMG channels are selected to measure the muscle activity and they are used to determine the joint torque by knowing weight value for particular EMG signal. This weight depends on upper limb anatomy or result of experiment [20]. The essential tremor is a rhythmic motion and its vibrational component is extracted by using a band pass filter in the controller. Also, the user intention is extracted by using a low pass filter.

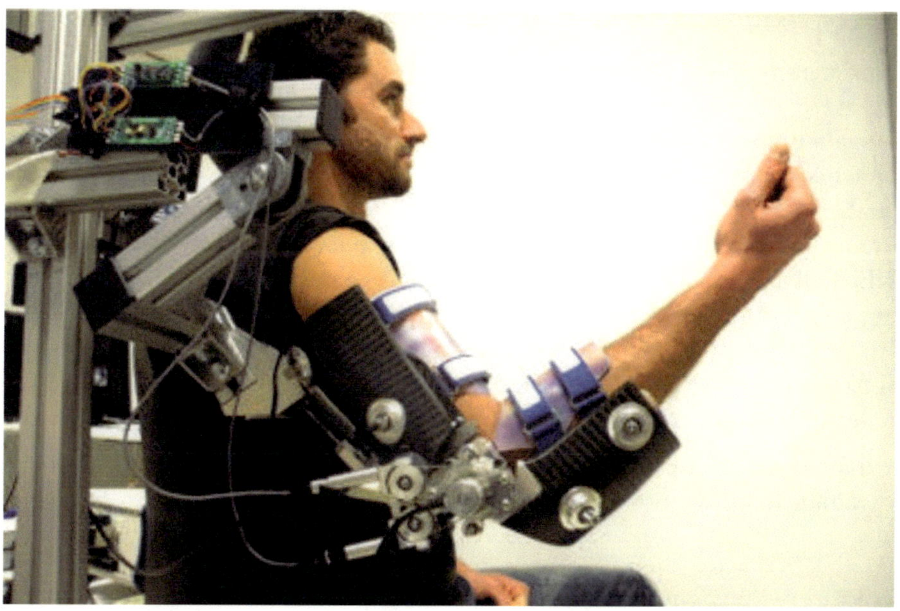

Figure 14. NEUROExos with a subject [10]

The desired hand position is then obtained considering the summation of the above two amplitudes. Therefore X_{avrg} represents the desired hand motion while suppressing the tremor.

$$X_{avg} = X_{usr} - X_{tre} \tag{2}$$

Where X_{avg}, X_{user} and X_{tre} are desired hand position, rhythmic motion and user intention respectively.

Further, a muscle-model matrix modifier is defined to take the changes of hand posture and minimize the effect of variation of EMG signal and hence torque variation. Also the amount of tremor is not uniform to all; therefore training of the muscle-model matrix is needed prior to use with the subject. Especially, in case of tremor, the training of the muscle-model matrix does not become easy, because the pattern of tremor is not uniform to all.

4.1.7. EMG based proportional control method of NEUROExos

NEUROExos [27] is an upper limb assistive robot designed to be controlled by EMG signals. The robot is shown in Fig. 14. Carrozza *et al* pointed the importance of understanding the accurate torque estimate for assistive robots. They have developed an EMG based proportional control method to estimate the required torque to operate the NEUROExos. [27]. In the control method, Raw EMG signals were processed to obtain the linear envelope (LE) profiles which resemble the muscle tension waveforms during dynamic changes of isometric forces [27]. These LEs were obtained on-line through full-wave rectification of band passed EMG signals and post-filtering by means of a second-order low-pass Butterworth filter with a cut-off frequency of 3 Hz [27].

The block diagram of EMG based proportional control method of NEUROExos is shown in Fig. 15. As in Fig. 15, two proportional controllers, K_{bic} (gain for bicep) and K_{tric} (gain for triceps) are set one after other starting from biceps. Both gains are initially set to zero and gradually increased while the subject moves the arm freely. This gain is increased until the subject feels a comfortable level of assistance. Once K_{bic} is set, the subject is instructed to repeat the same procedure for K_{tric} too. The experimental results of proportional EMG based control method of the NEUROExos shown in [27] are proved that the exoskeleton provides extra torque indicating effective reduction of effort spent by the subject for movement generation [27]. Therefore, proportional control of the EMG is one appropriate method to estimate the torque required to move the assistive robot. However, the amount of assistance given by the exo-skeleton depends on the subject.

The neuro-fuzzy modifier proposed by Kiguchi *et al* [6] can be applied with modifications for effective training for different subjects and hence it may possible to perform a task in minimum time.

4.1.8. EMG based fuzzy-neuro control method of W-EXOS

The W-EXOS is a 3DOF exoskeleton robot and its control method is an EMG based fuzzy-neuro control. The control method is illustrated in Fig.16. Surface EMG signals of muscles and sensors

http://dx.doi.org/10.5772/56174

17

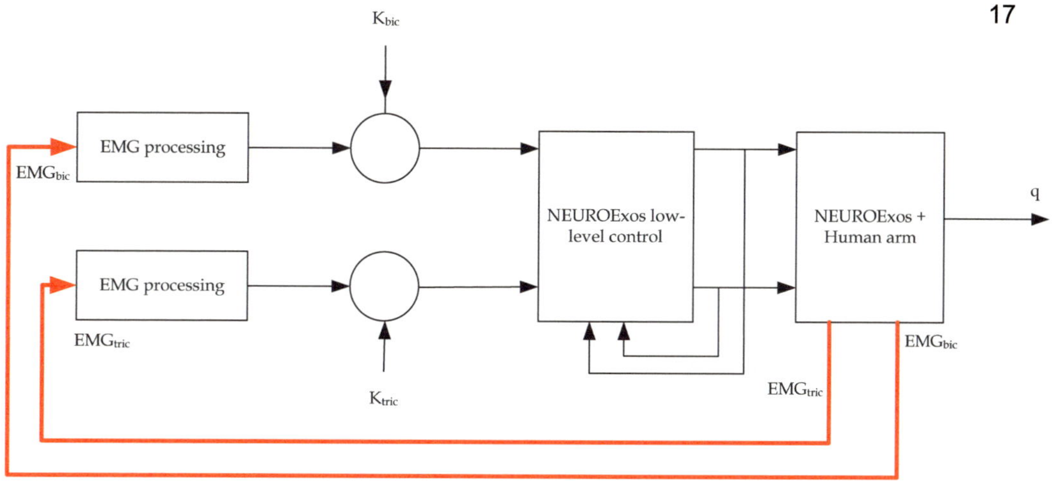

Figure 15. Proportional control block diagram of NEUROExos [27].

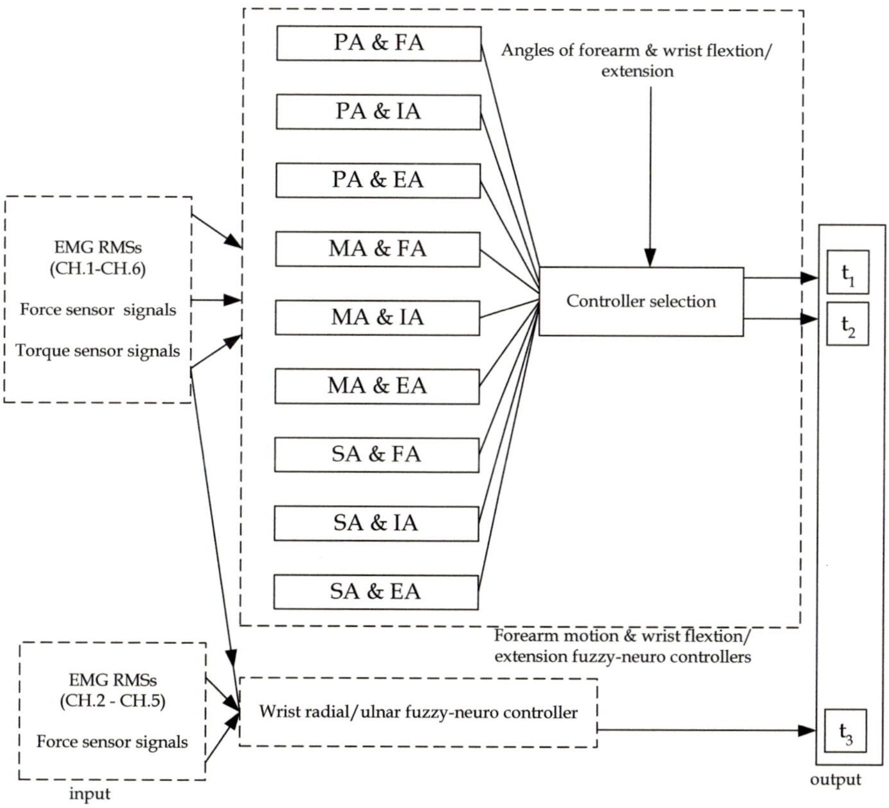

Figure 16. EMG-based fuzzy-neuro control method [35].

of the exoskeleton (hand force and forearm torque) robot [35] are used as input information to the controller. This fuzzy-neuro control method consists of a flexible fuzzy control and adaptive neural network control which is used to obtain natural and flexible motion assist. Fuzzy if-then rules have been constructed to determine the required torque to the motor according to the motion intention of the human. In total, nine fuzzy-neuro controllers are used and this allows operating the exoskeleton robot flexible with EMG signals. Depending on the subject and nature of power-assistance, training of the fuzzy-neuro controller is performed.

The main drawback of this kind of control method is the difficulty of defining the fuzzy if-then control rules when the controller is applied for exoskeleton robots with higher DoF. Further, training of the controller is essential even when the physical and psychological conditions change in the user.

4.2. EMG based control methods of upper-limb prostheses

This section reviews recent EMG based controllers of upper-limb prostheses. Controlling of a prosthetic device using EMG signals is cumbersome task compared to controlling an exoskeleton device using EMG signals, since already the person who wears the device has lost the best site of the body to get the required EMG signals for the controlling of the prosthesis. It makes the number of inputs for the control system to be less and obviously causes to underperform a conventional control system. So far researchers [21-23] have proposed different control methods to control prosthetic devices. In addition, the introduction of more advanced technologies such as targeted muscle reinnervation and implantable electrodes marks new boundaries in prosthesis controlling. The ensuing subsections review EMG based control methods of upper-limb prostheses. The logic for selecting a particular control method is its significance and novelty.

4.2.1. Control method of Saga university prosthetic arm

Saga University prosthetic arm is developed for the realization of 5DoF upper limb motions for a transhumeral amputee. The hand is controlled using a combination of an EMG based controller (EBC) and a task oriented kinematic based controller (KBC). Figure 17 shows an experimental setup of an EMG signal based controller of a Saga prosthetic arm. In a transhumeral amputee a part of the biceps and triceps are remaining. EMG signals of the amputee's biceps and triceps are used as the input information for the EBC to control elbow flexion/ extension and hand grasp/release. Forearm supination/pronation, wrist flexion/extension and ulnar/radial deviation get controlled from the KBC. Motion intention of the amputee is identified via a task classifier using shoulder and prosthesis elbow kinematics. For the scope of this context only the EBC will be considered. EMG based fuzzy controller is the base for EBC. It proportionally controls the torque of the elbow and hand actuator according to the amount of the EMG signal. The activation of biceps generates the elbow flexion and the activation of triceps generates the elbow extension. Hand grasp is realized when both triceps and biceps are activated simultaneously. The release position of the hand is achieved when the both muscles are not working.

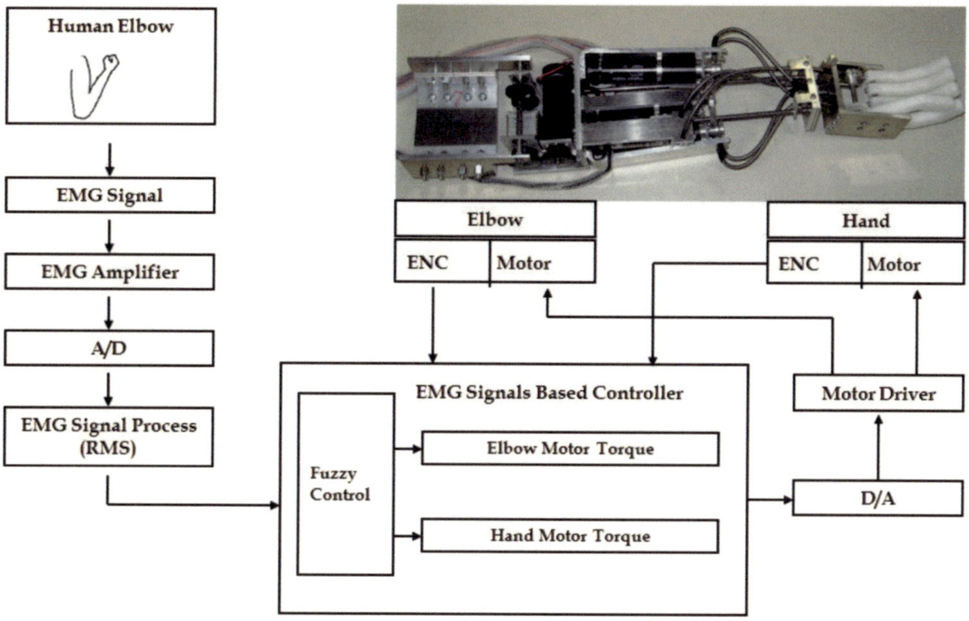

Figure 17. Experimental setup of EMG signals based Controller of Saga prosthetic arm [22]

Information from the raw EMG signals is extracted by taking the RMS value of the raw EMG signals. The RMS is determined as,

$$RMS = \sqrt{1/N \sum_{i=1}^{N} v_i^2} \tag{3}$$

where v_i is the voltage value at i^{th} sampling and N is the number of samples in a segment.

The EBC is provided with four EMG RMSs. Three kinds of fuzzy linguistic variables for each input were defined. Ten kinds of fuzzy if-then rules for elbow joint torque control and seven kinds of if-then rules for hand torque control were prepared. In addition, details on the KBC can be found in [22].

Even though the prosthetic arm is capable of catering to the human motion intension to a certain degree, still some improvements can be made. Since the KBC is trained to offline Vicon data for a given set of daily activities, the orientations of the limbs other than those trained for cannot be achieved using the KBC. Therefore, an inertial measurement unit (IMU) can be fixed to the stem arm of the amputee and used as an interface to read the real time kinematic data. By using the real time kinematic data as an input to the controller it can be improved to reach almost all the orientations of daily activities. In addition a hybrid control method - EMG coupled with EEG - can be used to enhance the performance of the controller by obtaining correct human motion intention.

4.2.2. EMG based control method with targeted muscle reinnervation

Targeted muscle reinnervation (TMR) is a surgical procedure which is developed to increase the number of psychologically appropriate control inputs available for use with a prosthetic device [42]. A surgical procedure is used to transfer the motor neurons of the residual limb to a remaining set of muscles. After denerverting, the target muscles motor nerves can be reinnervated. These reinnervated muscles are capable of providing EMG to a prosthesis controller with more accurate motion intention. For a transhumeral amputee, the goal is to transfer the median and distal radial nerves to target muscle segments creating hand open and close signals. For the shoulder/humeral neck disarticulated amputees all four brachial plexus nerves are transferred to the target muscles [42]. It should be noted that for cases with left shoulder disarticulation the interference of electrocardiogram (ECG) causes an effect to the TMR EMG signals [42]. This could be eliminated using a second-order high pass filter with 60Hz cutoff frequency, which results in 80% elimination of the ECG signals and 20% elimination of the EMG signals producing an improved law signal-to-noise ratio output.

Boston Digital arm [43], Otto Bock electric wrist rotator [44] and an electric terminal device (hook or hand, depending on subject preference) are fitted to six TMR subjects, three transhumeral (TH) amputees, two shoulder disarticulation (SD) amputees and one humeral neck transhumeral amputee. After attaching the patient with the prosthetic device the patient should be guided and continuously monitored to achieve better outcome from the TMR. Even though the training process of the prosthetic user with TMR EMG control is much more easily compared to the pre-TMR, EMG controlling since the TMR itself provides an initiative to the user for training. The control algorithm of the system is comprised of proportional controlling of velocity according to the amplitude of the EMG signal. Table 2 shows summary of information of TMR subjects in the experiment [42].

Even though TMR is capable of providing more sites to extract EMG signals, it is a surgical process and involves invasive procedures, which may cause user discomfort. Therefore, TMR should be replaced by a hybrid control mechanism developed using other signals such as EMG of residual muscles and the EEG signals.

4.2.3. EMG based control of prosthetic finger

Rami *et al* [16] have proposed an improved control algorithm for a control of a prosthetic finger. Using the developed controller different finger postures of the prosthetic hand can be controlled. The main EMG pattern recognition setup is shown in Fig. 18. The controller is mainly developed considering the main ten motions of the hand; flexion of each finger, pinching of thumb combined with each and every finger and clenching of the fist..

Data was collected using two EMG channels. For the feature extraction the windowing was done using a disjoint windowing scheme, which consumes less computer resources due to its simplicity. Various feature sets have been extracted; Waveform length, Hjoth Time Domain (TD) Parameters, Slope Sign Changes, Number of Zero Crossings, Sample Skewness and Auto Regressive (AR) Model parameters were selected [46]. The two feature sets from the two channels resulted in a large one feature set. Dimensionality reduction of the feature set has been done using Linear Discriminant Analysis (LDA) and it provides nine features for the collected EMG data set. Then both k-Nearest Neighbor (kNN) and Library Support Vector Machine (LIBSVM) have been used for the classification. Use of majority voting technique has resulted in providing smoothed classification accuracies.

Subject identifier	Level of amputation	Elbow flexion	Elbow extension	Hand close	Hand open	Wrist rotation
SD-A	Shoulder Disartic.	Musculocutaneous N. to P.Major, Clav.Head	Redial N. to P.head Major, inf. Stemal	Median N. to upper stemal head	Median N. to upper stemal head*	Toggle between Hand Open/Close control using socket-mounted FSR
SD-B	Shoulder Disartic.**	Musculocutaneous N. to P.Major, Clav.Head	Native remnant triceps	Median N.to P.Major, stemal head and P.Minor	Distal Radial N. to Thoracodorsal N (Serratus Anterior)	Two-site control with two socket mounted FSRs
SD-C	Shoulder Disartic.	Musculocutaneous N. to P.Major, Clav.Head	Native remnant triceps/post. Deltoid	Ulnar N.to remnant P.Major stemal head segment	Radial N to P.Minor	Single-site control with one socket mounted FSR
TH-A	Trans-humeral	Native Biceps, long head	Native Triceps	Median N. to Biceps, short head	Distal Radial N. to Brachialis	Single-site control with harness linear potentiometer
TH-B	Trans-humeral	Native Biceps, long head	Native Triceps	Median N. to Biceps, short head	Distal Radial N. to Brachialis	Single-site control with harness linear potentiometer
TH-C	Trans-humeral	Native Biceps, long head	Native Triceps, long and medial head	Median N. to Biceps, short head	Distal Radial N. to Brachialis, lateral head	Single-site control with harness linear potentiometer

*Unexpected result: subject indicates opening hand with a movement of thumb abduction, a median nerve function

**Humeral neck level amputation clinically fit as a shoulder disarticulation level amputee

Table 2. Summary of TMR subjects including level of amputation, surgical sites used as inputs and any other prosthetic controls implements in the post-TMR prosthetic fitting [42]

4.2.4. EMG based control method of manus hand

Manus hand shown in Fig. 19 as a replacement to a lost hand for an amputee is capable of generating 3DoF, reproducing the grasping function for the user [23]. The hand is controlled via EMG signal of the residual muscle of the user. The simultaneous operation of the joints has been realized. It is achieved using a differently approached pattern recognition technique [23]. In this technique, single muscle EMG signal is used to generate the grasping commands. In order to do this a command language comprising of three EMG bits has been developed. Each bit has defined three digital levels. Accordingly, an input comprises of three muscle contractions to generate three EMG levels and 27 different commands. From the practical point of view, 18 out of 27 commands were selected for the implementation. However, no information relevant to the pattern recognition has been published by the authors. Table 3 shows the main commands of the 3-bit command language extracted from [45]. According to the controller mechanism no simultaneous operation could be realized using the MANUS hand. Therefore instead of the 3-bit command language it would be better to use a proper pattern recognition method with a higher number of EMG inputs. This could also be coupled with an EEG or other biological signal, in order to achieve higher effectiveness from the controller.

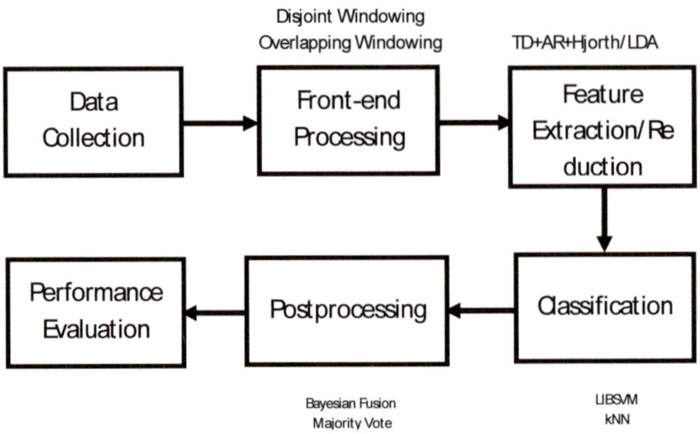

Figure 18. Block diagram of experimental evaluation of the EMG-pattern recognition system [46]

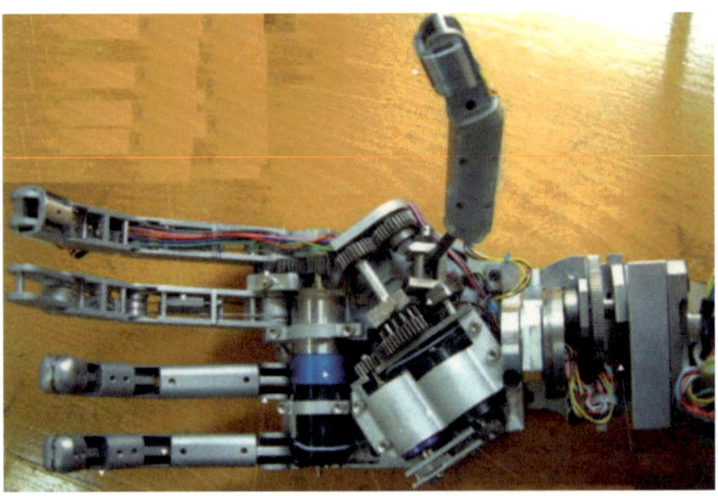

Figure 19. MANUS hand [23]

Functional command	3-bit pattern	Remarks
Stop	100	Constant, pre-set, compulsory
Default position	200	Constant, pre-set, compulsory
Calibration	212	Constant, pre-set, compulsory
Rotate to right, until "Default" or until "Stop"	210	Individually adapted, recommended "preset"
Close, gripping mode "1", Preset 0 to 250 gr. Total pressure, or until "Stop"	211	Individually adapted
Close, gripping mode "1", Preset 251 to 500 gr. Total pressure, or until "Stop"	221	Individually adapted
Close, gripping mode "1", Preset total pressure.500gr., or until "Stop"	222	Individually adapted
Rotate to left, until "Default" or until "Stop"	101	Individually adapted, recommended "preset"
Close, gripping mode "2", Preset 0 to 250 gr. Total pressure, or until "Stop"	120	Individually adapted
Close, gripping mode "2", Preset 251 to 500 gr. Total pressure, or until "Stop"	121	Individually adapted
Close, gripping mode "1", Preset total pressure.500gr., or until "Stop"	122	Individually adapted
Close, gripping mode "3", Preset 0 to 300 gr. Total pressure, or until "Stop"	201	Individually adapted
Close, gripping mode "4", Preset: arch, or until "Stop"	202	Individually adapted
Available	111	
Available	112	

Table 3. Summary of TMR subjects including level of amputation, surgical sites used as inputs and any other prosthetic controls implements in the post-TMR prosthetic fitting [45]

4.2.5. EMG based ANN controller for a transhumeral prosthesis

The EMG based Artificial Neural Network (ANN) controller was developed to realize elbow flexion/extension and forearm supination/pronation based on the artificial neural network (ANN) techniques using EMG signals as the input. Fig. 20 shows the basic concept of the design of the controller. EMG signals are fed into the controller from seven muscles: brachialis, biceps, medial head of triceps, posterior deltoid, anterior deltoid, clavicular and pectoralis major. Raw EMG signals from the muscles are amplified, alternating current coupled, low-pass filtered and recorded. Recorded EMG signals are processed offline. They are filtered, windowed and features extracted. Several features are extracted from 320 samples, 128ms sample time rectangular windows with 50 percent overlap between adjacent segments which provides a sample time of 64ms. The features, mean absolute value, waveform length, number of zero crossing and number of slope sign changes are extracted from each window, which generate a four-element feature set for each EMG channel. Simultaneously motion capturing data from the Optotrak Certus motion capture system is resampled such that its sample time matched that of the EMG data and average joint angles were extracted.

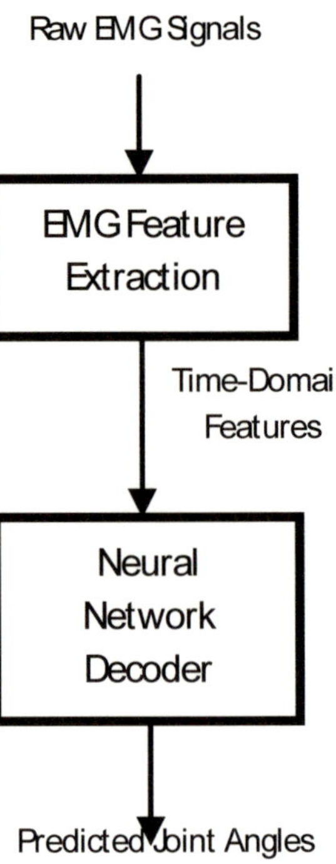

Figure 20. Block diagram of control strategy [36]

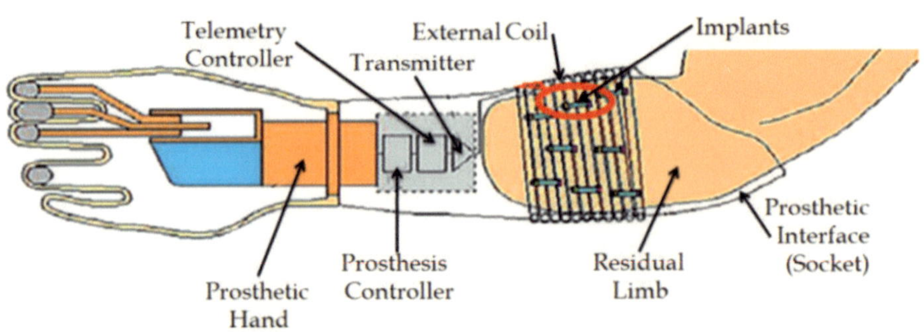

Figure 21. Schematic of the implantable myoelectric sensor system[8]

4.2.6. iEMG controlled prosthetic device

iEMG is capable of providing accurate EMG data to the control system. Use of implantable myoelectric sensor (IMS) would result in nullifying the problem of multiple-component EMGs, an inborn problem of surface EMG recording, as well as the nullifying the considerable amount of environmental effects caused for the changes in regular sEMG signal supply. Here the IMS receives commands and power from an external telemetry controller [8]. It drives a coil attached to the prosthetic socket as shown in Fig. 21. EMG data and digital information transmit between the implants and the telemetry controller forming a magnetic link through the coil. The data is then converted into analog form at the controller and can be used to control the prosthetic device. When the results from iEMG are compared with sEMG for the same user, iEMG results show a drastic improvement in providing the same motion of the natural hand. Even though iEMG is capable of providing better signals, it is an invasive process and may cause discomfort to the user. Therefore, a hybrid control method, EMG coupled with EEG would result in providing a better control for the prosthetic device. Further, it will not cause discomfort to the user.

5. Conclusion and future directions

In this chapter, recent EMG based control methods of assistive robots were comprehensively reviewed. As assistive robots, upper-limb exoskeleton robots and upper-limb prostheses were mainly considered here. At first, the detection and processing of the EMG was explained discussing available EMG extraction systems. Then ways of categorization of EMG based control methods as input information to the controller, architecture of the control algorithm, output of the controller and other ways were discussed. EMG based control methods were categorized based on structure of the control algorithm as pattern recognition based control and non-pattern recognition based control. Even though assistive robots with pattern recognition based control can be commonly found, control methods that belong to non-pattern recognition based control are hardly found. Recent EMG based control methods of upper-limb exoskeleton robots and prostheses were reviewed separately. In the review recent EMG based control methods of upper-limb exoskeleton robots and upper-limb prostheses were compared considering their features.

In addition to EMG signals, EEG, EOG and MMG signals also represent the human motion intention and these can be used as input signals to the controller of the assistive robots. Accordingly, in the future a hybrid control algorithm can be developed with a combination of two or more biological signals as inputs to the controller. Assistive robots are expected to function and appear as their biological counterparts. That is, an exoskeleton should ideally act as a second skin for the human and a prosthetic device the same as the natural limb. Accordingly, control methods of devices should be improved in the future.

Actuator technology also plays an important role of control methods of exoskeleton robot and prostheses. Actuators drive a robot interacting with human according to control inputs. Linearity, stability, correspondence between human motion and actuator actions are important terms for successful function of actuators and hence the control system too. New actuator technologies can be successfully used with exoskeleton robots and prostheses to improve its function.

In future developments, the aspect of control systems of the assistive robot can be extended to take the effect of microclimate conditions present around the user and take suitable control efforts to provide comfort to the user. Since exoskeleton robots and prostheses closely interact with the human, safety conditions should be guaranteed at a maximum level. Although some safety features are connected with mechanical design through stoppers and emergency shutdown systems in an electrical system, proper software locks can be implemented in the control system of the robot to improve the safety features. Further, intelligent safety methods can be introduced to the assistive robot with the help of a feedback system of its control method. One of the human biological signals generated by eye ball movement called electrooculogram (EOG) can be used to generate the feedback signal to the controller. Therefore, when a person feels any unsatisfactory motion of the robot, a particular eye ball movement can be traced and used as a feedback signal and further it can be used to switch off the function of the robot. Since this type of safety method is directly connected with human function it gives maximum protection to the user.

The performance of the control methods is not only based on the controller; it may vary on selection of different components in the control loop. This includes selection of final control elements or actuators, instrumentation for feedback signal, disturbance rejection (inside control loop or outside to the loop), input signals etc. Therefore selection of actuators and sensors play an important role in exoskeleton and prosthesis control systems. In case of sensors, Micro-Electro-Mechanical System (MEMS) inertial sensors are very suitable to detect the changes in velocity, orientation and location of above assistive robots. This technology has made miniaturized sensors and provides low power consumption, low cost, low size and weight which can be used to enhance the function of control method of assistive robots.

Acknowledgements

The authors gratefully acknowledge the support provided by national research council (NRC), Sri Lanka from the research grant (no 11-067). The authors would also like to extend their sincere gratitude to Mr. Nilhan Niles for his cooperation.

Author details

R. A. R. C. Gopura, D. S. V. Bandara, J. M. P. Gunasekara and T. S. S. Jayawardane

University of Moratuwa, Sri Lanka

References

[1] Population Division, DESA, United Nations, Magnitude and Speed of Population Ageing, World Population Ageing 1950-2050, www.un.org/esa/population/ publication ns/worldageing19502050/ (accessed 20 April 2012).

[2] Population Division, DESA, United Nations, Demographic Determinants of Population Ageing, World Population Ageing 1950-2050, www.un.org/esa/ population/ publications/worldageing19502050/ (accessed 20 April 2012).

[3] Mosher RS. Handyman to Hardiman [Internet]. Warrendale, PA: SAE International; 1967 Feb. Report No.: 670088. Available from: http://papers.sae.org/670088/

[4] Cloud W. Man Amplifiers: Machines that Let You Carry a Ton. Popular Science, vol. 187, no. 5, p70–73, 1965.

[5] Oskoei MA, Hu H. Myoelectric control systems—A survey. Biomedical Signal Processing and Control. 2007 Oct; 2(4):275–94.

[6] Gopura RARC, Kiguchi K, Li Y. SUEFUL-7: A 7DOF upper-limb exoskeleton robot with muscle-model-oriented EMG-based control. IEEE/RSJ International Conference on Intelligent Robots and Systems, 2009. IROS 2009. Oct. page 1126–31.

[7] Kiguchi K, Hayashi Y, Asami T. An upper-limb power-assist robot with tremor suppression control. IEEE Int Conf Rehabil Robot. 2011; 2011:5975390.

[8] Merrill DR, Lockhart J, Troyk PR, Weir RF, Hankin DL. Development of an Implantable Myoelectric Sensor for Advanced Prosthesis Control. Artificial Organs. 2011;35(3):249–52.

[9] Anon, Robots - The Big Picture - Boston.com, http://www.boston.com /bigpicture/ 2009/03/robots.html (accessed September 28, 2012).

[10] Yanco HA. A Robotic Wheelchair System: Indoor Navigation and User Interface. Lecture notes in Artificial Intelligence: Assistive Technology and Artificial Intelligence. Springer-Verlag; 1998. page 256–68.

[11] Hudgins B, Parker P, Scott RN. A new strategy for multifunction myoelectric control. IEEE Transactions on Biomedical Engineering. Jan.; 40(1):82–94.

[12] Farina D, Merletti R. Comparison of algorithms for estimation of EMG variables during voluntary isometric contractions. Journal of Electromyography and Kinesiology. 2000 Oct; 10(5):337–49.

[13] Schultz AE, Kuiken TA. Neural interfaces for control of upper limb prostheses: the state of the art and future possibilities. PM R. 2011 Jan; 3(1):55–67.

[14] Silva J, Heim W, Chau T. A Self-Contained, Mechanomyography-Driven Externally Powered Prosthesis. Archives of Physical Medicine and Rehabilitation. 2005 Oct; 86(10):2066–70.

[15] Christoph Guger WH. Prosthetic Control by an EEG-based Brain- Computer Interface (BCI): 2–7.

[16] Fukuda O, Tsuji T, Ohtsuka A, Kaneko M. EMG-based human-robot interface for rehabilitation aid. IEEE International Conference on Robotics and Automation, 1998. Proceedings. May. page 3492–3497 vol.4.

[17] Nishikawa D, Yu W, Yokoi H, Kakazu Y. EMG prosthetic hand controller using real-time learning method. 1999 IEEE International Conference on Systems, Man, and Cybernetics, 1999. IEEE SMC '99 Conference Proceedings. page 153–158 vol.1.

[18] Kiguchi K, Tanaka T, Fukuda T. Neuro-fuzzy control of a robotic exoskeleton with EMG signals. IEEE Transactions on Fuzzy Systems. Aug.;12(4):481–90.

[19] DiCicco M, Lucas L, Matsuoka Y. Comparison of control strategies for an EMG controlled orthotic exoskeleton for the hand. 2004 [cited 2013 Mar 10]. Available from: http://dx.doi.org/10.1109/ROBOT.2004.1308056

[20] Kiguchi K., Hayashi Y., Asami T., An Upper limb power assist robot with tremor suppression control: 2011 IEEE International Conference on Rehabilitation Robotics (ICORR). 2011. Page 1-4.

[21] Anon, Dean Kamen's "Luke Arm" Prosthesis Readies for Clinical Trials - IEEE Spectrum. Available at: http://spectrum.ieee.org/biomedical/bionics/dean-kamens-luke-arm-prosthesis-readies-for-clinical-trials [Accessed September 17, 2012].

[22] Kundu S, Kiguchi K. Design and Control Strategy for a 5 DOF Above-Elbow Prosthetic Arm. International Jounral of ARM. 2008;9(3):61–75.

[23] Pons JL, Rocon E, Ceres R, Reynaerts D, Saro B, Levin S, et al. The MANUS-HAND Dextrous Robotics Upper Limb Prosthesis: Mechanical and Manipulation Aspects. Autonomous Robots. 2004;16(2):143–63.

[24] Mulas M, Folgheraiter M, Gini G. An EMG-controlled exoskeleton for hand rehabilitation. International Conference on Rehabilitation Robotics, 2005. ICORR 2005. June-1 July. page 371–4.

[25] Rechy-ramirez EJ, Hu H. Stages for Developing Control Systems using EMG and EEG Signals: A survey. 2011; Available from: http://130.203.133.150/viewdoc/summary; jsessionid=05255194140389CDB76E5767700A934C?doi=10.1.1.229.3184

[26] Wege A, Zimmermann A. Electromyography sensor based control for a hand exoskeleton. IEEE International Conference on Robotics and Biomimetics, 2007. ROBIO 2007. Dec. page 1470–5.

[27] Lenzi T, De Rossi SMM, Vitiello N, Carrozza MC. Proportional EMG control for upper-limb powered exoskeletons. Conf Proc IEEE Eng Med Biol Soc. 2011;2011:628–31.

[28] Moon I, Lee M, Chu J, Mun M. Wearable EMG-based HCI for Electric-Powered Wheelchair Users with Motor Disabilities. Proceedings of the 2005 IEEE International Conference on Robotics and Automation, 2005. ICRA 2005. April. page 2649–54.

[29] Felzer T, Freisleben B. HaWCoS: the "hands-free" wheelchair control system. Proceedings of the fifth international ACM conference on Assistive technologies [Inter-

net]. New York, NY, USA: ACM; 2002 [cited 2013 Mar 10]. page 127–34. Available from: http://doi.acm.org/10.1145/638249.638273

[30] Zhang X, Wang X, Wang B, Sugi T, Nakamura M. Finite State Machine with Adaptive Electromyogram (EMG) Feature Extraction to Drive Meal Assistance Robot. IEEJ Transactions on Electronics, Information and Systems. 2009;129(2):308–13.

[31] Anon, NIHON KOHDEN, http://www.nihonkohden.com/ (accessed September 23, 2012).

[32] Anon, Surface EMG Systems and Sensors, http://www.delsys.com/ (accessed September 23, 2012).

[33] Anon, Biosemi EEG ECG EMG BSPM NEURO amplifier electrodes, http://www.bio semi.com/ (accessed September 23, 2012).

[34] Anon, CED Products, http://www.ced.co.uk/pru.shtml (accessed September 23, 2012).

[35] Gopura RARC, Kiguchi K. Electromyography (EMG)-signal based fuzzy-neuro control of a 3 degrees of freedom (3DOF) exoskeleton robot for human upper-limb motion assist. Journal of the National Science Foundation of Sri Lanka [Internet]. 2009 Dec 31 [cited 2013 Mar 10];37(4). Available from: http://www.sljol.info/index.php/ JNSFSL/ article/view/1470

[36] Pulliam CL, Lambrecht JM, Kirsch RF. Electromyogram-based neural network control of transhumeral prostheses. The Journal of Rehabilitation Research and Development. 2011;48(6):739.

[37] Kiguchi K, Kariya S, Watanabe K, Izumi K, Fukuda T. An exoskeletal robot for human elbow motion support-sensor fusion, adaptation, and control. IEEE Transactions on Systems, Man, and Cybernetics, Part B: Cybernetics. Jun;31(3):353–61.

[38] Kiguchi K, Iwami K, Yasuda M, Watanabe K, Fukuda T. An exoskeletal robot for human shoulder joint motion assist. IEEE/ASME Transactions on Mechatronics. March; 8(1):125–35.

[39] Kiguchi K, Esaki R, Tsuruta T, Watanabe K, Fukuda T. An exoskeleton for human elbow and forearm motion assist. 2003 IEEE/RSJ International Conference on Intelligent Robots and Systems, 2003. (IROS 2003). Proceedings. Oct. page 3600–3605 vol.3.

[40] Benjuya N, Kenney S. Myoelectric Hand Orthosis: JPO: Journal of Prosthetics and Orthotics [Internet]. [cited 2013 Mar 10]. Available from: http://journals.lww.com/ jpojournal/Fulltext/1990/01000/Myoelectric_Hand_Orthosis.11.aspx

[41] Gopura RARC, Kiguchi K. An Exoskeleton Robot for Human Forearm and Wrist Motion Assist. Journal of Advanced Mechanical Design, Systems, and Manufacturing. 2008;2(6):1067–83.

[42] Miller LA, Stubblefield KA, Lipschutz RD, Lock BA, Kuiken TA. Improved Myoelectric Prosthesis Control Using Targeted Reinnervation Surgery: A Case Series. IEEE Transactions on Neural Systems and Rehabilitation Engineering. Feb.;16(1):46–50.

[43] Anon, Boston Digital Arm System | Liberating Technologies, Inc., http://www. liberatingtech.com/products/LTI_Boston_Arm_Systems.asp (accessed September 30, 2012).

[44] Anon, Ottobock – Rotator, http://www.ottobockus.com/cps/rde/xchg /ob_us_en/ hs.xsl/16562.html?id=16638 (accessed September 30, 2012).

[45] Pons JL, Ceres R, Rocon E, Levin S, Markovitz I, Saro B, et al. Virtual reality training and EMG control of the MANUS hand prosthesis. Robotica. 2005;23(03):311–7.

[46] Khushaba RN, Kodagoda S, Takruri M, Dissanayake G. Toward improved control of prosthetic fingers using surface electromyogram (EMG) signals. Expert Systems with Applications. 2012 Sep 15;39(12):10731–8.

Chapter 13

Simulator of a Myoelectrically Controlled Prosthetic Hand with Graphical Display of Upper Limb and Hand Posture

Gonzalo A. García, Ryuhei Okuno and Kenzo Akazawa

Additional information is available at the end of the chapter

http://dx.doi.org/10.5772/55503

1. Introduction

Three types of prosthetic hand are currently available: cosmetic, body-powered, and myoelectric (Laschi *et al.*, 2000). Cosmetic prostheses are passive, and designed to look like the natural hand, with solely an aesthetic purpose. Body-powered prostheses are powered and controlled by body movements, generally of the shoulder or of the back. Myoelectric hands are electrically powered and controlled by electromyographic (EMG) signals; *i.e.*, small electric potentials produced by contracting muscles. Myoelectric hands are typically controlled in switched or simple proportional mode, according to the amplitude of the EMG signals (Stein and Walley, 1983; Näder, 1990; Sears and Shaperman, 1991; Bergman *et al.*, 1992; Kyberd and Chappell, 1994). The switched control is the simplest one, as it consists of only two states: on or off. Although much progress has been made in myoelectric hands, their motor functions are still not comparable with those of a natural hand, partly because they have been designed to provide only the most basic functions of a natural hand, such as grasping and holding.

Akazawa's Lab has developed a myoelectric prosthetic hand (*Osaka Hand*) that simulates fundamental dynamic properties of the neuromuscular control system of the human hand, mainly the viscoelastic properties of muscles, which depend on their stiffness (Akazawa *et al.*, 1987). This hand can be used by an amputee subject with almost the same subconscious control that he/she had prior amputation (Okuno *et al.*, 1999).

The current design of the *Osaka Hand* requires the user to be fitted for and to wear a handmade fiberglass or thermoplastic socket into which the stump is comfortably and tightly inserted. The *Osaka Hand* is attached to the other tip of the socket via a screw. This socket is expensive to produce and requires weeks to manufacture after measurements are taken (Sears, 1991).

An additional initial problem is that shortly after an amputation atrophy of the remnant muscles occurs, and their EMG signal becomes very weak. As that EMG signals are used to control the prosthesis, users wanting to wear the *Osaka Hand* (or any other myoelectric hand) must undergo a training phase in which their remnant muscles are strengthened and at the same time they re-learn how to perform fine, detailed muscles contractions, which are needed for a precise control of the prosthetic hand.

In order to solve the two problems mentioned above, we developed a graphic simulator system for the *Osaka Hand* that eliminates the need of a socket for attachment of that prosthetic hand to the stump and it is also used for physical training of myoelectric patients.

A number of works on prosthesis simulators have been already described, each of them fitting the specific requirements of a given prosthesis. Yamada *et al.* (1983) employed six different bi-dimensional (2D), fix images appearing on the screen depending on the frequency and amplitude pattern of three EMG signals in order to evaluate their proposed control method for a theoretical prosthetic hand. Daley *et al.* (1990) developed a simple 2D graphical simulator for operator performance comparison when using different myoelectric control strategies. Abul-Haj and Hogan (1987) performed an emulation with a combination of software and hardware for elbow-prosthesis prototypes evaluation. Perlin *et al.* (1989) developed a simulation program for their Utah/MIT 16-joint, four-finger *Dextrous Hand*.

Several works describe simulators operated by shoulder movement; Zahedi and Farahani (1995), for example, used a graphical simulator for a fuzzy EMG classifier; Durfee *et al.* (1991) created a 2D graphic simulator to evaluate command channels trough which control an upper limb neural prosthesis; and Zafar and Van Doren (2000) employed a video-based simulator for a shoulder-activated neuroprosthesis for spinal cord injured persons. Lin and Huang (1997) made a computer simulation of a robotic hand to test its potential use as a prosthesis.

There are already some commercially available systems such as *MyoBoy* –from OTTO BOCK HealthCare GmbH (Duderstadt, Germany)- that is a software tool used for the evaluation, selection, training, and documentation of myoelectric patients. MOTION CONTROL Inc. (Utah, USA) has developed an EMG tester and trainer (*Myolab II*) that is used to locate intact muscle activity and to help patients in strengthening and relaxation tasks.

However, all the abovementioned simulators can be used only with prosthetic hands with a switched or single proportional mode, not for those with a more complex control mode as the one of the *Osaka Hand*.

The goal of the present work was to develop an upper limb and hand graphic simulator system that solves the abovementioned problems, allowing amputee subjects to try virtually the myoelectric hand without needing the socket, and to perform the physical training required prior to use the real one. This simulator allows us also to easily identify the optimal electrode location for the EMG signals acquisition in each individual. In addition, the simulator allows physicians and related staff to recognize how easily the hand can be controlled and its advantages over other kinds of prosthesis.

The simulator that we have developed consists of a data acquisition system, a mathematical model that simulated the behavior of the *Osaka Hand* (including its model of the human neuromuscular control system dynamics), and a graphics display device.

2. Materials and methods

2.1. Structure of the *Osaka Hand*

A general overview of the system is shown in Figure 1. An exceptional feature of the *Osaka Hand* is that the user can control voluntarily the angle of its fingers and the stiffness of the grip (the resistance that the fingers oppose to change their angle) by the EMGs of flexor and extensor muscles of the wrist (see details in Akazawa *et al.*, 1987).

To obtain such a control, the *Osaka Hand* mimics the properties of both muscle viscoelasticity and the gain of the stretch reflex (both varying linearly with muscle activity). The dynamics of this neuromuscular control system were determined by analyzing the tension responses of finger muscle to mechanical stretch (Akazawa *et al.*, 1999). The dynamics are quite complex, due to the non-linearity and time delay of the stretch reflex; however, we used a simple model representing the dynamics as a first approximation. Once that model was introduced in the prosthetic hand, it was proved that a sound-limbed subject and an amputee subject were able to accurately control finger angle and stiffness of the prosthetic hand (Okuno *et al.*, 1999).

As shown in Figure 1, for each subject a pair of surface electrodes were put on the *flexor carpi radialis* (wrist flexor muscle) and another pair on their *extensor carpi radialis brevi* (wrist extensor muscle) to measure their EMG signal. The measured signal was amplified in differential mode, full-wave rectified, and then smoothed with a low-pass filter to obtain its envelope, the amplitude of which is approximately proportional to the force exerted by the muscle (Basmajian and Deluca, 1985). Therefore, the resultant signal corresponded to the isometric contractile force (torque) of each muscle: A_f being the torque of the flexor muscle, and A_e the torque of the extensor muscle.

From those two calculated torques, the desired finger angle $\tilde{\Theta}_H$ of the end effector (the target angle the user wants to achieve) was calculated as

$$\tilde{\Theta}_H(s) = \{P_H(s) + A_e(s) - A_f(s)\} / G_x(s) \tag{1}$$

where P_H is the grip force exerted by the fingers of the *Osaka Hand*, and was measured by strain gauges (KYOWA DENGYO Co., Ltd. (Yokohama, Japan), model KFG-1N) attached to its thumb, index, and middle fingers. $G_x(s)$is the transfer function that represents the dynamics of human neuromuscular control system (Akazawa *et al.*, 1987; Okuno *et al.*, 1999), and is given by:

$$G_x(s) = K\frac{1+\tau_2 s}{1+\tau_1 s} \tag{2}$$

where the time constants were calculated to be τ_1=0.12s and τ_2=0.25s, and the gain K corresponds to the stiffness of the prosthesis fingers, which is not constant, but time-varying as:

$$K(t) = K_0 + a\left[A_f(t) + A_e(t)\right], \tag{3}$$

in proportion to the contraction level of the extensor-flexor muscles pair. The user can regulate the stiffness of the hand fingers angle by varying the level of contraction of each of those muscles. The stiffness at resting state K_0 is 0.1 Nm/rad, and the coefficient a is 0.98 rad^{-1}. A software program implementing this model was introduced in the microprocessor that controls the end effector.

The position control system (see Figure 1) consists of a DC motor (MINIMOTOR SA, Croglio, Switzerland, type 2233), its servo controller (Figure 1(c2)), and a one degree-of-freedom end effector with three fingers (Figure 1(c3)). Index and middle fingers are bound between them and are endorsed with an open-close movement with respect to the thumb. This movement is produced by the DC motor, the servo controller of which works to nullify the difference between the commanded angle $\tilde{\Theta}_H$ and the actual motor rotational angle $\hat{\Theta}_H$ as measured by an optical encoder.

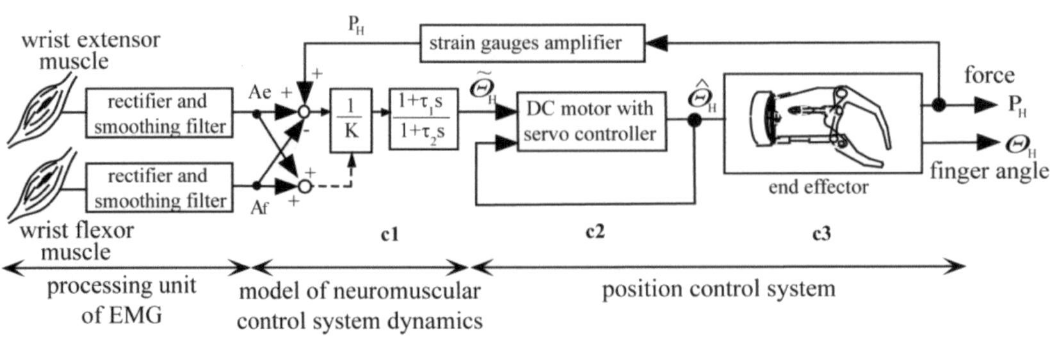

Figure 1. Block diagram of the *Osaka Hand*. The model of the human neuromuscular control system dynamics (labeled as c1) takes the processed EMG signals A_e and A_f from the subject's forearm and calculates the target angle $\tilde{\Theta}_H$; the servo controller (c2) works to nullify the difference between $\tilde{\Theta}_H$ and the actual motor rotational angle $\hat{\Theta}_H$. The end effector (c3) has one opening-closing degree-of-freedom Θ_H.

http://dx.doi.org/10.5772/55503

2.2. Composition and operation of the simulator

Figure 2 shows the components of the simulator system, which can be divided into three main sub-systems: data acquisition (EMG and video), processing, and display. Ten light emitter diode (LED) markers and two pairs of surface electrodes are attached to the subject's upper limb as shown in Figure 2(a) and 2(b). Those LEDs and electrodes provide the inputs for the processing sub-system, which is implemented in the graphic workstation (Figure 2(c)).

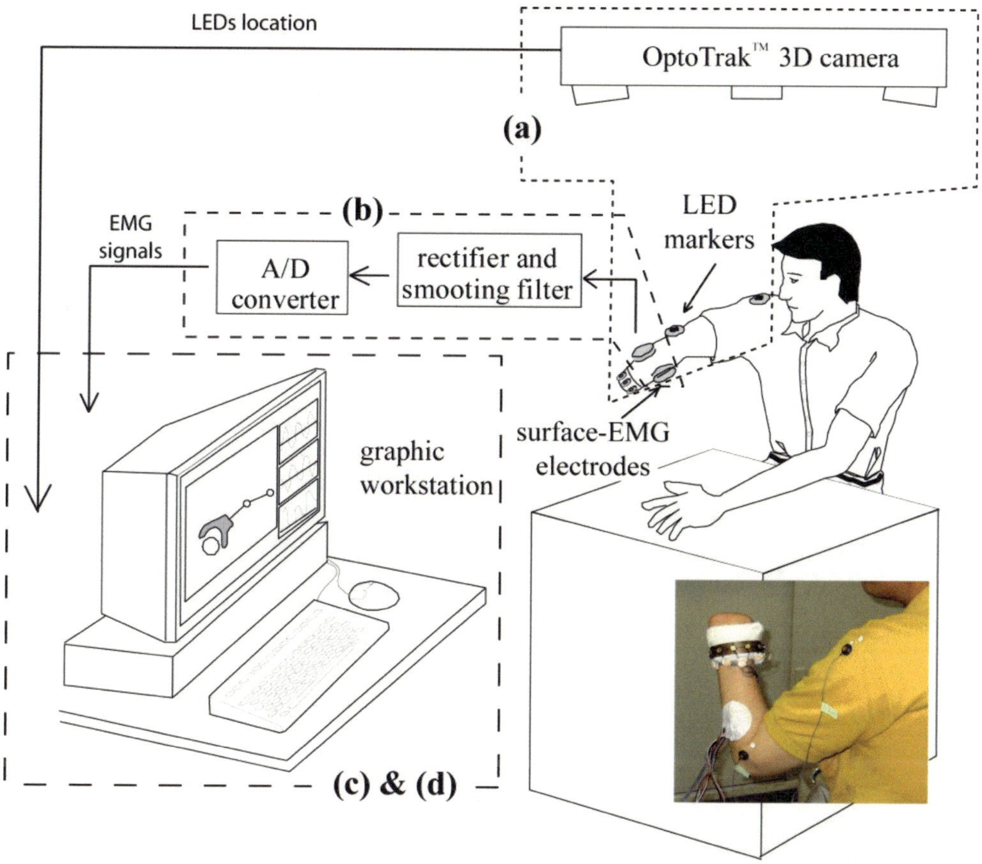

Figure 2. Overview of the simulator components. The graphic workstation (GW) receives the 3D location of the LED markers (a) attached to the subject's arm and the processed EMG signals from two surface electrodes placed on the subject's forearm (b). From these data, the GW calculates and displays (c and d) the finger angle and the arm posture. Inset: detail of LED markers attachment.

Figure 3 shows the block diagram of the simulator, illustrating how the processing system (Figure 3(c)) determines the position of the upper limb from the three-dimensional (3D) location of the markers on the shoulder, elbow, and wrist detected with an OPTOTRAK™ 3D camera (NORTHERN DIGITAL Inc., Ontario, Canada) (Figures 2(a) and 3(a)). The processing system determines the desired finger angle from the processed surface EMGs of both wrist flexor and extensor muscles of the subject (Figures 2(b) and 3(b)). The virtual upper limb and hand are ultimately presented on the 3D graphic workstation (display system, Figure 3(d)).

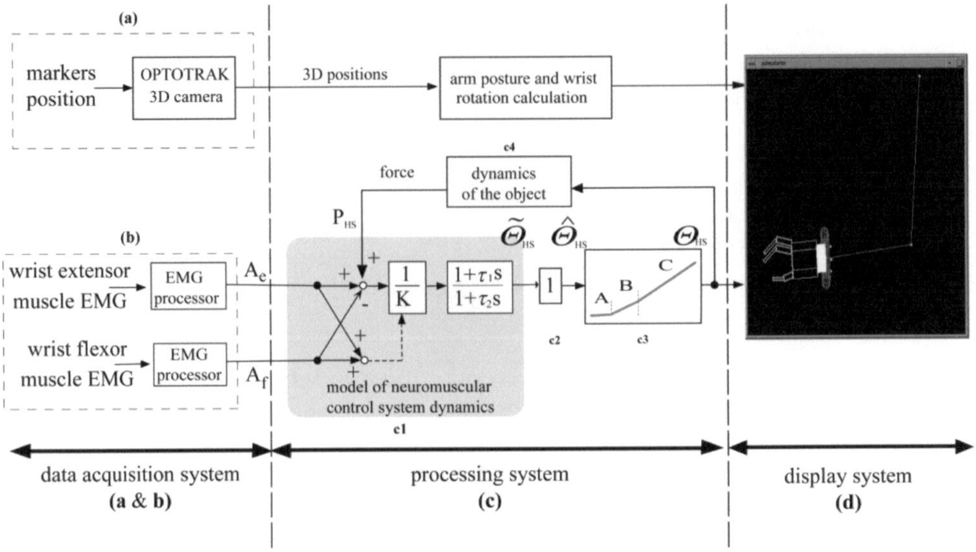

Figure 3. Simulator block diagram. With the 3D markers position obtained from the Optotrak 3D camera (block a), the processing system (c) calculates subject's arm posture and wrist rotational angle. From the processed EMG signals A_e and A_f (b), the model of the human neuromuscular control system dynamics (c1) calculates a first approximation of the desired angle $\tilde{\Theta}_{HS}$. The dynamics of the servo control system (c2) can be regarded as the identity, $\tilde{\Theta}_{HS}=\hat{\Theta}_{HS}$. Non-linear characteristics of the relationship between $\hat{\Theta}_{HS}$ and Θ_{HS} are inserted in block c3. The virtual arm and prosthetic hand are displayed in the display system (d).

2.2.1. Data acquisition system

The OPTOTRAK 3D camera (Figure 2(a) and Figure 3(a)) detects the position of the LED markers attached to the user's shoulder, elbow, and wrist. The marker on the shoulder is attached to the point where the movement of the *acromion* of the scapula is smallest during the motion of the arm. The marker on the elbow is fixed in the external palate of the humeral. The arm posture is calculated from those LEDs locations.

To measure the rotational angle of the wrist during an external pronation of the arm, eight LEDs are placed on the external side of a bracelet-like device attached to the wrist (shown in the inset of Figure 2).

The EMG signals of wrist muscles are picked up with surface electrodes (Figure 2(b) and Figure 3(b)). These signals are then amplified (gain 58.8 dB, CMRR 110 dB) to the range ±5 V, full-wave rectified, smoothed with a second order low-pass filter (cut-off frequency 2.7 Hz), and then sampled at a frequency of 25 Hz, 12 bits per sample (resolution of ±2.4 mV, less than 0.01% of the maximum value) with an OPTOTRAK Data Acquisition Unit (NORTHERN DIGITAL Inc., Ontario, Canada).

http://dx.doi.org/10.5772/55503

2.2.2. Processing system

The location of the LEDs and the processed EMG signals are collected by a graphics workstation (GW, SILICON GRAPHICS, Inc., California, USA) that holds the processing system software (Figure 2(c) and Figure 3(c)).

The angle that the user wants to achieve with the prosthesis fingers (the target angle) is given by Eqs. (2) and (3) using the current value of user's EMG signals A_e and A_f. Those equations are calculated in the real *Osaka Hand* by a Z-transform that gives in discrete time their solution, originally expressed in the frequency domain (see Figure 3(c1)). In the case of the processing system of the simulator, the sampling frequency is not high enough to allow using that transform. Therefore, we used the Runge-Kutta-Gill approximation method for differential equations in order to implement the transfer function $G_x(s)$ (Eqs. (2) and (3)).

Dynamics of the DC motor servo system of the actual prosthetic hand were calculated in terms of the relationship between target angle $\tilde{\Theta}_H$ and rotational angle $\hat{\Theta}_H$ of the motor shaft (see Figure 1). In the steady case, we assumed $\hat{\Theta}_H = \tilde{\Theta}_H$, with zero time delay (Figure 3(c2)).

In order to model the relationship between $\hat{\Theta}_H$ and final finger angle Θ_H of the real *Osaka Hand* (see Figure 1), we performed the following measurements by attaching two LEDs to the prosthesis chassis and one on each fingertip as shown in Figure 4. The hand finger angle Θ_H was defined as the angle formed between the vectors $\overrightarrow{M_1M_3}$ and $\overrightarrow{M_1M_4}$, *i.e.*, the angle between the fingertips with respect to the chassis. The operation range of this angle is from 0° to 110°. The relationship between $\hat{\Theta}_H$ and final finger angle Θ_H (see Figure 1) was modeled with a piecewise approximation calculated by a least squares method. The error was always below 8% with an average of 1.7%, standard deviation (s.d.) 1.36. We roughly divided the operation range into three areas, as shown in Figure 3(c3).

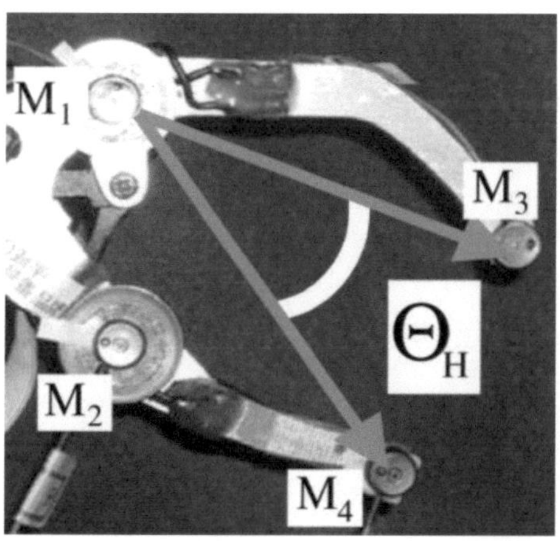

Figure 4. Finger angle Θ_H is defined as the angle formed between the vectors $\overrightarrow{M_1M_3}$ and $\overrightarrow{M_1M_4}$. M_1 to M_4 are LED markers attached to the prosthetic hand.

2.2.3. Display system

The tasks depicted in Figure 3(c1) to (c4) were implemented in a program that used OpenGL graphical library to represent the virtual arm and prosthetic hand by the wire-frame drawing shown in Figure 3(d). The refresh rate was 25 frames/s, which was sufficient to give the impression of smooth motion. In addition, the GW displayed the processed EMG signals used as input. During the experiments, supplementary information was displayed to guide the subject to achieve the proposed goal.

2.3. Common experimental set-up

To test the performance, validity, and controllability of the simulated hand, several experiments were carried out with three male, able-bodied subjects aged 22, 24, and 32; and a 43-years-old male who had both hands amputated 18 years earlier after a traffic accident. All of them gave their informed consent.

The amputee subject uses a body-powered hook at the end of the right upper limb and a body-powered hand at the end of the left upper limb. He had worn a myoelectric prosthetic hand on the right upper-limb until four years before the experiment. Since then, he has not been actively using his forearms muscles; for this reason, he suffered from muscular atrophy (very weak muscles) in both forearms. Consequently, his EMG signals corresponding to the maximal voluntary contraction (MVC) had a value of less than 20% of the average MVC of the three non-amputee subjects (0.65V/3.51V). In addition, he exhibited a slightly higher level of involuntary co-contraction (simultaneous contraction of antagonist muscles) in his wrist flexor and extensor muscles.

All subjects performed the same protocol composed of four sessions. One session consisted of two different tasks: angle and position control. Subjects repeated these tasks from three to five times in each session.

The subject sat barefoot in a chair, with one foot on a steel sheet on the floor in front of the chair and with sleeves rolled up to expose the forearm. The steel sheet was used as reference voltage for the EMG processing unit. The subject was instructed to sit in a relaxed position in a chair, with the forearm and the arm forming an angle of about 15°. The forearm of the right-hand was cleaned with SkinPure skin abrasion gel (NIHON KOHDEN Corp., Tokyo, Japan) and ethanol. A pair of bipolar, surface electrodes (Ag-AgCl, 1 cm in diameter; NIHON KOHDEN Corp., Tokyo, Japan. Type NS-111U) was attached, with a centre-to-centre distance of about 2 cm, following the muscle fiber direction of the wrist flexor muscle (*flexor carpi radialis*), and another pair was positioned on the wrist extensor muscle (*extensor carpi radialis brevi*). Gelaid electrode paste (NIHON KOHDEN Corp., Tokyo, Japan) was placed in the contact area between the skin and the electrodes to ensure good electric conductivity between them. The subject was then given a brief explanation of how the system functions.

Before starting the experiments, the subject was instructed to exert for 1 second his maximal contraction of each target muscle from which the EMG signals were taken. The simulator calculated the MVC amplitude value for each muscle as the average around its EMG peak (the maximum detected value). The EMG signals of each subject were normalized to the range of 0-1 by their respective MVC values.

To familiarize the subject with the equipment and functioning of the simulator, the subject was firstly instructed to freely move the virtual hand contracting his forearm muscles. When he felt comfortable with the system, the different sessions of experiments were performed. In order to avoid fatigue, a rest was scheduled between tasks, and the subject was not asked to keep any of the postures for more than a few seconds (Basmajian and Deluca, 1985; Kampas, 2001).

After the experiments, a short questionnaire was given to the amputee volunteer to gather feedback on the *Osaka Hand* and on its simulator. Some questions were based on the surveys described by Sears and Shaperman (1998) as well as Atkins *et al.* (1996). This gathered information allowed us to plan the direction of our future research.

3. Experiments and results

Two types of experiments were carried out; the ones of the first block (3.1) were oriented to check whether the behavior of the simulator corresponded to the behavior of the *Osaka Hand*. The experiments of the second block (3.2) checked the controllability of the simulator.

3.1. Behavior of the simulator system

3.1.1. Validation of the input-output relationship

EMG signals were acquired from one subject as explained in the previous section and given as input to the simulator and, simultaneously, to the *Osaka Hand*. In this way, we were able to compare their respective output, which is the angle of the fingers, when both were given the same input.

Figure 5 shows the result of one of these experiments, carried out with a non-amputee subject freely moving the simulated hand. Figure 5(a) shows the inputs of the system: processed EMG signals of the wrist extensor muscle (dashed line) and those of the wrist flexor muscle (solid line). Figure 5(b) shows a comparison between the finger angle of the *Osaka Hand* (thick line) and the one given by the simulator (thin line). The average of the error (difference between the angle given by the simulated hand and that of the real *Osaka Hand*) was 0.85° (s.d. 0.39), with a maximum of 3.54°, which we consider acceptable for our purpose.

3.1.2. Variable stiffness

As one of the main features of the *Osaka Hand* is that the subject can control its stiffness by antagonist muscles co-contraction, we performed another experiment to corroborate that the stiffness of the virtual hand fingers can be controlled in that same way.

To simulate different levels of co-contraction, we fed the simulator with different levels of A_e and A_f under the condition ($A_e = A_f$) (see Figure 3(b) and (c1)). We sinusoidally modulated the

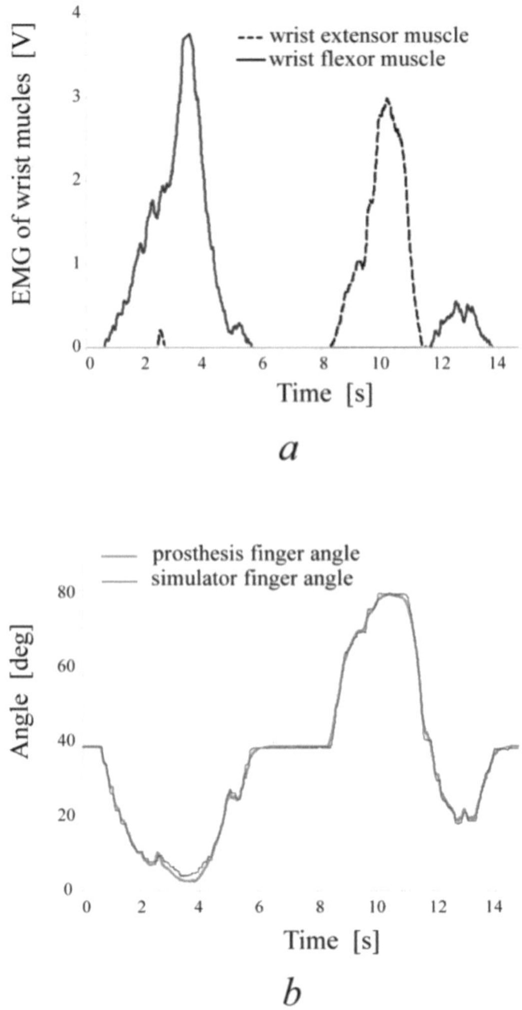

Figure 5. Comparison between simulator and actual *Osaka Hand* finger angles. (a) Same inputs given to both the simulator and the prosthetic hand. (b) Simulator output (thin line) and prosthesis actual finger angle (thick line).

applied grip force P_{HS} (see Figure 3(c4)) at a frequency of 0.2 Hz and a range between -0.08 V and 0.08 V, which corresponds to the actual output amplitude of the strain gauges. Figure 6 shows that as $A_e + A_f$ increased –that is, as the level of co-contraction increased-, in response to the same perturbation P_{HS}, the finger angle displacement decreased; that is, the stiffness increased. When there was no co-contraction ($A_e + A_f$ = 0V), the perturbation caused the total opening of the hand (110° is its maximal aperture), but when the level of co-contraction was maximum ($A_e + A_f$ = 10V), the perturbation had nearly no effect on the angle of the hand fingers. Therefore, the simulator behaves like the *Osaka Hand* also in stiffness.

3.1.3. *Effect of force feedback*

We carried out a preliminary experiment to study the simulator behavior when a subject grasped a virtual object (a sphere). The mechanical dynamics of the object were modeled in a simple fashion as a spring (Figure 3(c4)). The exerted force P_{HS} was calculated then as

$$P_{HS} = K_s \cdot (\Theta_{HS} - \Theta_{HS0}) \tag{4}$$

where K_s is the spring constant; Θ_{HS0} is the finger angle when the contact with the object occurs, and Θ_{HS} is the current angle. The inputs A_e and A_f to the simulator were given as sinusoidal waves. Figure 7(a) compares the fingers angle when grasping the sphere: continuous line curve corresponds to the experiment carried out without P_{HS} feedback; and the dashed line curve when P_{HS} was calculated as explained above.

The first contact fingers-sphere occurred at $t = 9.5s$ (marked in the graph as A), when the fingers angle was around 43°. The maximal grasping force occurs when the fingers angle without P_{HS} was 3°. Therefore, there is a difference of approximately 40° in Θ_{HS} providing or not P_{HS} feedback, practically the third part of the whole simulated fingers angle range (110 °).

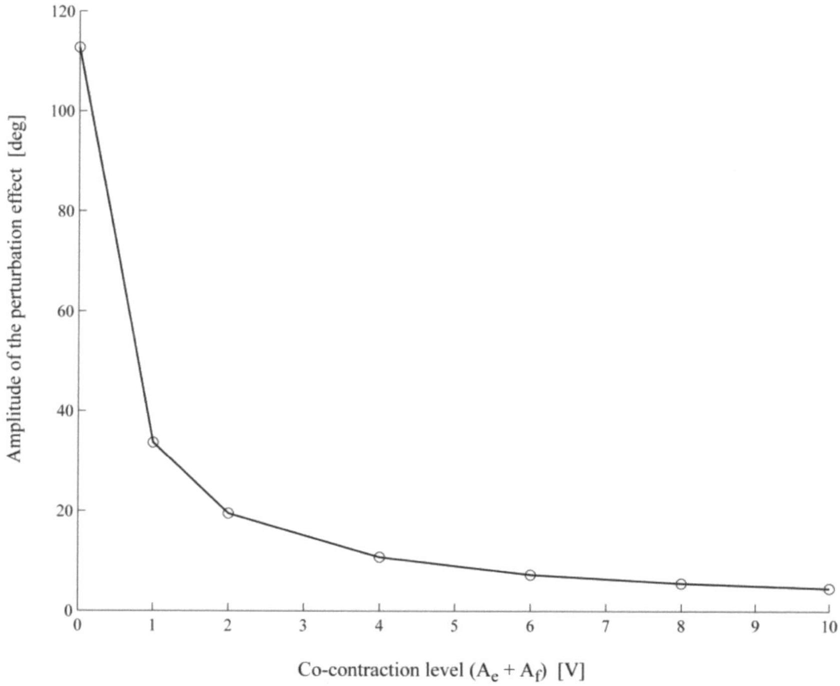

Figure 6. Stiffness (resistance to perturbations) control experiment. In response to the same simulated perturbation, an increase of co-contraction level decreases the amplitude of the perturbation effect (increase of the stiffness).

Figure 7(*b*) shows the value of the calculated P_{HS}. When it reaches its maximal value, approximately 25 mV (roughly one third of its maximum), the difference between the fingers target angle with and without pressure feedback is nearly 10°. Therefore, as it happens with the real prosthetic hand (Okuno *et al.*, 1999), P_{HS} gives self-control to the hand over the exerted force when grasping objects, producing a smoother grasping motion.

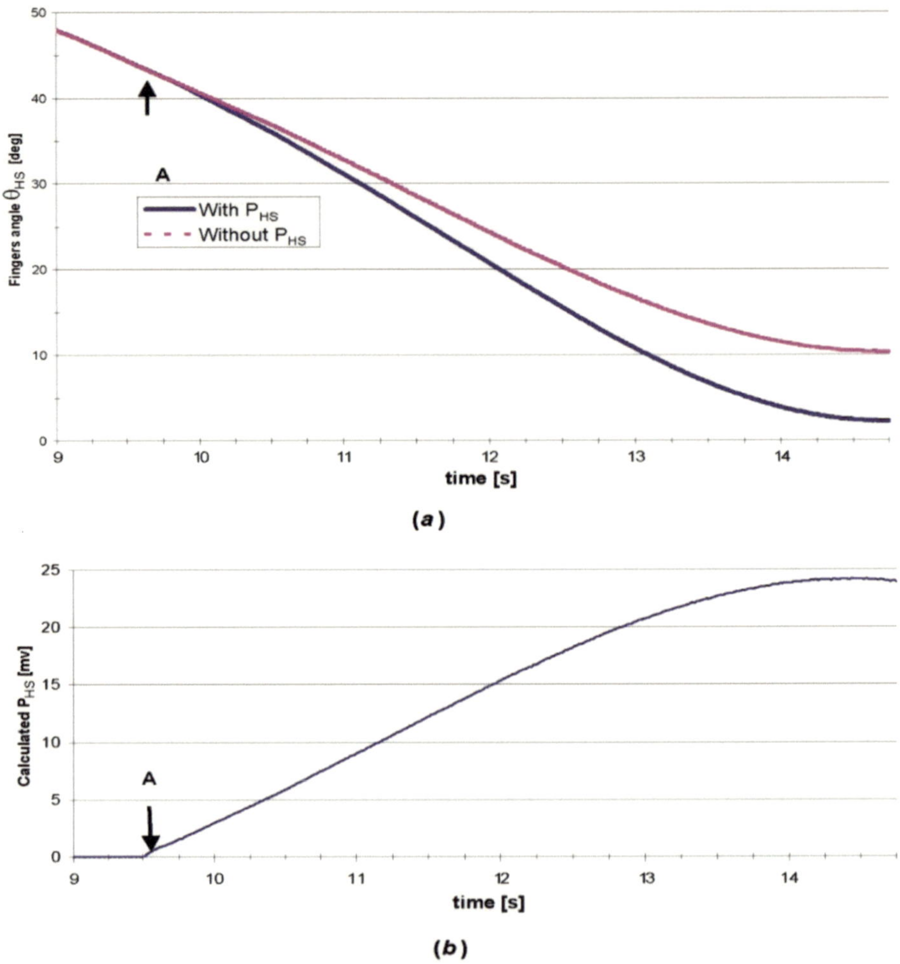

Figure 7. Soften effect (*a*) obtained when a simulated pressure feedback P_{HS} (*b*) was given to the simulator.

3.2. Control experiments

3.2.1. Finger angle control

We ran a control experiment to determine how accurately the subjects could control the finger angle of the simulator hand. The effects of using the simulator were also investigated by comparing the performance of the subjects before and after two trails. In this finger angle control task, the subject was asked to achieve a series of eight different angles (from 0° to 110°) showed on the screen of the GW.

Figure 8 shows the typical results obtained, where the target angle to achieve was 55° (thick horizontal line). Figures 8(a) and 8(c) (left column) show the results of the first trial of two different subjects; (a) a sound-limbed subject and (c) the amputee subject. Both subjects needed more than 4 s to be able to keep the angle within the acceptable range, and were able to maintain it there for only less than 2 s (period between points *A* and *B*).

Figure 8(b) shows the results obtained by the sound-limbed subject after several trials for a period of about 40 min, and Figure 8(d) for the amputee subject after a similar period. In this case, both achieved the angle in just approximately 1 s (point *A*), and held it until they were asked to relax the muscles (point *B*).

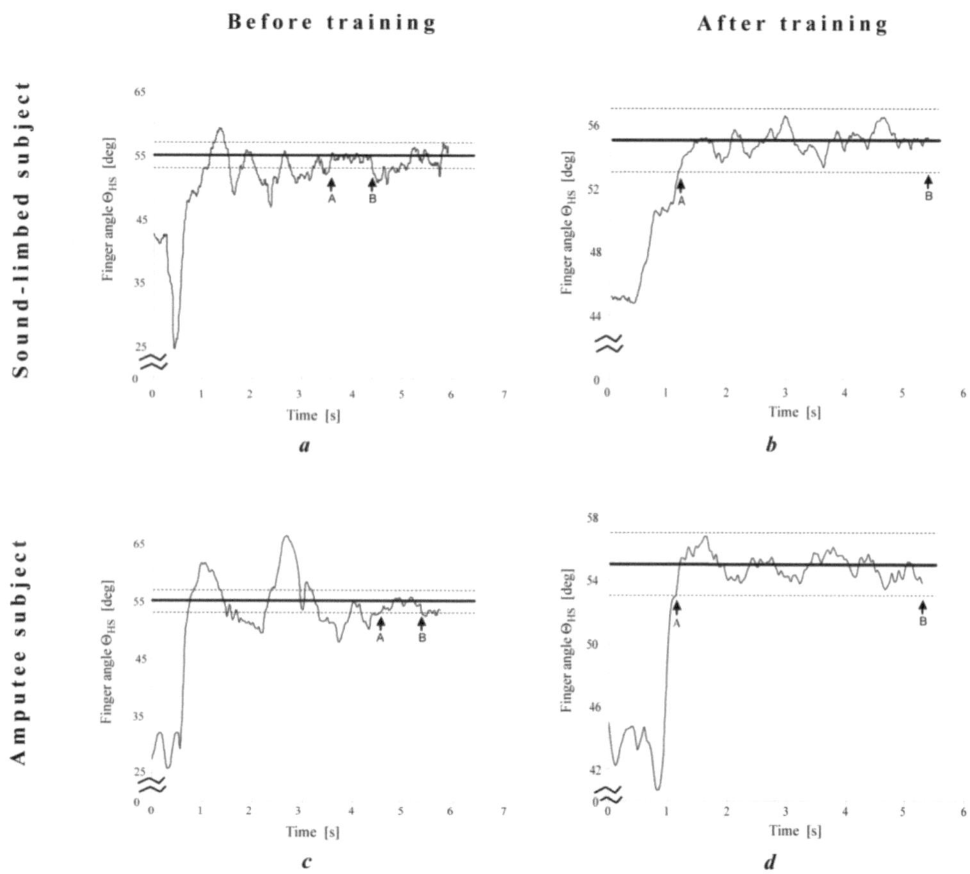

Figure 8. Effect of training on position control (step response). The target angle was 55°, marked by a thick horizontal line. We defined the acceptable error range as ±2° (dashed horizontal lines). (a) shows the result of the first session by the sound-limbed subject ((c), amputee subject). (b) shows his result after training ((d), amputee subject).

To measure how accurately the subjects performed the task, we calculated the mean square error ε made while trying to keep a constant target angle Θ_{target} as

$$\varepsilon = \frac{1}{N}\sum_{n=1}^{N}\sqrt{(\Theta_{HS}[n]-\Theta_{target})^2} \tag{5}$$

where $\Theta_{HS}[n]$ is the hand simulator finger angle in the sample n, and N is the number of samples between the points A and B. We defined ±2° as the acceptable range of error (dashed horizontal lines in Figure 8).

The average of the error ε was 1.19° (s.d. 0.67) for the three non-amputee subjects and 1.78° (s.d. 0.54°) for the amputee subject.

3.2.2. Grasping control

An additional control experiment was carried out to examine whether the subjects were able to grasp a virtual object using the simulator hand. In this grasping control task, six spheres with different diameters (from 2 mm to 10 cm) were depicted one at a time on a fix position on the simulator screen. The subject was instructed to grasp them with the virtual hand. To give some feedback to the subjects about the virtual force exerted over the sphere, a second index finger was drawn (with a very faint color) in the position the simulated index finger would have been if there was not a solid object in its way.

The results of this experiment were very similar to the ones shown in Figure 8. In this case, we defined the error as the distance between the index fingertip and the surface of the sphere. The average error while subjects tried to hold onto the sphere in the last two trails of each subject was 1.32 mm (s.d. 0.47). For the amputee subject, the average error was 1.77 mm (s.d. 0.63). In conclusion, subjects were able to grasp the object, and to do it in a smooth, natural way. These results prove that the simulator developed in this work is a valid tool for rehabilitation.

4. Conclusion

In this study, we have introduced a simulator of our biomimetic, myoelectric prosthetic hand (*Osaka Hand*), which is operated by the subject's EMG signals, and displays in 3D a virtual arm and a prosthetic hand.

We have demonstrated that the simulator output agrees sufficiently for practical use with the finger angle of the prosthetic hand when both are given the same input.

Usefulness of the simulator has been shown in the experiments of controlling angle and stiffness of the hand. After a short period of training, subjects were able to control quite accurately the simulated hand. The precision achieved by an amputee subject was nearly as good as the precision obtained by the three non-amputee subjects, even though the amputee had not actively used his forearm muscles for four years.

This kind of powered myoelectric prostheses is not yet widely known. For example, in Japan only 350 units have been sold in the last 30 years (report of the Ministry of Health, Labour and Welfare of Japan). Our simulator could be accessible to physicians and related staff and be used to offer the opportunity to a wider group of amputees to try a myoelectrically controlled prosthesis.

The simulator can also be used for EMG signal processing and modeling. For example, when new features are added to the *Osaka Hand*, such as a new control program, the simulator can help in the design and testing phases, since it is easier and less expensive to make modifications in the model than in the actual prosthesis.

This simulator could be easily adapted to any myoelectric prosthesis, by performing just a few simple modifications on its software.

Acknowledgements

This work was partially funded by the Ministry of Education, Culture, Sports, Science, and Technology of Japan. G.A.G. was funded by a grant from the same Ministry (*Monbusho*). This work was carried out at Akazawa's Laboratory, Graduate School of Information Science and Technology, Osaka University (Osaka, Japan).

G.A.G. thanks Professor Pedro García Teodoro (Granada University, Granada, Spain) for encouragement and scientific support during the first stages of this project.

Authors would like to thank as well Dr. Sandra Rainieri (AZTI Foundation, Bilbao, Spain) and Professor Antonio Peinado (Granada University, Granada, Spain) for useful comments and input on the original manuscript.

Author details

Gonzalo A. García[1], Ryuhei Okuno[2] and Kenzo Akazawa[2]

1 Freelance, Bilbao, Spain

2 Department of Electrical and Electronic Engineering, Setsunan University, Osaka, Japan

References

[1] Abul-Haj, C., and Hogan, N. (1987): 'An emulator system for developing improved elbow-prosthesis designs', *IEEE Trans. Biomed. Eng.*, 34, pp. 724-737

[2] Akazawa, K., Okuno, R., and Kusumoto, H. (1999): 'Relation between intrinsic viscoelasticity and activation level of the human finger muscle during voluntary isometric contraction', *Frontiers Med. Biol. Engng.*, 9, pp. 123-135

[3] Akazawa, K., Hayashi, Y., and Fujii, K. (1987): 'Myoelectrically controlled hand prosthesis with neuromuscular control system dynamics'. Proc. 9th Int. Symp. On External Control of Human Extremities, Dubrovnik, Yugoslavia.

[4] Atkins, D. J., Heard, D. C. Y., and Donovan, W. H. (1996): 'Epidemiologic overview of individuals with upper-limb loss and their reported research priorities', *Journal of Prosthetics and Orthotics*, 8(1), pp. 2-12

[5] Basmajian, J. V., and Deluca, C. J. (1985): 'Muscle alive. Their functions revealed by electromyography. Fifth edition, (Williams and Wilkins, Baltimore).

[6] Bergman, K., Ornholner, L., Zackrisson, K. and Thyberg, M. (1992): 'Functional benefit of an adaptive myoelectric prosthetic hand compared to a conventional myoelectric hand', *Prosthet. Orthot. Int.*, 16, pp. 32-37

[7] Daley, T. L., Scott, R. N., Parker, P. A., and Lovely, D. F. (1990): 'Operator performance in myoelectric control of a multifunction prosthesis simulator', *Jour. Rehab. Res. Dev.*, 27, pp. 9-20

[8] Durfee, W. K., Mariano, T. R., and Zahradnik, J. L. (1991): 'Simulator for evaluating shoulder motion as a command source for FES grasp restoration systems', *Arch. Phys. Med. Rehabil.*, 72, pp. 1088-1094

[9] Kampas, P., (2001): "The optimal use of myoelectrodes", Translation of: *Med. Orth. Tech.* 121, pp. 21-27

[10] Kyberd, P. J., and Chappell, P. H. (1994): 'The Southampton hand: an intelligent myoelectric prosthesis', *J. Rehabil. Res. Dev.*, 31, pp. 326-334

[11] Laschi, C., Dario, P., Carrozza, M. C., Guglielmelli, E., Teti, G., Taddeucci, D., Leoni, F., Massa, B., Zecca, M. and Lazzarini, R. (2000): 'Grasping and manipulation in humanoid robotics'. First IEEE-RAS Workshop on Humanoids - Humanoids 2000, Boston, Massachuset.

[12] Lin, L., and Huang, H. (1997): 'Mechanism and computer simulation of a new robot hand for potential use as an artificial hand', *Artificial Organs*, 21(1), pp. 59-69

[13] Ministry of Health, Labour and Welfare of Japan: http://www.mhlw.go.jp

[14] Motion Control Inc (Utah, USA) '*Myolab II*'. http://www.utaharm.com/products.htm

[15] Näder, M. (1990): 'The artificial substitution of missing hands with myoelectrical prostheses', *Clin. Orth. & Rela. Res.*, 258, pp. 9-17

[16] Okuno, R., Yoshida, M., and Akazawa, K. (1999): 'Biomimetic myoelectric hand with voluntary control of finger angle and compliance', *Frontiers Med. Biol. Engng.*, 9, pp. 192-210

[17] Otto Bock HealthCare GmbH (Duderstadt, Germany): '757M10 *MyoBoy*', http://www.ottobockus.com/products/op_myoboy.htm

[18] Perlin, K, Demmel, J. W, & Wright, P. K. (1989). Simulation Software for the Utah/MIT Dextrous Hand, *Robotics & Computer-Integrated Manufacturing*, 5, 281-292.

[19] Sears, H. H., and Shaperman, J. (1998): 'Electric wrist rotation in proportional-controlled systems', *Journal of Prosthetics and Orthotics*, 10(4), pp. 92-98

[20] Sears, H. H. (1991): 'Approaches to prescription of body-powered and myoelectric prostheses', *Physical Medicine and Rehabilitation Clinics of North American*, 2(2), pp. 361-371

[21] Sears, H. H., and Shaperman, J. (1991): 'Proportional myoelectric hand control', *Am. J. Phys. Med. Rehabil.*, 10, pp. 20-28

[22] Stein, R. B., and Walley, M. (1983): 'Functional comparison of upper extremity amputees using myoelectric and conventional prosthesis', *Arch. Phys. Med. Rehabil.*, 64, pp. 243-248

[23] Yamada, M., Niwa, N., and Uchiyama, A. (1983): 'Evaluation of a multifunctional hand prosthesis system using EMG controlled animation', *IEEE Trans. Biomed. Eng.*, 30, pp. 759-763

[24] Zafar, M., and Van Doren, C. L. (2000): 'Effectiveness of supplemental grasp-force feedback in the presence of vision', *Med. Bio. Eng. Comp.*, 38, pp. 267-274

[25] Zahedi, E., and Farahani, H. (1995): 'Graphical simulation of artificial hand motion with fuzzy EMG pattern recognition'. Proceedings RC IEEE-EMBS & 14th BMESI, 3.43

Chapter 14

Biofeedback with Pelvic Floor Electromyography as Complementary Treatment in Chronic Disorders of the Inferior Urinary Tract

B. Padilla-Fernandez, A. Gomez-Garcia,
M. N. Hernandez-Alonso, M.B. Garcia-Cenador,
J. A. Mirón-Canelo, A. Geanini-Yagüez,
J. M. Silva-Abuin and M. F. Lorenzo-Gomez

Additional information is available at the end of the chapter

http://dx.doi.org/10.5772/56237

1. Introduction

Chronic inflammatory disorders of the female urinary tract are common and often impact negatively on the quality of life of the affected individual. The management of these disorders, which encompass infectious and non-infectious conditions presenting with pain, is evolving as a result of current research. These changes are reflected in recent changes in the commonly used management guidelines.

Pelvic floor biofeedback with electromyography is used as a primary or adjuvant treatment for these disorders. In this chapter we present the experience gathered in our unit with this treatment modality.

1.1. Definitions

The Association for Applied Psychophysiology and Biofeedback, Inc. (http://www.aapb.org) defines biofeedback as: "the process of gaining greater awareness of many physiological functions primarily using instruments that provide information on those same systems, with a goal of being able to manipulate them at will." In their website it is further stated that: "Biofeedback is a process that enables an individual to learn how to change physiological activity for the purposes of improving health and performance". Precise instruments measure physiological activity such as brainwaves, heart function, breathing, muscle activity, and skin temperature. These instruments rapidly and accurately "feed back" information to the user. The presentation of this information —often in conjunction with changes in thinking, emotions, and behavior— supports desired physiological changes. Over time, these changes can endure without continued use of an instrument.

Also, biofeedback techniques have been defined as the use of instrumentation to help a person to instantly and better perceive the information of a specific physiological process which is under the control of the nervous system control but that is not correctly perceived (Miller 1974). Many physiological responses which are purely anatomical can be modified under voluntary control. The mechanisms for many of these responses include the relaxation of smooth or striated muscles or both (Repariz and Salinas 1995).

Programs for bladder re-education in women with bladder instability have opened new therapeutic perspectives for the various micturition dysfunctions (Frewen 1972 ; Cardozo, Abrams et al. 1978; Jarvis and Millar 1981; Cardozo and Stanton 1984)

Bladder sphincter re-education using surface electrodes was described for adults and children in 1979 and has since been widely applied (Maizels, King et al. 1979; Wear, Wear et al. 1979).

Electronic instrumentation allows the translation of normal or abnormal physiological processes (often unconscious) to visual or auditory signals. The method involves the manipulation of unconscious or involuntary events modifying these signals. Thus the technique is at the same time behavioural therapy and a learning process which aims at creating awareness of an unconscious function that is incorrectly performed, and to correct it. Biofeedback has allowed going from subjectivity to objectivity.

Individuals know little about their perineal region, and therefore control its functions (bladder, anorectal and sexual functions) poorly. Biofeedback permits a progressive and active awareness of these functions, creating a "ring" or "communication cycle" between patient and computer. The instructor serves as a guide in this Learning process.

Biofeedback with electromyography (BFB-EMG) was approved by the Food and Drug Administration in the USA in 1991. It has been effectively used since 1992 without secondary effects or complications (Perry 1994).

For biofeedback to be successful, it is important to have a single instructor conducting the sessions with a given patient. The following are also important for success: 1) A friendly attitude of the instructor; 2) A receptive and confident patient with sufficient cognitive ability; 3) Effective teaching technique 4) Patient's willingness to reproduce at home what was learned during the sessions; 5) A relaxed working atmosphere free of interruptions; 6) Patient friendly equipment 7) Adequate length and frequency of the sessions 8) A system of rewards to encourage the patient, 9) Confidence in success of the treatment.

The conditions listed below can benefit from biofeedback with EMG:

- Cauda equina syndrome with neurogenic bladder.
- Anal sphincter spasm.
- Atonic bladder.

- Extrinsic urethral sphincter's deficiency.
- Urethral instability.
- Muscle atrophy or weakness due to disuse.
- Fecal incontinence.
- Specific and non-specific acute urinary retention.
- Incomplete bladder emptying.
- Urgency urinary incontinence..
- Female stress urinary incontinence.
- Female and male mixed urinary incontinence.
- Urinary incontinence without voiding desire.
- Post-micturition dribling.
- Nocturnal enuresis.
- Continuous leakage and urinary frequency.

1.1.1. Existing protocols for perineal electromyography

Many protocols have been used to treat pelvic floor dysfunction. No single protocol is applicable to all patients given individual variations. We favour a personalized approach or "therapist guided method" in which one therapist carries out the entire treatment (Lorenzo Gómez, Silva Abuín et al. 2008).

Variations in described protocols include frequency and duration of the sessions. For example: Three 20-minutes sessions per week over a seven-week period (Amaro, Gameiro et al. 2006); twice weekly for 8 weeks (Voorham-van, Pelger et al. 2006); stimulator is activated on demand only by a sudden increase in intra-abdominal pressure (Nissenkorn, Shalev et al. 2004); 30 minutes per session, twice a week for 6 weeks ; 12 weeks training (Di-Gangi-Herms, Veit et al. 2006);and six weeks, two training sessions per week (Seo, Yoon et al. 2004).

1.1.2. Scientific evidence supporting the use of biofeedback with electromyography (BFB-EMG)

The main component of the pelvic floor musculature is the levator ani. The contraction of the levator compresses the urethra and helps continence (DeLancey 1990). The aim of pelvic floor re-education is to improve muscle function, which can significantly reduce stress incontinence. Success rates vary between 21 and 84%, but the subjective improvement is always greater than the objective results.

Several studies have demonstrated the efficacy of BFB-EMG for the treatment of pelvic floor dysfunction in women with stress urinary incontinence (Burgio, C et al. 1986; Aukee, Immonen et al. 2002).

In the elderly, pelvic exercises with biofeedback in the office is more effective than pelvic floor exercises alone (Burns, Pranikoff et al. 1990).

The first study using rehabilitation assisted with pelvic floor muscles EMG for the treatment of vulvovaginal pain was published in 1995 by Glazer et al. These authors reported a cure rate greater than 50% with an average subjective improvement of 83%. Only changes in the electromyographic signal at rest preceded improvement of pain. These findings confirmed that the efficacy of the treatment depended on muscle stabilization (Glazer, Rodke et al. 1995).

1.2. Chronic inflammatory disorders of the lower urinary tract in females

In the following section we shall discuss common conditions, both infectious and non-infectious that can benefit from biofeedback.

1.2.1. Recurrent urinary tract infections

Urinary tract infections (UTIs) are the second most common infections in humans (Foxman 2002). A UTI is the presence of microorganisms in the urine (not due to contamination) which can invade the urinary tract or adjacent structures. It is well established the route of infection is ascending in most cases of infections with enteric bacteria which explains why UTIs are more common in females. The development of a UTI is determined by the balance between bacterial virulence, size of the inoculum, local defence mechanisms and anatomical or functional alterations of the urinary tract (Andreu, Cacho et al. 2011).

It is estimated that the prevalence of UTIs in sexually active young women is 0.5-0.7 episodes per year. One fourth of these will recur. Eighteen out 10000 of these women will develop pyelonephritis and 7% will require hospitalization (Andreu, Cacho et al. 2011). This is despite the fact that most young women with UTI have normal urinary tracts (Hooton 2001). The development of infection is determined by the balance between bacterial virulence, size of the inoculum, local defence mechanisms and anatomical or functional alterations of the urinary tract.

Recurrent UTIs are defined as 3 or more culture-documented infections in 1 year or 2 or more in 6 months in women without structural or functional abnormalities. (Grabe, Bjerklund-Johansen et al. 2011).

Risk factors that predispose to UTIs abnormalities of the urinary tract (such as urinary incontinence or obstruction), sexual behaviour, use of contraceptives, postmenopausal hormonal deficiency, asymptomatic bacteriuria and past urinary tract surgery (Grabe, Bjerklund-Johansen et al. 2011). Risk factors for recurrent UTIs in postmenopausal institutionalised women include atrophic vaginitis, incontinence, cystocele and post-voiding residual urine and a history of UTI before menopause (Nicolle 1997). Collagen diseases represent another extra-urogenital risk factor.

Systemic diseases, mainly diabetes mellitus and chronic renal failure are also important risk factors (Sharifi, Geckler et al. 1996). Women with diabetes mellitus are prone to UTIs. UTI in both diabetic men and women is more likely to progress to pyelonephritis. Patients with type

1 diabetes and UTIs can develop renal damage with time. This is more likely in the presence of proteinuria and peripheral neuropathy. Risk factors for renal damage in women with type 2 diabetes mellitus and recurrent UTIs include old age, proteinuria and low body mass index (Geerlings, Stolk et al. 2000). In addition, autonomic neuropathy may cause bladder dysfunction(Korzeniowski 1991).

In the presence of risk factors, bacterial strains of low virulence can cause UTIs. These risk factors predispose to recurrence but do not affect outcome.

Prevention of recurrent UTIs should avoid the use antibiotics given the alarming rise in antibiotic resistance observed worldwide (Fihn 2003; Grabe, Bjerklund-Johansen et al. 2011).Antibiotic prophylaxis should only be used after counselling and behaviour modification has been attempted (Grabe, Bjerklund-Johansen et al. 2011). Other measures to prevent recurrences include immune active prophylaxis (Lorenzo-Gómez, MF et al. 2013), probiotics and cranberry juice.

1.2.2. Non-infectious chronic cystitis — Painful bladder syndrome

Over the years much of the focus for chronic pelvic pain has been on peripheral-end-organ mechanisms, such as inflammatory or infective conditions (Engeler, Baranowski et al. 2012).

A peripheral stimulus such as infection may initiate the beginning of chronic pelvic pain, and the illness may become self-perpetuating as a result of modulation of the central nervous system, independent of the original cause (Engeler, Baranowski et al. 2012).

Chronic pelvic pain mechanisms may involve on-going acute pain mechanisms, such as those associated with inflammation or infection, which may involve somatic or visceral tissues (Linley, Rose et al.). Nevertheless in most cases, inflammation or infection is not present (van de Merwe, Nordling et al. 2008). However, conditions that produce recurrent trauma, infection or inflammation may result in chronic pelvic pain in a small proportion of cases (van de Merwe, Nordling et al. 2008). Therefore such factors should be ruled out early.

Central sensitisation is responsible for a decrease in threshold and increase in response duration and magnitude of dorsal horn neurons. For instance, with central sensitisation, stimuli that are normally below the threshold may result in a sensation of fullness and a need to void (Nazif, Teichman et al. 2007) and other non-painful stimuli may be interpreted as pain and noxious stimuli may be magnified with an increased perception of pain. Also, somatic tissue hyperaesthesia is associated with recurrent bladder infection.

The increased perception of stimuli in the viscera is known as visceral hyperalgesia, and the underlying mechanisms are thought to be responsible, among, others for bladder pain syndrome and dysmenorrhoea.

Chronic bladder pain may be associated with the presence of Hunner's ulcers and glomerulation on cystoscopy, whereas other bladder pain conditions may have normal cystoscopic findings. Recent reports about prevalence of bladder pain syndrome show higher figures than earlier ones, ranging from 0.06% to 30% (Parsons and Tatsis 2004).

The conditions associated with the painful bladder include interstitial cystitis, bladder pain syndrome or BPS. The European Urological Association (EUA), the International Society for the study of BPS (ESSIC), the International Association for the Study of Pain (IASP) and several other groups now prefer the term bladder pain syndrome (BPS). Terms that end in "itis" in particular should be avoided unless infection and/or inflammation is proven and considered to be the cause of the pain (Abrams, Baranowski et al. 2006). Chronic pelvic pain may be subdivided into conditions with well-defined classical pathology, such as infection, and those with no obvious pathology.

BPS is the occurrence of persistent or recurrent pain perceived in the urinary bladder region, accompanied by at least one other symptom, such as pain worsening with bladder filling and day-time and/or night-time urinary frequency. There is no proven infection or other obvious local pathology. BPS is believed to represent a heterogeneous spectrum of disorders. There may be specific types of inflammation as a feature in subsets of patients (Engeler, Baranowski et al. 2012).

Pelvic floor muscle pain syndrome is the occurrence of persistent or recurrent episodic pelvic floor pain. It is often associated with symptoms suggestive of lower urinary tract dysfunction (Engeler, Baranowski et al. 2012).

BPS should be diagnosed on the basis of pain, pressure or discomfort associated with the urinary bladder, accompanied by at least one other symptom, such as daytime and/or night-time increased urinary frequency, the exclusion of confounding diseases as the cause of symptoms, and if indicated, cystoscopy with hydrodistension and biopsy (van de Merwe, Nordling et al. 2008). Hunner's lesion and inflammation is referred to as BPS type 3. Current thought implicates an initial unidentified insult to the bladder, triggering inflammatory, endocrine and neural phenomena (Warren, Wesselmann et al.).

No infection aetiology has been implicated since BPS patients and controls have equal UTI frequency (Nickel, Shoskes et al. ; Warren, Brown et al. 2008). Of interest however is the fact that UTI and urgency are significantly more frequent during childhood and adolescence in patients who later develop BPS in adulthood (Peters, Killinger et al. 2009).

Cystoscopic and biopsy findings in both ulcer and non-ulcer BPS are consistent with defects in the urothelial glycosaminoglycan (GAG) layer. Urinary uronate, and sulphated GAG levels are increased in patients with severe BPS (Lokeshwar, Selzer et al. 2005).

The physiopathologic relationship between interstitial cystitis and rheumatic, autoimmune, and chronic inflammatory diseases has been investigated. (Lorenzo Gomez and Gomez Castro 2004).

Biological markers have been explored as an attractive idea to support or, even better, to confirm the clinical diagnosis and prognosis (Lokeshwar, Selzer et al. 2005).

The therapeutic modalities currently available for BPS include the following:

Medical management: Analgesics, corticosteroids, anti-allergic medications, Amitriptyline, Pentosan polysulphate sodium.Immunosuppressants such as Azathioprine, Cyclosporin A,

Methotrexate, Gabapentin, Pregabalin, Suplatast tosilate (IPD-1151T), Quercetin. Antibiotics have a limited role in the treatment of BPS. Cimetidine, prostaglandins, L-Arginine, anticholinergic drugs have also been used (Engeler, Baranowski et al. 2012).

Intravesical therapy: Local anaesthetic (lidocaine), Pentosan polysulphate sodium, intravesical heparin, hyaluronic acid (hyaluronan, chondroitin sulphate, dimethyl sulphoxide (DMSO), bacillus Calmette Guérin (BCG) and vanilloids which disrupt sensory neurons such as Resiniferatoxin (Engeler, Baranowski et al. 2012).

Interventional management: Bladder distension with or without electromotive drug administration, transurethral resection (TUR) coagulation and laser, Botulinum toxin A (BTX-A), Hyperbaric oxygen (HBO), neuromodulation (Engeler, Baranowski et al. 2012).

Non-pharmacological: Behavioural bladder training techniques (Parsons and Koprowski 1991), physiotherapy (Karper 2004), electrical stimulation (de-Oliveira-Bernardes and Bahamondes 2005). Physiotherapy with pelvic floor biofeedback (Borrego-Jiménez, Lorenzo-Gómez et al. 2009 Jan).

Surgical: When all efforts fail to relieve disabling symptoms, surgical removal of the diseased bladder is the ultimate option (Loch and Stein 2004).

1.2.2.1. Urethral pain syndrome

Urethral pain syndrome is the occurrence of chronic or recurrent episodic pain perceived in the urethra, in the absence of proven infection or other obvious local pathology (Parsons 2011). There pathogenesis of urethral pain syndrome is unknown but it may part of the spectrum of BPS. Some have postulated that neuropathic hypersensitivity can develop following urinary a UTI (Kaur and Arunkalaivanan 2007). The same authors suggested that behavioural therapy including biofeedback and bladder training can be helpful (Kaur and Arunkalaivanan 2007).

1.2.2.2. Other causes of chronic pelvic pain

Pelvic organ prolapse is often an asymptomatic condition, unless it is so marked that it causes back strain, vaginal pain and skin excoriation (Roovers, van der Vaart et al. 2004).

In the past few years, non-absorbable mesh has been used in the pelvic organ prolapse surgery. Although they may have a role in supporting the vagina, they are also associated with several complications including bladder, bowel and vaginal trauma (Niro, Philippe et al. 2010).A subset of these patients may develop chronic pain because mesh insertion causes nerve and muscle irritation (Daniels, Gray et al. 2009).

Most patients can be treated by surgical removal of the mesh (Margulies, Lewicky-Gaupp et al. 2008). If appropriate, multidisciplinary pain management strategies can be applied. Another cause of pain is previous surgery for incontinence with transoburator tapes. Chronic perineal pain at 12 months after surgery was reported by 21 trials and meta-analysis of these data showed strong evidence of a higher rate in women undergoing transobturator insertion (7%) compared to retropubic insertion (3%)(Barber, Kleeman et al. 2008; Lorenzo-Gómez, B et al. 2013).

Vulvovaginal pain can developed after bacterial vaginal infections or bacterial vaginosis. Infections change the vaginal ecosystem. Oestrogen deficiency in peri- and post-menopausal women can also lead to vulvar tissue atrophy and a subsequent irritation. Contact with irritanting agents such as soaps, detergents and topical preparations as well as vulvar trauma associated with accidents or surgery can lead to vulvar irritation and the development of vulvovaginal pain (White, Jantos et al. 1997 Mar).

1.3. Urinary incontinence

Urinary incontinence is an extremely common complaint worldwide. It causes a great deal of distress and embarrassment, as well as significant costs, to both individuals and societies (Lucas, Bosch et al. 2012). The standardization committee of the International Continence Society (ICS) has defined the female urinary incontinence as the involuntary urine loss, objectively demonstrable, which represents a social or hygienic problem (Abrahams, Blaivas et al. 1988).

At least one out of four women in Europe suffers from a disorder associate with incontinence which often has been present for several years before consultation (Thomas, Plymat et al. 1980). In geriatric hospitals, the incidence of urinary incontinence I in women is 43% and as high as n 91% in psychogeriatric patients.

Patients with 'complicated incontinence' are those with co-morbidities, a history of previous pelvic surgery, past surgery for incontinence, radiotherapy and associated genitourinary prolapse (Lucas, Bosch et al. 2012). Urinary incontinence is more common in women with UTIs and is also more likely in the first few days following an acute infection (Moore, Jackson et al. 2008).

In women with incontinence, diagnosis of a UTI by positive leucocytes or nitrites using urine test strips had low sensitivity but high specificity (Semeniuk and Church 1999; Buchsbaum, Albushies et al. 2004).

Incontinent women with symptoms of lower urinary tract or pelvic floor dysfunction and pelvic organ prolapse have a higher risk of of incomplete bladder emptying (elevated post void residual urine volume) compared to asymptomatic patients. Therefore it is suggested that the presence of post void residual should be ruled out in this patients (Fowler, Panicker et al. 2009).

In the elderly incontinence can be caused or worsened by underlying diseases including diabetes (Lee, Cigolle et al. 2009). A higher prevalence of incontinence was associated with higher age and body mass index (Sarma, Kanaya et al. 2009). A recent meta-analysis showed that systemic oestrogen therapy for post-menopausal women was associated with the development and worsening of urinary incontienece (Cody, Richardson et al. 2009). Obesity appears to confer a four-fold increased risk of UI (Chen, Gatmaitan et al. 2009).

1.3.1. Physical therapies for the urinary incontinence

The treatment of lower urinary tract's disorders with pelvic floor exercises with or without biofeedback represents a risk-free option which can be applied in a great number of women. The correct function of the female pelvic floor depends on the position and mobility of the urethra and the urethrovesical junction. Pelvic floor muscle training increases urethral closure pressure and stabilises the urethra, preventing downward movement during moments of increased physical activity. There is evidence that increasing pelvic floor strength may help to inhibit bladder contraction in patients with an overactive bladder. This training may be augmented with biofeedback (Bidmead 2002).

The evidence published in the guidelines regarding urinary incontinence suggests that UTI treatment does not correct the UI. It is unclear if improving the incontinence helps decrease recurrence rate of UTI.

Valid methods to evaluate the morphologic and electromyographic abnormalities of the levator ani muscle are necessary in order to better select women or the treatment with pelvic floor training and biofeedback (Bo, Larsen et al. 1988; Espuña-Pons 2002).

The most recently published systematic review in 2010 found that medication was less effective than behavioural therapy in a comparative effectiveness trial (81% vs. 69% reduction in UI episodes) (Goode, Burgio et al. 2010), therefore pelvic floor physiotherapy must always be the first line of treatment for stress incontinence and overactive bladder. Drugs must be prescribed if pelvic floor physiotherapy fails (Bidmead 2002).

1.3.1.1. RTUI after surgical correction of UI or pelvic organs prolapses

In 1995 the tension-free transvaginal tape (TVT) was introduced to treat UI (Ulmsten and Petros 1995). In 2001 another technique, the suburethral transobturator tape (TOT), was introduced (Delorme 2001). The main advantages were that the tape lays at a more anatomic position than in TVT, the needle does not cross the retropubic space, no abdominal incisions are made, there is a lower risk of vesical or intestinal injury and no cystoscopy is required (Sola Dalenz, Pardo Schanz et al. 2006; Delorme and Hermieu 2010).

The simplicity of these techniques and their reproducibility has dramatically increased their use, by both Urologists and Gynaecologists (Castiñeiras-Fernández 2005).

When surgical treatment is indicated, the TOT procedure is the procedure of choice, absent contraindications. This recommendation is supported by the establishment of TVT as a worldwide validated and proven procedure for the surgical correction of urinary stress incontinence.

2. Our experience with the treatment of bladder pain syndrome

In the following sections we describe the experience with biofeedback and electromyography obtained at our academic unit.

2.1. Method and tools used

We conducted a retrospective study of 548 women diagnosed with inflammatory, infectious and non-infectious disorders of the lower urinary tract treated between March 2003 and May 2012.

Patients were divided into 2 groups according to whether or not they had UTIs. Each group received conventional treatment and were further divided into 2 subgroups, one receiving biofeedback with electromyography and the other not.

Group A consisted of 270 patients with repeated urinary tract infections managed with prophylactic Sulfamethoxazole/Trimethoprim 40/200mg/day for a period of 6 months versus sublingual bacterial vaccine Uromune® for a period of 3 months.

Subgroup A1 (n=112) no biofeedback.

Subgroup A2 (n=158) treatment was supplemented with biofeedback and electromyography.

Group B consisted of 278 patients with non-infectious chronic inflammatory diseases of the inferior urinary tract who were managed with Perphenazine 2mg/ Amitriptyline 25 mg orally daily and intravesical Hyaluronic acid weekly for 4 weeks.

Subgroup B1 (n= 99) received no biofeedback.

Subgroup B2 (N=179) treatment was supplemented with biofeedback and electromyography.

Age, secondary diagnoses, concomitant treatments, medical and surgical background, response to treatment, answers to the King's Health Questionnaire (Kelleher, Cardozo et al. 1997 Dec) and SF-36 QoL Questionnaire Spanish Version (Vilagut, Ferrer et al. 2005 Mar-Apr) were recorded. The interpretation of results of the questionaires was as follows:for of Kings Health questionnaire the range varied between 25 points (normal status, healthy) to 97 points (critical illness perception). For the SF-36 questionnaire the range varied from 149 points (normal status, healthy) to 36 points (critical illness perception).

For subgroups A2 and B2, the program of biofeedback with electromyography (BFB-EMG) consisted of 20 sessions of therapy. Two surface electrodes were placed on the perineum over the pelvic floor musculature and a neutral or ground electrode was placed on the inner aspect of the thigh.

In the first 3 sessions the electrodes were placed near anal external sphincter. In the subsequent sessions the electrodes were placed closer and closer to the urethra. We considered the correct position of the electrodes very important (Figure 1).

The contractions lasted 3-5 seconds followed by a relaxation period of 8-10 seconds Patients were trained to manage the signal in the screen by using the appropriate perineal muscles. The goal was to bring the two perineal electrodes closer together. The weekly session lasted 20 minutes.

Sessions took place at the urodynamics office with Medicina y Mercado™ equipment. The patient lay supine, with light flexion of the hips and protection of the lumbar lordosis in order

http://dx.doi.org/10.5772/56237

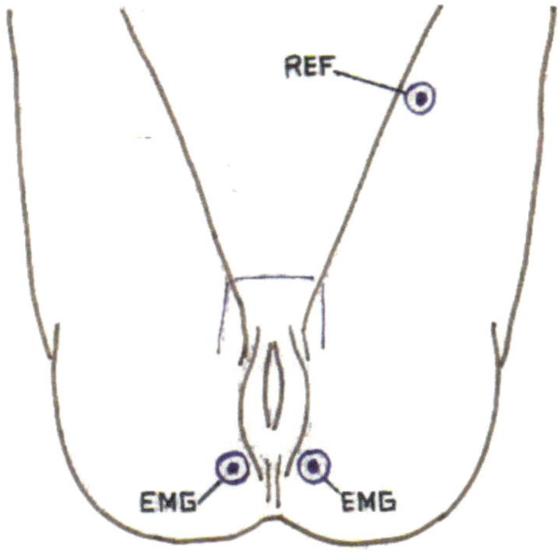

Figure 1. Position of electrodes for BFB-EMG session.

to avoid fatigue (figure 2). In this position the patient could see the screen of the biofeedback equipment (figures 3 and 4). The electrodes used were paediatric pre-gelled electrodes. After explaining the anatomy and physiology of the pelvic floor, the patient was instructed to contract the perineal musculature during 3-5 seconds and relaxing to relax it during 6-8 seconds. Each signal was recorded continuously with a polygraph the power, muscle tone and the duration were recorded in the perineal electromyography (figures 2-4).

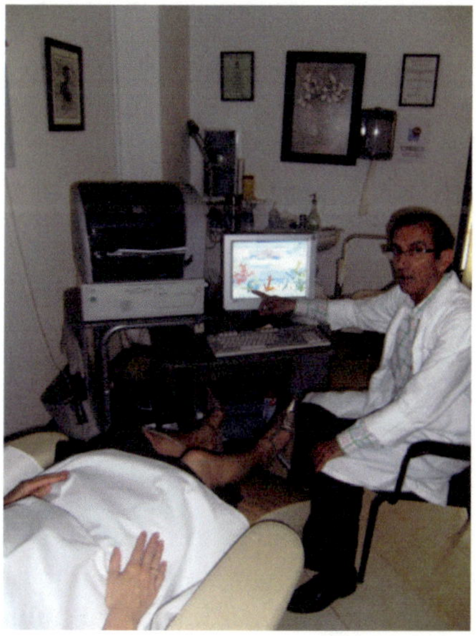

Figure 2. BFB session.

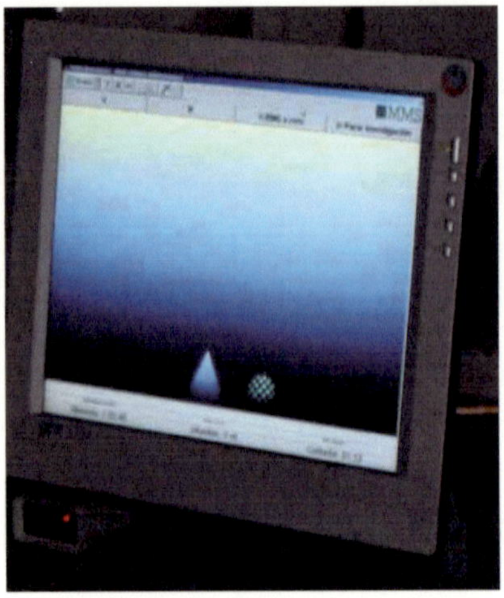

Figure 3. Screens showing several scenes for BFB-EMG.

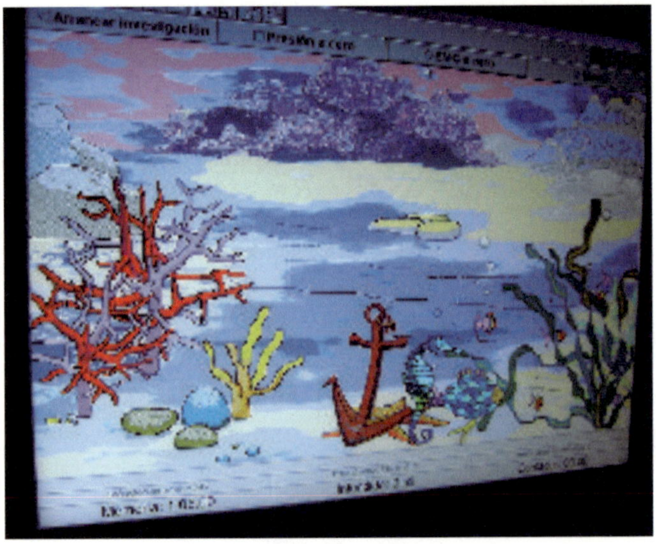

Figure 4. Screens showing several scenes for BFB-EMG.

Figure 5 shows fragments of the graphics obtained from the EMG activity registry at a biofeedback session.

Statistical analysis was as follows: Results from the answers in Kings´Health and SF-36 QoL questionnaires yielded qualitative and quantitative variables which were analysed by NCSS-2000™ statistic program. Descriptive and inferential studies included analysis of cross tabulation, Fisher exact test, Chi-square, Student's t-test, Pearson correlation test. $p<0.05$ was accepted as statistically significant.

http://dx.doi.org/10.5772/56237

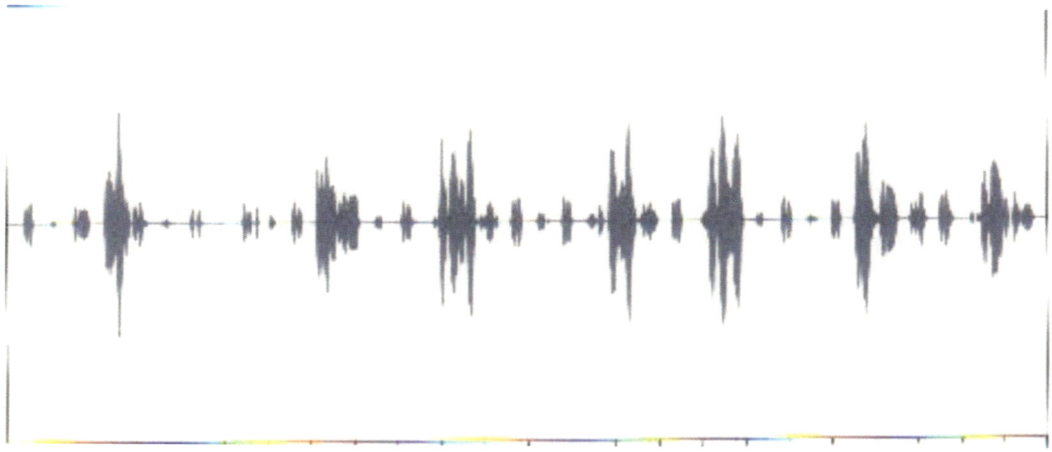

Figure 5. EMG registry at BFB session.

2.2. Results

There were no difference in the age (p=0.2615), medical history of diabetes (p=2365), arterial hypertension (p=0.1629), smoking, alcohol and caffeine consumption (p=0.8317), obesity (p=0.6732), occupation (p=0.4319) and marital status (p=0.0729) between the four groups. Median age were Group A

Table 1 shows the prevalence of urinary incontinence (UI) grade 1, 2 and 3, cystocele>2, cystocele>2+rectocele, colpocele, cystocele>2+UI, rectocele in the 4 groups:

Pelvic floor condition	Subgroup A1 (n= 112)	Subgroup A2 (n= 158)	Subgroup B1 (n= 99)	Subgroup B2 (n= 179)
Incontinence grade 1	4	6	10	6
Incontinence grade 2	11	8	2	3
Incontinence grade 3	8	13	1	2
Cystocele"/>2	11	20	11	10
Rectocele and cystocele	9	15	1	2
Colpocele	7	11	3	15
Cystocele and Incontinence	8	10	3	12
Rectocele	6	5	1	5
SIGNIFICANCE	*p*=0.4507		*p*=0.7886	

Table 1. Pelvic floor conditions in the inferior urinary tract chronic inflammations (Incontinence grade 1: uncontrollable urine leakage, dripping (< 50 cc); grade 2: uncontrollable leakage of moderate urine quantities (50-120 cc); grade 3: uncontrollable leakage of big urine quantities (> 200 cc).

The results of the questionaires before and after treatment are shown in the figures below.

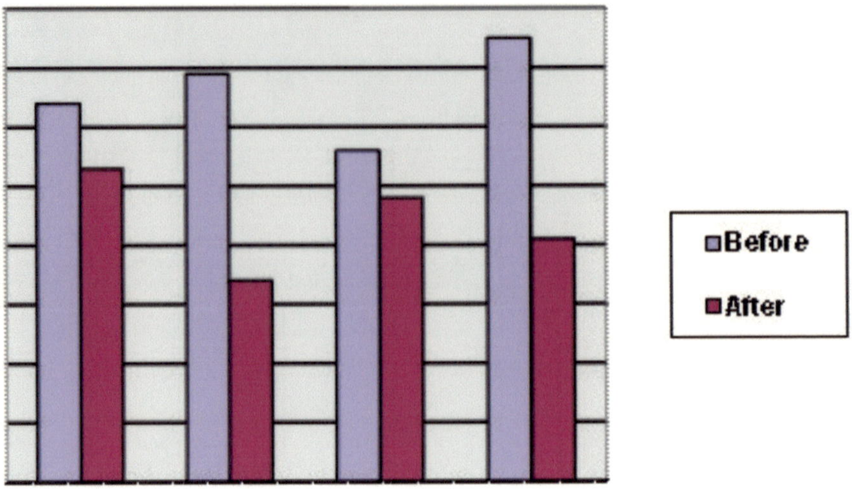

Graphic 1. King´s Health Test before and after treatment.

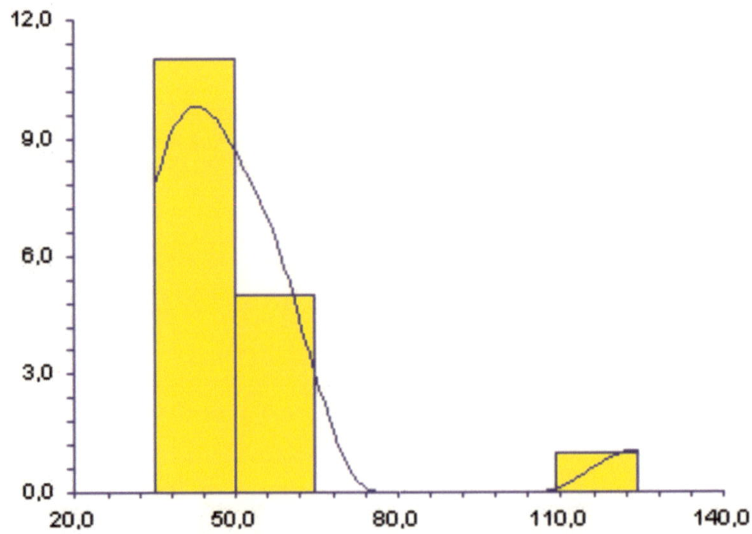

Graphic 2. Histogram showing Group B1 King´s score after treatment.

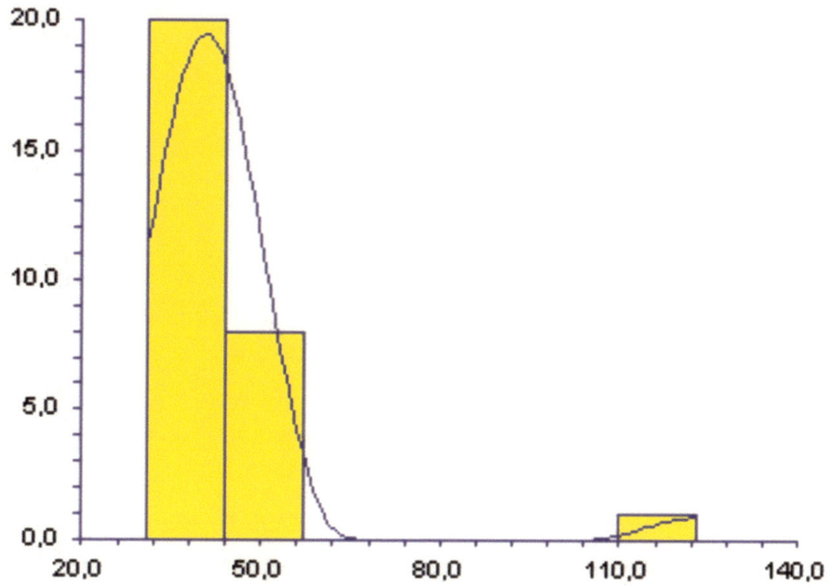

Graphic 3. Histogram showing Group B2 King´s score after treatment.

In the King´s Health Questionnaire, Group B2 shows better results compared with Group B1 (p<0.0003). Group A2 shows better results than group A1 (p<0.0042). Group B2 shows the best results. We found similar findings in the SF-36 questionnaire.

3. Discussion

Pelvic floor dysfunction can lead to urinary incontinence and to other lower urinary tract symptoms (LUTS). A neuromuscular disorder has been found in women with incontinence or traumatic delivery, with a good response to the functional treatment of the pelvic floor (Gunnarsson, Ahlmann et al. 1999).

In our unit, we decided to combine the BFB-EMG program for patients with LUTS who were refractory to conventional treatments. We have not found any adverse effects caused by the treatment, but we have recorded surprisingly good results with the quality of life tests test we systematically performed.

Regarding the patient allocation between antibiotic treatment and immunological modulators (bacterial vaccines), there was an homogeneous distribution of treated recurrent UTIs between both groups, but patients treated with bacterial vaccine showed a better response than those treated with suppressive antibiotic protocol ($p<0.001$).

Pelvic floor exercises are an essential part of the bladder-sphincter re-education. Pelvic floor's functional treatment with or without BFB has been used to treat stress urinary incontinence with an efficacy ranging between 17 and 84% (Cammu, van Nylen et al. 1991 Oct; Workman, Cassisi et al. 1993 Jan; Lorenzo-Gómez, Silva-Abuín et al. 2008).

We wish to emphasize the benefit that the BFB-EMG gives to patients with chronic lower urinary tracts disorders, whether of an infectious nature or not. Several explanations can be offered. There is a demonstrated benefit in the collagen type changes that the pelvic floor's muscles after BFB-EMG, which increases the contractile capability of the levator ani and strengthen the type I (slow contraction, high resistance) and type II fibres (quick contraction, quick fatigue) (Arlandis-Guzmán and Martínez-Agulló 2002). In addition the detrusor activity is inhibited by the voluntary perineal contraction (activating the Mahony's reflex #3 or perineal-detrusor reflex (Mahony, Laferte et al. 1977 Jan) in a more natural and physiological manner than with other more aggressive therapeutic methods.

Until now, UTI and chronic cystitis have not been included within the specific pathologies of the pelvic floor. However, we find that in clinical practise patients have frequent concomitant UTI.

In this study, we investigated the relationship between UTI and incontinence. Scientists agree that UTI facilitates the development of incontinence. Recurrent UTI is defined as at least three episodes of uncomplicated infection documented by culture in a 12-month period in women with no structural/functional abnormalities(Naber 1999). This assertion is maybe challenged since many women diagnosed with recurrent UTI have urethral hyper-motility, stress or urgency incontinence, voiding urgency or subclinical cystocele.

BFB-EMG has shown to be of benefit for women with painful bladder using the same protocol (Borrego Jiménez, Lorenzo Gómez et al. 2007), but also in women with vaginism, pelvic floor myalgia and other similar conditions. (Arlandis-Guzmán and Martínez-Agulló 2002).

There is little information about the importance of the anatomy of the pelvic floor in patients with incontinence. It has been postulated that the irritative voiding symptoms in patients with incontinence can be aggravated by a higher tonicity of the pelvic floor muscles (Griebling and Takle 1999). BFB-EMG program can be an useful adjuvant to the treatment of patients with incontinence (Borrego Jiménez, Lorenzo Gómez et al. 2007). On the other hand, neuromodulation is still finding its role in pelvic pain management. There has been growing evidence in small case series or pilot studies but more detailed research is required (Fariello and Whitmore). Published papers show an important role of BFB for impotence, premature ejaculation, perineal pains and vaginism treatment. For these reasons, a consensus was reached in our Pelvic Floor Unit in order to use BFB-EMG as an adjuvant treatment in patients with chronic inflammatory diseases, both infectious and non-infectious, of the lower urinary tract. Results have been satisfactory.

These findings are in agreement with the experts' opinion contained in the European Association of Urology's guidelines, relating to the design of individual therapeutic protocols for each patient (Grabe, Bjerklund-Johansen et al. 2012).

Biofeedback-EMG is an essential element in the functional treatment of the pelvic floor, providing information about other hidden muscular functions. It has been shown that giving only verbal or written instructions, fewer than half of the patients could correctly and effectively contract their pelvic floor muscles and in 25% of the case the symptoms worsened. (Theofrastous, Wyman et al. 2002; Gray and David 2005 Jul-Aug) likely due to the strengthen of the antagonist muscles (Llorca-Miravet 1990).

The somatic and the vegetative (with the sympathetic and the parasympathetic components) nervous system are implicated in the micturition cycle. There is an inhibition-excitation balance at any time in this system, the so called "balancing" principle by Schimdt, which explains the hypo-contractile detrusor of women with urethral hyper-activity. In the conscious component of the voiding cycle, the periurethral muscles can influence this balance, re-establishing the correct voiding cycle, and this is the principle for the conservative techniques in voiding re-education (González-Chamorro and Lledó 2001).

Biofeedback can be helpful in the treatment of pelvic floor pain in the process of recognising the muscles' action. EMG is one of the most used input methods for biofeedback (Romanzi, Polaneczky et al. 1999). A study in patients with chronic pelvic pain syndrome participating in a pelvic floor BFB re-education program reported a correlation between the decline in EMG values and symptoms relief (Cornel, van Haarst et al. 2005).

In a study among patients with levator ani syndrome, biofeedback was found to be the most effective therapy. Other modalities used were electrostimulation and massage. Adequate relief was reported by 87% in the biofeedback group, 45% for electrostimulation, and 22% for massage (Chiarioni, Nardo et al.).

Treating the pelvic floor muscles is recommended as the first line of treatment in patients with chronic pelvic pain syndrome. In patients with an overactive pelvic floor, BFB is recommended as adjuvant therapy to muscle exercises (Engeler, Baranowski et al. 2012).None of the present existing treatments have effect on any BPS subtypes or phenotypes. Bladder training may be effective in patients with predominant urinary symptoms and little pain.

Multimodal behavioural, physical and psychological techniques should always be considered alongside pharmacological or invasive treatments. Manual and physical therapy should be considered as a first approach (Engeler, Baranowski et al. 2012).

Investigations on chronic spams of the pelvic floor muscles in patients with chronic pelvic pain syndrome revealed that all patients had significant voiding symptoms (urgency, frequency, incontinence due to final dripping) and ureteral hypersensitivity concomitant to chronic pain at the perineal area. Up to the 44.3% of patients had previous voiding problems in childhood (enuresis, constipation and retarded urination habit learning) (Bo, Larsen et al. 1988).

Verbal or written instructions for patients using practise equipment at home can be less effective because patients cannot exactly remember the training given at the office or they can have problems following the treatment protocol (Aukee, Immonen et al. 2002).

The main limitations shown by the BFB-EMG are that minimum muscular activity intensity is needed in order to register and visualize any activity at the BFB screen. It is an active technique that requires motivation and a minimum intellectual level that is not suitable for patients with mental problems or retarded. High-quality, reliable and valid equipment is necessary to avoid interference present in machines of lesser quality. The instructor is a integral part of the method and must evaluate and study how to reach the patient and to devise the therapeutic protocol.

From our experience, the following lower urinary tract inflammatory disorders are eligible for combined treatment including BFB-EMG:

- Infectious:
- Repeated urinary tract infections: more than 3 per year or more than two every 6 months in women without risk factors.
- Repeated urinary tract infections in women with urinary incontinence.
- Urinary tract infections in patients previously treated of urinary incontinence or pelvic floor prolapse.
- Non-infectious: bladder pain syndrome or interstitial cystitis, non-infectious chronic cystitis (follicular, eosinophilic), chronic pain after surgical treatment of urinary incontinence or pelvic floor prolapse.

4. Conclusions

BFB-EMG is a basic and essential technique for the perineal-sphinteric re-education. EMG-guided BFB gives faster and more reliable information, it allows the development of awareness and a faster learning of the perineal work, both contracting and relaxing.

A BFB-EMG therapeutic protocol is very useful as a coadjuvant treatment for chronic inflammatory pathologies of the lower urinary tract, both infectious and non-infectious.

Author details

B. Padilla-Fernandez[1], A. Gomez-Garcia[2], M. N. Hernandez-Alonso[3], M.B. Garcia-Cenador[4], J. A. Mirón-Canelo[5], A. Geanini-Yagüez[3], J. M. Silva-Abuin[1] and M. F. Lorenzo-Gomez[1,4]

1 Department of Urology, Universitary Hospital of Salamanca, Spain

2 Family and Community Medicine, Department of Surgery. University of Salamanca, Spain

3 Department of Rehabilitation, Universitary Hospital of Salamanca, Spain

4 Department of Surgery, University of Salamanca, Spain

5 Department of Preventive Medicine and Public Health, University of Salamanca, Spain

References

[1] Abrahams, P, Blaivas, J, et al. (1988). The standarization of terminology of lower urinary tract function." Scan J Urol Nephrol Supple: , 114-115.

[2] Abrams, P, Baranowski, A, et al. (2006). A new classification is needed for pelvic pain syndromes--are existing terminologies of spurious diagnostic authority bad for patients?" J Urol , 175(6), 1989-1990.

[3] Amaro, J, Gameiro, M, et al. (2006). Intravaginal electrical stimulation: a randomized, double-blind study on the treatment of mixed urinary incontinence." Acta Obstet Gynecol Scand , 85(5), 619-622.

[4] Andreu, A, Cacho, J, et al. (2011). Microbiological diagnosis of urinary tract infections]." Enferm Infecc Microbiol Clin , 29(1), 52-57.

[5] Arlandis-guzmán, S, & Martínez-agulló, E. (2002). Alternativas terapéuticas para la disfunción miccional crónica. Neuromodulación: Una nueva alternativa terapéutica para los tratornos del tracto urinario inferior. E. Ediciones. Madrid, Asociación Española de Urología.

[6] Aukee, P, Immonen, P, et al. (2002). Increase in pelvic floor muscle activity after 12 weeks' training: a randomized prospective pilot study." Urology , 60(6), 1020-1023.

[7] Barber, M. D, Kleeman, S, et al. (2008). Risk factors associated with failure 1 year after retropubic or transobturator midurethral slings." Am J Obstet Gynecol 199(6): 666 e, 661-667.

[8] Bidmead, J. (2002). Urinary incontinence: A Gynaecologist´s Experience." Eur Urol: , 21-24.

[9] Bo, K, Larsen, S, et al. (1988). Knowledge about and ability to correct pelvic floor muscle exercise in women with urinary stress incontinence." Neurol Urodyn , 7, 261-262.

[10] Borrego-jiménez, P. S, Lorenzo-gómez, M. F, et al. (2009). Jan). "Fisioterapia y personas con discapacidad: papel de la fisioterapia coadyuvante en la discapacidad física y psicosomática causada por la cistopatía intersticial." Fisioterapia , 31(1), 3-11.

[11] Borrego JiménezP. S., M. F. Lorenzo Gómez, et al. ((2007). Actuación fisioterápica tras la valoración pericial de las lesiones de columna vertebral." Rev Iberoam Fisioter Kinesol , 10(1), 38-43.

[12] Buchsbaum, G. M, Albushies, D. T, et al. (2004). Utility of urine reagent strip in screening women with incontinence for urinary tract infection." Int Urogynecol J Pelvic Floor Dysfunct discussion 393., 15(6), 391-393.

[13] Burgio, K. L, et al. (1986). The role of biofeedback in Kegel exercise training for stress urinary incontinence." Am J Obstet Gynecol. , 154(1), 58-64.

[14] Burns, P, Pranikoff, K, et al. (1990). Treatment of stress incontinence with pelvic floor exercises and biofeedback." J Am Geriatr Soc , 38(3), 341-344.

[15] Cammu, H, Van Nylen, M, et al. (1991). Oct). "Pelvic physiotherapy in genuine stress incontinence." Urology , 38(4), 332-337.

[16] Cardozo, L, Abrams, P, et al. (1978). Idiopathic bladder instability treated by biofeedback" Br J Urol , 50(7), 521-523.

[17] Cardozo, L, & Stanton, S. year review." Br J Urol 56(2): 220., 5.

[18] Castiñeiras-fernández, J. (2005). Técnicas de cintas sin tensión. Incontinencia de esfuerzo y reparación del suelo pélvico: Atlas de técnicas quirúrgicas. J. González and J. Angulo. Madrid, Boehringer Ingelheim: 276.

[19] Chen, C. C, Gatmaitan, P, et al. (2009). Obesity is associated with increased prevalence and severity of pelvic floor disorders in women considering bariatric surgery." Surg Obes Relat Dis , 5(4), 411-415.

[20] Chiarioni, G, Nardo, A, et al. Biofeedback is superior to electrogalvanic stimulation and massage for treatment of levator ani syndrome." Gastroenterology , 138(4), 1321-1329.

[21] Cody, J. D, Richardson, K, et al. (2009). Oestrogen therapy for urinary incontinence in post-menopausal women." Cochrane Database Syst Rev(4): CD001405.

[22] Cornel, E. B, Van Haarst, E. P, et al. (2005). The effect of biofeedback physical therapy in men with Chronic Pelvic Pain Syndrome Type III." Eur Urol , 47(5), 607-611.

[23] Daniels, J, Gray, R, et al. (2009). Laparoscopic uterosacral nerve ablation for alleviating chronic pelvic pain: a randomized controlled trial." Jama , 302(9), 955-961.

[24] de-Oliveira-bernardes, N, & Bahamondes, L. (2005). Intravaginal electrical stimulation for the treatment of chronic pelvic pain." J Reprod Med 2005 Apr;50(4):267-72 50(4): 267-272.

[25] Delancey, J. (1990). Anatomy and physiology of the urinary continence." Clin Obstet Gynecol , 33(2), 298-307.

[26] Delorme, E. (2001). Transobturator urethral suspension: mini-invasive procedure in the treatment of stress urinary incontinence in women]." Prog Urol , 11(6), 1306-1313.

[27] Delorme, E, & Hermieu, J. F. (2010). Guidelines for the surgical treatment of female urinary stress incontinence in women using the suburethral sling]." Prog Urol 20 Suppl 2: S, 132-142.

[28] Di-gangi-herms, A, Veit, R, et al. (2006). Functional imaging of stress urinary incontinence." Neuroimage. , 29(1), 267-275.

[29] DiPiroJ. ((2000). Infectious diseases. Pharmacotherapy handbook. B. Wells, J. DiPiro, T. Schwinghammer and C. Hamilton. New York, Stamford: , 544-557.

[30] Engeler, D, Baranowski, A, et al. (2012). Guidelines on Chonic Pelvic Pain. European Association of Urology Guidelines. Arnhem, The Netherlans.

[31] Espuña-pons, M. (2002). Criterios para la indicación de tratamiento conservador de la incontinencia urinaria de esfuerzo y tipos de tratamiento. La Opinión de los expertos. Barcelona: , 12-14.

[32] Fariello, J. Y, & Whitmore, K. Sacral neuromodulation stimulation for IC/PBS, chronic pelvic pain, and sexual dysfunction." Int Urogynecol J , 21(12), 1553-1558.

[33] Fihn, S. (2003). Clinical practice. Acute uncomplicated urinary tract infection in women." N Engl J Med , 349(3), 259-266.

[34] Fowler, C. J, Panicker, J. N, et al. (2009). A UK consensus on the management of the bladder in multiple sclerosis." J Neurol Neurosurg Psychiatry , 80(5), 470-477.

[35] Foxman, B. (2002). Epidemiology of urinary tract infections: incidence, morbidity, and economic costs." Am J Med 113(Suppl 1A): 5S-13S.

[36] Frewen, W. (1972). Urgency incontinence. Review of 100 cases." J Obstet Gynaecol Br Commonw , 79(1), 77-79.

[37] Geerlings, S, Stolk, R, et al. (2000). Asymptomatic bacteriuria may be considered a complication in women with diabetes. Diabetes Mellitus Women Asymptomatic Bacteriuria Utrecht Study Group." Diabetes Care , 23(6), 744-749.

[38] Glazer, H, Rodke, G, et al. (1995). Treatment of vulvar vestibulitis syndrome with electromyographic biofeedback of pelvic floor musculature." J Reprod Med , 40(4), 283-290.

[39] González-chamorro, F, & Lledó, E. (2001). La Neuromodulación como tratamiento de la disfunción miccional." Revisiones en Urología II 1: 26.

[40] Goode, P. S, Burgio, K. L, et al. (2010). Incontinence in older women." Jama , 303(21), 2172-2181.

[41] Grabe, M, Bjerklund-johansen, T, et al. (2012). Guidelines on Urological Infections. European Association of Urology Guidelines. ArnHem, The Netherlans: 110.

[42] Grabe, M, Bjerklund-johansen, T, et al. (2011). Guidelines on Urological Infections. European Association of Urology." http://www.uroweb.org/gls/pdf/15_Urological_Infections.pdf.

[43] Gray, M, & David, D. J. (2005). Jul-Aug). "Does biofeedback improve the efficacy of pelvic floor muscle rehabilitation for urinary incontinence or overactive bladder dysfunction in women?" J Wound Ostomy Continence Nurs Review., 32(4), 222-225.

[44] Griebling, T, & Takle, T. (1999). Prevalence of genital organ prolapse in women with interstitial cystitis. 29th Annual General Meeting of International Continence Society, Denver. USA., American Urological Association.

[45] Gunnarsson, M, Ahlmann, S, et al. (1999). Cortical magnetic stimulation in patients with genuine stress incontinence: correlation with results of pelvic floor exercises." Neurourol Urodyn discussion 444-435., 18(5), 437-444.

[46] Hooton, T. (2001). Recurrent urinary tract infection in women." Int J Antimicrob Agents , 17(4), 259-268.

[47] Jarvis, G, & Millar, D. (1981). The treatment of incontinence due to detrusor instability by bladder drill." Prog Clin Biol Res 78(341-3).

[48] Karper, W. B. (2004). Exercise effects on interstitial cystitis: two case reports." Urol Nurs , 24(3), 202-204.

[49] Kaur, H, & Arunkalaivanan, A. S. (2007). Urethral pain syndrome and its management." Obstet Gynecol Surv quiz 353-344., 62(5), 348-351.

[50] Kelleher, C, Cardozo, L, et al. (1997). Dec). "A new questionnaire to assess the quality of life of urinary incontinent women." Br J Obstet Gynaecol , 104(12), 1374-1379.

[51] Korzeniowski, O. (1991). Urinary tract infection in the impaired host" Med Clin North Am , 75(2), 391-404.

[52] Lee, P. G, Cigolle, C, et al. (2009). The co-occurrence of chronic diseases and geriatric syndromes: the health and retirement study." J Am Geriatr Soc , 57(3), 511-516.

[53] Linley, J. E, Rose, K, et al. Understanding inflammatory pain: ion channels contributing to acute and chronic nociception." Pflugers Arch , 459(5), 657-669.

[54] Llorca-miravet, A. (1990). Tratamiento funcional en la incontinencia urinaria. Incontinencia Urinaria: Conceptos Actuales. E. Martínez-Agulló. Valencia., Graficuatre: , 629-649.

[55] Loch, A, & Stein, U. (2004). Interstitial cystitis. Current aspects of diagnosis and therapy." Urologe A , 43(9), 1135-1146.

[56] Lokeshwar, V. B, Selzer, M. G, et al. (2005). Urinary uronate and sulfated glycosaminoglycan levels: markers for interstitial cystitis severity." J Urol , 174(1), 344-349.

[57] Lorenzo-gómez, M, et al. (2013). Evaluation of a therapeutic vaccine for the prevention of recurrent urinary tract infections versus prophylactic treatment with antibiotics." Int Urogynecol J , 24(1), 127-134.

[58] Lorenzo-gomez, M, Padilla-fernandez, B, et al. (2011). Recurrent urinary infection: Effectiveness of the bacterial individualized vaccine. International Conference on Global Health and Public Health Education., Hong Kong, China.

[59] Lorenzo-gómez, M, Silva-abuín, J, et al. (2008). Treatment of stress urinary incontinence with perineal biofeedback by using superficial electrodes." Actas Urol Esp , 32(6), 629-636.

[60] Lorenzo GómezM., J. Silva Abuín, et al. ((2008). Treatment of stress urinary incontinence with perineal biofeedback by using superficial electrodes]" Actas Urol Esp , 32(6), 629-636.

[61] Lorenzo GomezM. F. and S. Gomez Castro ((2004). Physiopathologic relationship between interstitial cystitis and rheumatic, autoimmune, and chronic inflammatory diseases." Arch Esp Urol , 57(1), 25-34.

[62] Lucas, M, Bosch, J, et al. (2012). Guidelines on Urinary Incontinence. European Association of Urology Guidelines. Arnhem, The Netherlans.

[63] Mahony, D. T, Laferte, R. O, et al. (1977). Jan). "Integral storage and voiding reflexes. Neurophysiologic concept of continence and micturition." Urology 91(95-106).

[64] Maizels, M, King, L, et al. (1979). Urodynamic biofeedback: a new approach to treat vesical sphincter dyssynergia." J Urol , 122(2), 205-209.

[65] Margulies, R. U, Lewicky-gaupp, C, et al. (2008). Complications requiring reoperation following vaginal mesh kit procedures for prolapse." Am J Obstet Gynecol 199(6): 678 e, 671-674.

[66] Miller, N. (1974). Editorial: Evaluation of a new technique." NEJM , 290(12), 684-685.

[67] Moore, E. E, Jackson, S. L, et al. (2008). Urinary incontinence and urinary tract infection: temporal relationships in postmenopausal women." Obstet Gynecol 111(2 Pt 1): 317-323.

[68] Naber, K. G. (1999). Experience with the new guidelines on evaluation of new anti-infective drugs for the treatment of urinary tract infections." Int J Antimicrob Agents 11(3-4): 189-196; discussion , 213-186.

[69] Nazif, O, Teichman, J. M, et al. (2007). Neural upregulation in interstitial cystitis." Urology 69(4 Suppl): , 24-33.

[70] Nickel, J. C, Shoskes, D. A, et al. Prevalence and impact of bacteriuria and/or urinary tract infection in interstitial cystitis/painful bladder syndrome." Urology , 76(4), 799-803.

[71] Nicolle, L. (1997). Asymptomatic bacteriuria in the elderly." Infect Dis Clin North Am , 11(3), 647-662.

[72] Niro, J, Philippe, A. C, et al. (2010). Postoperative pain after transvaginal repair of pelvic organ prolapse with or without mesh." Gynecol Obstet Fertil , 38(11), 648-652.

[73] Nissenkorn, I, Shalev, M, et al. (2004). Patient-adjusted intermittent electrostimulation for treating stress and urge urinary incontinence." BJU Int , 94(1), 105-109.

[74] Parsons, C. L. (2011). The role of a leaky epithelium and potassium in the generation of bladder symptoms in interstitial cystitis/overactive bladder, urethral syndrome, prostatitis and gynaecological chronic pelvic pain." BJU Int , 107(3), 370-375.

[75] Parsons, C. L, & Koprowski, P. F. (1991). Interstitial cystitis: successful management by increasing urinary voiding intervals." Urology , 37(3), 207-212.

[76] Parsons, C. L, & Tatsis, V. (2004). Prevalence of interstitial cystitis in young women." Urology , 64(5), 866-870.

[77] Perry, J. (1994). General Letter for Insurance Appeals (Biofeedback) Pelvic Muscle Rehabilitation (EMG Biofeedback) For Urinary & Fecal Incontinence and Related Disorders Using Perry Vaginal TM and Perry Anal TM Sensors. National PerryMeter Home Trainer Rental Program. Petaluma. CA. USA.

[78] Peters, K. M, Killinger, K. A, et al. (2009). Childhood symptoms and events in women with interstitial cystitis/painful bladder syndrome." Urology , 73(2), 258-262.

[79] Repariz, M, & Salinas, J. (1995). Uncoordinated urinary syndrome. New aspects of an old problem]." Actas Urol Esp , 19(4), 261-280.

[80] Romanzi, L. J, Polaneczky, M, et al. (1999). Simple test of pelvic muscle contraction during pelvic examination: correlation to surface electromyography." Neurourol Urodyn , 18(6), 603-612.

[81] Roovers, J. P, Van Der Vaart, C. H, et al. (2004). A randomised controlled trial comparing abdominal and vaginal prolapse surgery: effects on urogenital function." Bjog , 111(1), 50-56.

[82] Sarma, A. V, Kanaya, A, et al. (2009). Risk factors for urinary incontinence among women with type 1 diabetes: findings from the epidemiology of diabetes interventions and complications study." Urology , 73(6), 1203-1209.

[83] Semeniuk, H, & Church, D. (1999). Evaluation of the leukocyte esterase and nitrite urine dipstick screening tests for detection of bacteriuria in women with suspected uncomplicated urinary tract infections." J Clin Microbiol , 37(9), 3051-3052.

[84] Seo, J, Yoon, H, et al. (2004). A randomized prospective study comparing new vaginal cone and FES-Biofeedback." Yonsei Med J , 45(5), 879-884.

[85] Sharifi, R, Geckler, R, et al. (1996). Treatment of urinary tract infections: selecting an appropriate broad-spectrum antibiotic for nosocomial infections." Am J Med 100(6A): 76S-82S.

[86] Sola DalenzV., J. Pardo Schanz, et al. ((2006). Minimal invasive surgery in female urinary incontinence: TVT-O]." Actas Urol Esp , 30(1), 61-66.

[87] Theofrastous, J. P, Wyman, J. F, et al. (2002). Effects of pelvic floor muscle training on strength and predictors of response in the treatment of urinary incontinence." Neurourol Urodyn , 21(5), 486-490.

[88] Thomas, T, Plymat, K, et al. (1980). Prevalence of urinary incontinence." Br Med J , 281, 1243-1245.

[89] Ulmsten, U, & Petros, P. (1995). Intravaginal slingplasty (IVS): an ambulatory surgical procedure for treatment of female urinary incontinence." Scand J Urol Nephrol , 29(1), 75-82.

[90] van de MerweJ. P., J. Nordling, et al. ((2008). Diagnostic criteria, classification, and nomenclature for painful bladder syndrome/interstitial cystitis: an ESSIC proposal." Eur Urol , 53(1), 60-67.

[91] Vilagut, G, Ferrer, M, et al. (2005). Mar-Apr). "The Spanish version of the Short Form 36 Health Survey: a decade of experience and new developments." Gac Sanit Review., 19(2), 135-150.

[92] Voorham-van, d, Pelger, Z. , R, et al. (2006). Effects of magnetic stimulation in the treatment of pelvic floor dysfunction." BJU Int , 97(5), 1035-1038.

[93] Warren, J. W, Brown, V, et al. (2008). Urinary tract infection and inflammation at onset of interstitial cystitis/painful bladder syndrome." Urology , 71(6), 1085-1090.

[94] Warren, J. W, Wesselmann, U, et al. Numbers and types of nonbladder syndromes as risk factors for interstitial cystitis/painful bladder syndrome." Urology , 77(2), 313-319.

[95] Wear, J, Wear, R, et al. (1979). Biofeedback in urology using urodynamics: preliminary observations." J Urol , 121(4), 464-468.

[96] White, G, Jantos, M, et al. (1997). Mar). "Establishing the diagnosis of vulvar vestibulitis." J Reprod Med , 42(3), 157-160.

[97] Workman, D. E, Cassisi, J. E, et al. (1993). Jan). "Validation of surface EMG as a measure of intravaginal and intra-abdominal activity: implications for biofeedback-assisted Kegel exercises." Psychophysiology , 30(1), 120-125.